DATE DUE

DEMCO 38-297

D1447325

A CELEBRATION OF MEDICAL HISTORY

The Henry E. Sigerist Supplements to the
Bulletin of the History of Medicine

New Series, no. 6
Editor: Lloyd G. Stevenson

Henry E. Sigerist, recruited by William H. Welch to be director of the Johns Hopkins Institute of the History of Medicine, was the founder of the *Bulletin of the History of Medicine* and also of the first series of supplements, which extended from 1943 to 1951. It was Sigerist's resolve that the *Bulletin* should provide the organ not only of the Johns Hopkins Institute but also of the American Association, and to this day it subserves both functions. It is therefore eminently suitable that the new series should bear the founder's name and perpetuate his scholarly interests. These interests were so broad and so varied that the supplements will recognize no narrow limits in range of theme and will publish historical essays of greater scope than the *Bulletin* itself can accommodate. It is not too much to hope that in time the Sigerist supplements will help to extend the purview of medical history.

Other Books in the New Series

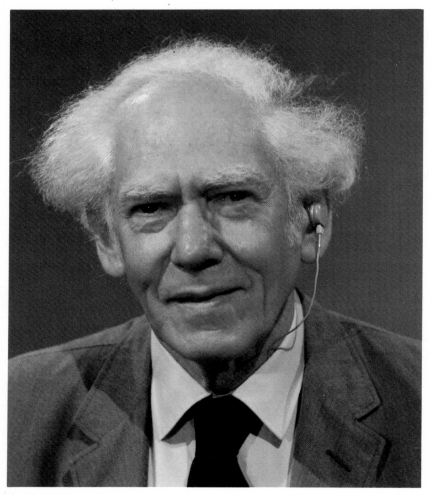

Owsei Temkin

A CELEBRATION OF MEDICAL HISTORY

The Fiftieth Anniversary
of The Johns Hopkins Institute of the History of Medicine
and The Welch Medical Library

Edited by
LLOYD G. STEVENSON

THE JOHNS HOPKINS UNIVERSITY PRESS
Baltimore and London

The Johns Hopkins University Press, Baltimore, Maryland 21218
The Johns Hopkins Press Ltd., London

Library of Congress Cataloging in Publication Data

Main entry under title:

A Celebration of medical history.

(The Henry E. Sigerist supplements to the Bulletin
of the history of medicine; new ser., no. 6)
    1. Medicine—History—Congresses.   2. Johns
Hopkins University. Institute of the History of
Medicine—Congresses.   3. William H. Welch Medical
Library—Congresses.   I. Stevenson, Lloyd G.
II. Johns Hopkins University. Institute of the
History of Medicine.   III. William H. Welch Medical
Library.   IV. Series. [DNLM: 1. History of medicine.
W1 HE896 no. 6/WZ 40 C392]
R131.A2C44   610'.9   81-17168
ISBN 0-8018-2733-7   AACR2

✿ CONTENTS

A CELEBRATION OF MEDICAL HISTORY

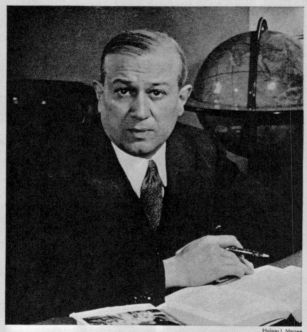
HENRY E. SIGERIST

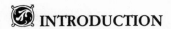

INTRODUCTION

Lloyd G. Stevenson

It was just over fifty years ago (17 and 18 October 1929) that The Johns Hopkins Institute of the History of Medicine was opened — shortly before the bottom fell out of the stock market and, for many people, out of the world. It is not suggested that there was any necessary connection between these two events. Had the opening of the Institute not occurred the stock market would not have been saved. What the Rockefeller Foundation built into the Institute would not, devoted to other ends, have shored up the American economy. This serves, however, to establish a time frame. It was the year of the market crash. It was ten years before World War II.

In that far-off time people were educated differently. Almost all of them learned to read. Dr. William H. Welch (already an old man, for he was born in 1850, a year after Osler) had actually aimed at education as a classicist and therefore knew some Greek and a great deal of Latin. This seems not to have hampered his subsequent medical education; it did not, of course, in itself provide (as decreasingly since the sixteenth century such training had provided) adequate support for medicine, which needed a great deal besides, but it gave him an essential key to many centuries' worth of medicine's past. Welch was in part a humanist, in part a scientist. He became the Hopkins's first professor of pathology and the first dean of its famous medical school, somewhat later the first director of the School of Hygiene, and at last the founder of the Institute of the History of Medicine and first professor of this novel discipline. At that point he was a highly valued advisor of the Rockefellers (he had played a considerable part in pointing the direction of their philanthropies) and the foundation wanted to do something nice for him in his old age. The university, for its part, wanted to strengthen the RF connection. Probably both foundation and university were surprised when their venerable activist took off at once for Europe to find his successor. His role, as he saw it, was to make broad the way.

Two of the essays read at the semicentennial (number three, by Janet B. Koudelka, and number ten, which happened not to be a paper but rather the banquet address, by Robert S. Morison) were concerned in large part with the genesis of the Institute, in the setting of the Welch Library, where it continues to this day to teach, to conduct research, and to edit and publish.

If Welch was the initiator of the Institute, it was another man who really established it, who put it on the map. This was the ebullient Swiss scholar

1

Henry E. Sigerist, whom Welch found in Leipzig, the world's primary center for medical historical studies. The Leipzig Institute was the creation of Professor Karl Sudhoff, the foremost of whose interests was that prophet known as the Luther of medicine, Paracelsus. The major scholarly enterprise of Sudhoff's domain at this time, however, was a new translation of the aphorisms of Hippocrates. As for Sigerist, he had been assigned to certain medieval studies and had become a notable medievalist. This may surprise those who knew him later as a modernist, a self-made medical sociologist, and a would-be reformer in the provision of medical care. To label him as either medievalist or modernist, however, would be misleading; whether as scholar or reformer he was a universalist. To his attainments in the classics he added a serious claim (largely through his studies in England) to Chinese and Sanskrit. His first Ph.D. candidate at Johns Hopkins worked in sinology; his last scholarly contribution was an ambitious parallel study of Greek medicine and the medicine of India. No language appeared to be so esoteric, no period so far off as to daunt him. But when he first came to the United States he sped around the country, indeed around the continent, lecturing with the zeal of an apostle. He was consumed with ardor for all things American and especially for American medicine, about which he wrote an enthusiastic book. When he assumed his duties at The Johns Hopkins Institute in 1932, this was his zealous state of mind. By 1939, when his picture appeared on the cover of *Time*, he was ready to proclaim that "history spirals toward socialization." A tour of Russia had kindled a new kind of ardor and he wrote a widely noticed book about Soviet medicine, which did little to win him the regard of the AMA. But his tour of America and his tour of Russia, with the books that followed, did not exhaust him. The same energy and the same capacity for appreciation (not always approval) were displayed in his other travels: to India, to South Africa, and regularly to Europe.

Meantime he wrote, lectured, edited, and entertained. His short, popular books, such as *Great Doctors* and *Civilization and Disease*, were to have been followed by a great eight-volume history of medicine. He retired to Switzerland in 1947 in order to write it, but only the first volume appeared before his death; a second, edited from incomplete copy and supplemented from his notes, was published posthumously.

An interregnum of about two years ended with the appointment as director of Professor Richard Shryock, who had taught American history at Duke and at the University of Pennsylvania and who had gained wide recognition and wide readership for a book entitled *The Development of Modern Medicine*. Most of Shryock's medico-historical writings, apart from this comprehensive survey volume, concerned the social history of American medicine. He was author, coauthor, or editor of a number of textbooks of American history, and for all his work became generally well known in departments of history all across the country. Not so familiar a figure in any of the medical schools (including even Johns Hopkins, perhaps) as Sigerist had been in

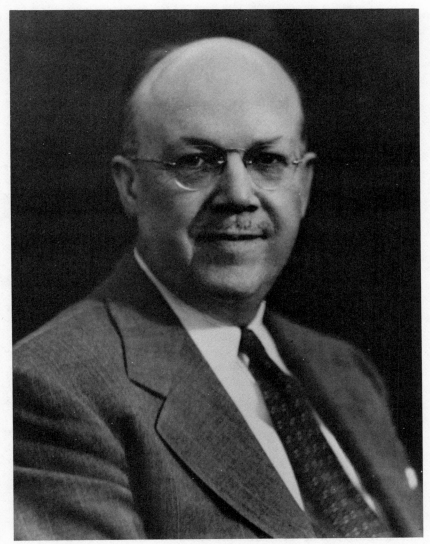

RICHARD SHRYOCK

many, Shryock was enormously better known to the American community of historians as a whole. For the Institute he had somewhat different aims than those of either his predecessors or his successors, for he hoped to gain a place for the history of science alongside the history of medicine. The ultimate development at Homewood of a Department of the History of Science precluded the sort of expansion of the Institute's role which Professor Shryock envisaged.

On Shryock's retirement his place was taken by Sigerist's Leipzig student and long-time colleague of both Sigerist and Shryock, Professor Owsei Temkin. Temkin is Russian-born but educated from an early age in Germany. He has been an American resident and citizen for nearly half a century. A popular teacher, a discerning editor, and, like his predecessors as director of the Institute, an active participant in the affairs of the American Association for the History of Medicine, Temkin is best known as a distinguished scholar — among learned, acute, and imaginative scholars, *facile princeps*. If he has a "period" it lies in late antiquity, on the one hand, and in the nineteenth century on the other; but as a matter of fact he is probably the supreme generalist among medical historians. He appears equally at home in many times, places, and particular fields, and in many languages, as exhibited in *The Falling Sickness*, a history of epilepsy, and in *The Double Face of Janus*, a comprehensive collection of essays selected from more than forty years of productive scholarly labor.

With Professor Temkin's achievement of emeritus status and his later retirement, his student, Professor Lloyd G. Stevenson, came from Yale to succeed him. A tight budget and the almost simultaneous withdrawal (from many departments) of NIH training grants, along with the discontinuance of the Macy Fellowships in the History of Medicine and Biology, have meant somewhat restricted possibilities, for Medical School and School of Hygiene programs, on the one hand, and graduate programs on the other. Work has nevertheless continued on both levels and additions have been made to the number of Hopkins-qualified historians across the continent, on East coast and West coast and from Canada down to the Gulf. The larger number of these appointments date from the Temkin era, but each of the directorates (except the first, when graduate study had not yet begun) has produced several. The first of the Ph.D.'s has recently retired and the latest has recently found employment; and this does not take account of the masters (the M.A.'s) who teach and write medical history either on a full-time basis or in conjunction with practice. The *Bulletin of the History of Medicine*, which will not be fifty years old until 1983, is the organ of The Johns Hopkins Institute and also of the American Association for the History of Medicine. Competition for a share of space in its pages grows ever stiffer, the doctors gradually overcoming their diffidence about the humanities, and the political, social, and economic historians their inhibitions about struggling with scientific and clinical technicalities. (Another solution, of course, has been to deny that any medical knowledge is required.) A clouded crystal ball does not permit us to see at all clearly what the future may hold, but peering into its sometimes murky depths we persuade ourselves that we can just discern a faint stirring of renewed medico-historical interest among physicians not yet retired: in fact among able physicians at the beginning of their professional careers desiring to qualify not as hobbyists but as historians. That means will be found to encourage and support this laudable ambition is, unfortu-

nately, improbable. The wishful vision is faint at best. Failing any development of this sort, there is some likelihood that medicine and its history will
be viewed increasingly from the outside, and perhaps viewed somewhat
coldly. Cool scrutiny need not be feared if it is also knowledgeable. But it is
precisely in this area that the greatest doubt arises. The history of medicine
seems likely, in fact, to become merely an aspect of social history. Medicine
in itself—the internal, the scientific, and the technical factors playing the
predominant role—once claimed the major share of attention. But no doubt
because it was dealt with, in considerable part, somewhat simplistically, the
social historians have moved in to fill a comparative void. During the fifty
years of the Institute's existence, the best of medical history has been intellectual and social history that has not disregarded medicine per se; or rather,
like *The Falling Sickness* and *The Double Face of Janus*, it has been *histoire
totale*, with medicine, health, and disease at its core. The tendency to shift
the core to the periphery and to see medicine at the edge of biological
science—health care being simply one among the welfare services—and at
the same time to adhere, although in much diminished degree, to some of
the inferior models of the past, has meant that the medical element, in the
better history, has shrunk, sometimes to the vanishing point. Current examples of good, scholarly medical history in the old style, and good, scholarly
medical history of a newer pattern (yet with medicine firmly fixed at its core)
make up, it is hoped, the substance of this volume.

Now that every tyro in history who has felt the neighborly impulse to explain to medical historians (in the introduction to an anthology, usually)
where they are going wrong has unfurled the banner which reads "Beyond
Great Doctors," some medical historians are falling back in disarray. They
should be of good courage. Professor Erwin H. Ackerknecht (one somehow
cannot imagine him dismayed by a charging anthologist) has given them the
good word. It is not surprising that the good word comes in French. Daremberg wrote it a hundred years ago: "Dans l'histoire de la médecine les
véritables personnages ce sont les maladies." To which Ackerknecht himself
has added: "The history of diseases is an ideal meeting ground for historians
and medical historians." And so it has proved to be. It is now more than
thirty years since *Malaria in the Mississippi Valley* demonstrated that while it
is by no means easy to explain history in terms of disease or to explain disease
in terms of history, neither task is impossible, and that the second, at least,
can carry us a long way toward conviction. And yet it is the historians, even
more than the medical historians, who have kept the book in print.

What about old theories of disease? Were they merely the fantasies with
which our childlike precursors kept themselves amused, or are such theories
a part of the history of diseases? "Certain theories reflect clearly the history
of diseases," proclaims Ackerknecht, "certain theories have had a strong influence on the further evolution of diseases" and what is more, they reflect
the society in which they were promulgated. After a workpersonlike survey

of the writings in this sphere of the past fifty years, Ackerknecht examines "causes and pseudocauses"—such as the psychological, hereditary, parasitic, indigent, and opulent—in his customary, fascinating way: all to the cheerful neglect of stars, miasms, contagia, and the rest of fusty standardized history. This is supplemented by Charles Rosenberg's forward-looking consideration of the prospects for the history of disease finding a place in "the canon of accepted historical subject matter." At once we hear the bugles of "the new social history" and are reassured to discover that "for a number of reasons disease has become a natural if not necessary part of that ill-defined but vigorous enterprise" which of course includes black history, women's history, and the histories of birth, life, and death. One can but admire the assurance with which the new social historians have assumed the mantles of epidemiology, demography, and genetics, as well as those of sociology, sociobiology, ecology, cultural anthropology, and even theology. "Nutrition, birth control, medical skills, and of course sickness and mortality are all relevant candidates for study." (On the same page we read that "one must of necessity evaluate such factors as diet, agricultural practice, family and household structure, work and religious belief, and of course morbidity and mortality.") It is understood that summaries of this kind touch only the peaks. The above-mentioned "canon of accepted historical subject matter" is obviously a comprehensive and elastic list. That disease has not been excluded from it does not mean that medical historians will now have to look around them for different themes. But however all-embracing the history of disease may become, it is nevertheless improbable that the shelf which holds *The Falling Sickness, Malaria in the Mississippi Valley*, and *The Cholera Years* will have to be lengthened very much very soon.

In Nikolaus Mani's learned and perceptive essay on aspects of Glisson and Wepfer, the historiographic review of the work on Glisson covers chiefly the last two decades and finds the contributions to be of increasing relevance. Described as "a highly theoretical and scholastic mind" Glisson was presumably of less appeal to the historians seen by Webster (earlier in the century and later in the day) as wickedly intent on science. Modern historical studies of Wepfer and his school begin somewhat earlier—a decade, in fact, before The Johns Hopkins Institute was to open—and have continued, in such hands as those of Buess and Eichenberger, in the post–World War II period. Mani sees Wepfer as "a clinical, morphological and experimental observer with a remarkable power of integration." And yet different as he finds his two protagonists, they appear to Mani to have had much in common. Both were early adherents of Harvey, by whom both, although particularly Wepfer, were much influenced. Wepfer's discovery of the true character of apoplexy was but the most famous instance of his concern with pathogenic mechanisms, not without effect on his disease management. Frank, in his interesting·commentary, avers: "It is only through scholarship such as Mani's, that attempts simultaneously to analyze the metaphysical, physiological, pathological, and clinical dimensions of medical thought, that we can have any hope of understanding such a crucial period in the history of medicine as the seventeenth century."

At a Joint Session for the Institute of the History of Medicine and the William H. Welch Medical Library, Janet B. Koudelka, whose knowledge and experience of both are unrivaled, astutely and knowledgeably outlined for us their beginnings; and the next day Robert S. Morison further surveyed, through a search of the Rockefeller Archives, the institution of the chair and of the Institute. If neither the foundation nor the university was very sure what it was doing with reference to the history of medicine, Welch knew what he intended. This point will reappear at the end of the Introduction. The joint session also considered library developments elsewhere in America.

The recent inauguration of HISTLINE has put the medical historians "on line," at least to a limited degree, along with the other users of MEDLINE, the young brother of MEDLARS. It is not long ago that the great NLM celebrated the one hundredth birthday of the *Index Catalogue*. Little more than a century ago, the *Index Catalogue* and *Index Medicus*, extraordinary tools for medical bibliography, constituted America's greatest contribution to medicine; or so said Dr. William H. Welch, who had as good a claim to a respectful hearing as anyone around. But with the coming of MEDLARS the greatest of medical libraries was equipped with the greatest of information retrieval systems. John Shaw Billings, first director of the Army Medical Library (afterwards the Armed Forces Medical Library, precursor of the National Library of Medicine) and the prophet of the *Index Catalogue*, had a distant successor in Dr. Frank B. Rogers, whose regime was marked, and will be forever marked, by the advent of MEDLARS. Seymour Taine and Frank B. Rogers, with the help of General Electric and Photon, set the system in operation in 1964. To have Rogers himself tell the graphic tale, modestly and straightforwardly though it be told, is like having the duke describe the battle. This is good oral history with all the essential background, including material on the Welch Project directed by Sanford V. Larkey. Larkey was Welch Library director and also a scholarly member of the Institute. His memory has been honored recently in a volume issued by his Oxford college, Pembroke; the first copy was presented to his widow, Geraldine Larkey Henderson, during the course of the semicentennial of library and Institute.[1]

Dr. Whitfield J. Bell, Jr., historian, librarian, and already (at the time of this fiftieth anniversary meeting in Baltimore) an administrator with heavy responsibilities to the American Philosophical Society, looked back with the rest of us to the far-off days when the Welch Library and the Institute of the History of Medicine were opened in 1929. He looked more especially at the initial day, devoted to a Conference on Medical Libraries which had been addressed by Sudhoff, Ashburn, Malloch, Francis, and Mackall, and which had been opened, after the dedicatory ceremonies, by Harvey Cushing's fine address on "The Binding Influence of a Library on a Subdividing Profession." The history of America's medical libraries, as Bell surveyed them in 1979, was various, glorious, and at the same time—like so many human endeavors which in the end have been fruitful—both paltry and frustrating. Some of his listeners were perhaps more than a little surprised to learn how early a scorn for libraries, or at any rate for all but the latest journals, matched enthusiasm for them among physicians. Even the great John Shaw Billings displayed a curious ambivalence. It was not, of course, until the marvelous bibliographical tools—which Billings did so much to supply—were well in place that library riches, including mighty accumulations of journals, were really put within reach of the profession. Meanwhile, however, the stupendous collectors—men like Lewis, Purple, Toner, and Chadwick—had been heaping up treasure, sometimes with a zeal that was almost blind, sometimes with the greatest discernment, and with unflagging ardor always. Perhaps the saddest aspect of the story is the very limited use made of many collections, whether meager or splendid. The great men of the early Johns Hopkins, however, were both collectors and users. Bell had several of them in mind when he confirmed Cushing's long-ago plea for the amateur historian among those professionals whose day was just dawning fifty years back. Hardly could Osler himself have spoken more warmly or more winningly of the medical bookmen of the time before that time than did Dr. Bell.

In taking up, with alacrity, knowledge, and insight, the organizers' invitation to look back at the transformation of medical history over the fifty-year period since the Institute was opened, Charles Webster gracefully indicated the links between Johns Hopkins and Oxford, links that were in fact forged even earlier. He then went beyond this to transatlantic associations of rather broader scope. His theme of "Medicine as Social History" turned out, happily, to be an inclusive one. Not only was social history in the usual sense embraced, but also sociology; and in a long and spirited passage, which perhaps surprised some part of his audience, he dealt very knowledgeably with demographic history. Cultural history was not specifically listed for attention but cropped up nonetheless: ideas on doctors and patients in the age of Shakespeare, after all, were ideas observed as changing in the minds of historians. That these ideas should be there at all Webster saw as the essential change; they had replaced, in some measure, an almost exclusive emphasis on science. "The pursuit of the history of medicine on an organized basis without respect to the history of science is still scarcely possible in Britain." This sentence presumably refers to the attempt to do something not yet tried in the United States, where the HSS and the AAHM have so far seemed sufficient, and where no society has yet been established solely for the social history of medicine. In both lands, however, there are apparently some who feel that science, having for long had all the heed, should now have almost none. Would it not be amusing to paraphrase Webster's statement about the history of medicine and the history of science in Britain by leaving out (twice) the three words, "the history of"? It would then read: "The pursuit of medicine on an organized basis without respect to science is still scarcely possible in Britain." Is one to assume that a more enlightened policy will some day limit history of medicine to its prescientific era? Recent medical history obviously has social aspects, but it is going to be hard to keep cultured hands quite unbesmirched with science if they handle anything much later than Shakespeare's era.

Most of the varied strands that Webster braids together to form social history have had something to do with practice, a term very broadly defined, and are often related therefore to institutional histories; apart from the history of science and of medical science it is institutional history that has had the most study in Britain. Webster appears to task Sir George Clark, author of the *History of the Royal College of Physicians*, with having adopted the viewpoint of the modern Fellows, or at any rate with having cherished much too narrow a view of the scope of practice in times past. Although Webster does not use the word, other recent historians have formed the habit of talking about "monopoly" and how it grew—a faintly pejorative word, monopoly, but of a faintness they endeavor to cure. Webster reminds us, quite rightly, that not a few in the medical establishment of Shakespeare's time were rather fearsome practitioners. Joined with a properly charitable impression of those outside the establishment this will be capable of adding to the revisionist doctrine, now growing in fashion, that a dash of science, like a few drops of holy water, was not necessarily the salvation of the medical orthodox, and that as a matter of fact there was no health in them. Fair enough, in a way, and altogether unsurprising. Perhaps, however, the time has almost come to remind ourselves that the old historians were in general quite right: that is, that uniform safety and effectiveness was to grow, if anywhere, inside the profession, however many genuine saviors cowered for a time in the hedges; that what the bumbling orthodox needed above all to transform them was indeed science, whether it came from surprising outside sources, or (more surprisingly still) from within the bounds of orthodoxy; and that the "monopoly" down the road was, for the customers, no bad thing. Nor have all the dirty words used for outsiders (mountebank, empiric, quack, etc.), the use of which Webster rather deplores, become meaningless with all the pupae sprouting wings and fluttering up out of the ditches.

While Webster warmly values the generalist, Osler, as well as the biographers, bibliographers, and the specialist historians, he is by no means unappreciative of medical history's veterans—of Creighton, Power, and the rest, and not least Singer. He takes it to be merely an effect of medical history's long-continued overemphasis on science that William Harvey has had a great deal of work devoted to him, Thomas Sydenham very little. This is a view not fully shared by Webster's discussant, Donald Bates, who is himself one of the few close students of Sydenham, and who feels that the scientists have had the spotlight to themselves because society in general has been deeply impressed by science, and because medicine has wanted to enter its own representative in the competition. To these observations it might be added that Harvey has always provided the best answer to those historians of science who regard medicine as nothing more than applied science, who see the physicians as trundling along behind the triumphal car of science to gather up and apply what they can. In what branch of biology, it is fair to ask, was the circulation of blood discovered? Was it not medicine's contribution to biology? Jerome Bylebyl has recently written of Harvey that "as the theory of circulation eventually took shape in his mind, it was indeed a startling new physiological principle, but one which owed a great deal to older pathological and therapeutic notions." Or, more briefly, to older medicine. That the discovery of the circulation had both a professional and a social context was persuasively shown in a symposium presented in Kansas City before the American Association for the History of Medicine in May 1978, a celebration in which Charles Webster, together with Jerome Bylebyl and Robert Frank, took prominent part: Webster in the social sector with an essay afterwards hailed as masterly by Professor Erna Lesky.

In Peter Niebyl's discussion of L. J. Rather's stimulating paper on metaphorical language in the history of Western medicine, and at the very end of his brief comment, he suggests that "a case could be made for the assertion that all language is ultimately metaphorical in origin." It is curious indeed that in an age when so much of philosophy is permeated, if not generated and formed, by linguistic considerations (what is known, particularly, as analytic philosophy) we should wait for the final paragraph of this section of the program, the section on the source and development of metaphorical language, to hear a fleeting reference to the linguists. And yet Rather is sensitive to language and is deeply interested (which is what makes his essay deeply interesting) in the source and also in the development of metaphorical language in the history of Western medicine. Professor Temkin is so often found to be the precursor of what appear to be innovations in the writing of medical history—and is again so here. Ackerknecht and Niebyl, too, have long been in the field, although in a narrower and more specific sense; and more recently, of course, Susan Sontag has made an interesting contribution, one which assumes the character of a special tract. But the most comprehensive of such surveys (among those that indeed stick to medicine), and the most clearly developmental, is the present essay by Rather.

It was in the domain of public health (and in the management—not yet the control—of epidemics, the practice of inoculation, and the choice and distribution of mineral waters) that what Jean-Pierre Goubert calls medicalization was first substantially achieved. "Ample opportunity to deploy the technical proficiency, the scientific zeal, and the ambition of the medical profession was opened up by the development of the public health sector," which gave rise to a "whole medical bureaucracy, working in close cooperation with that of the intendant and his subdelegates as well as with the network of parish priests." "Epidemics," we are assured, "propelled the physician into the public arena, instilled him with epistemological zeal, and strengthened his ambition to be 'useful to society.' " Inoculation represents "the first instance and the first victory of the physician's direct fight against disease and death" and the first preventive weapon. Unsurprisingly, hostility prevented early triumph. Of mineral waters we are told: "As in the case of epidemics the state of the art was patently inadequate"; but, on the other hand, "extraordinarily modern overtones...betray the trend toward medicalization." This seems to mean, chiefly, that a measure of authority was given to physicians.

Goubert declares that "the utopia of a medicalized society found a first expression in the medical discourse during the last years of the Ancien Régime." And again: "Thanks to the improved social position of the medical profession, thanks to the urban network it deployed, and because of an alliance concluded between the medical profession and the public authorities much rather than by virtue of any particular breakthrough in medical knowledge, this utopia had spawned a small number of accomplishments." All this and more was necessary, says Goubert, before "the physician, a new Caesar, could crown himself." With this crowning, one seems meant to conclude, medicalization was accomplished.

Some of the other prominent features of Dr. Goubert's paper can be referred to in considering his commentator's critique. Although Dr. Caroline Hannaway does not use the word Whiggish to describe Dr. Goubert's approach to certain aspects of the Ancien Régime in France (it is strictly speaking unsuitable outside the Anglo-American context) this is clearly what she has in mind. The place ascribed by Goubert to the Société Royale de Médecine is a principal case in point. Because the society was in essence an institution of the Ancien Régime—an agency, in fact, of the royal government—"it is not accurate to portray the society's activities as a self-expression of bourgeois professionalism or as an autonomous expression of medical dominance. It was the servant of an absolutist state." But there are other aspects we should not forget. "It is a mistake to underestimate the value which the early members attached to the scientific function of the society and make this subservient to purely professional goals. The image of the eighteenth-century Parisian savant is the more dominant image than that of the proto-nineteenth-century physician in the provinces." What about the question of professional autonomy? "Far from contributing to the autonomy of the medical profession, in the eyes of many physicians the Société Royale de Médecine and its proposals represented a distinct threat." An alliance with the royal government was not what was wanted. As for the rural aspect of Goubert's argument, Hannaway sees the society's concern with medical care in the countryside as "part of an agronomic vision of medicine and society....The unification of medicine that was of primary concern to Vicq d'Azyr [who was nonmedical] was the unification of human and animal medicine."

"In short," the commentator sums up, "what Dr. Goubert sees as a monolithic professional imperialism is composed in my view of a number of complex strands: administrative response to social and economic crisis, professional insecurity, and a well-articulated scientific program." It is at this point that one is forced to recall Goubert's invocation, at the beginning, not so much of Bloch and the early *Annales* group fifty years back as of Michel Foucault. Has he reduced almost everything to pattern in the Foucault manner? Possibly he is right about the kind of picture he is drawing and it is in fact more nearly contemporary, at any rate more fashionable, than Hannaway's. If her view of the state of things medical at the end of the Ancien Régime is initially the more convincing of the two, it remains for period scholars to choose between them or to discard both; to adopt both would be, as the saying goes, the neatest trick of the week. It is interesting that terms like medicalization, bureaucracy, and so forth, with the image of the physician as a new Caesar, have something of a pejorative, political character no longer unfamiliar in America.

In meticulous and patient detail Professor Loris Premuda has traced for us the role of Trieste and the role of his own Padua in the development of medical teaching and, more especially, medical research as they unfolded within these two cities and as they extended from them. But this he has not done vauntingly, for at the time of which he writes these great centers were subsidiary to a greater, having long been parts of the Austrian empire and for a long time satellites of Vienna. This was a Vienna, however, that had so much of cultural and scientific value to impart that cities well outside of its political orbit showed themselves eager to share in its cultural largesse. Professor Premuda has demonstrated most convincingly how Trieste and Padua absorbed and transmitted this pervasive influence. As Dr. Bylebyl has remarked, Professor Premuda's is "a most unchauvinistic piece of historical research." A great many medical historians, European and American alike, have characteristically limited their work to blowing their own horns, to exalting their own centers to the skies. It has been a captivating experience to listen to this chastened and unruffled account of the onetime colonial status and onetime vital transmitting role of these two great cities.

"Onetime" is a crucial word. At a much earlier period the capable and the ambitious of Europe had flocked to Padua for medical instruction and it was the influence of Padua itself that radiated from the Venetian republic. But to put the matter in the terms suggested by Sir William Osler, Minerva medica has set up her temple in a succession of different cities, and it was Leiden that proved to be next in the sequence; it was Leiden, too, that gained most, perhaps, from the example of Padua. Leiden, in turn, became a major center of influence and established its intellectual sway, in no small measure, in Vienna. So that when Padua began, in part because of the cur-

rent political situation, to exhibit that strong evidence of Viennese inspiration which Professor Premuda has demonstrated for us, the circle was at last
complete. This rounding of the circle has been shown very neatly by his
commentator, Dr. Bylebyl.

At the very end of a two-day meeting came what was in some ways the
crowning touch, a banquet speech on "The Foundation Interest" by Dr.
Robert S. Morison. It began, however, in a slightly disquieting way. This
was because Dr. Morison's thorough review of the material relating to The
Johns Hopkins Institute of the History of Medicine in the Rockefeller Archives revealed, at the beginning, something apparently unique in the history of Rockefeller grants: "Nowhere is there a formal memo by a member of
the staff of either the Rockefeller Foundation or the General Education
Board setting forth the reasons for believing that the History of Medicine
should be supported on such a substantial scale." At the end of the address
is a further admission: "Although there may have been, and probably was, a
general recognition among the officers of the two foundations that the growing emphasis on medicine's scientific base ought to be balanced by more attention to its social and historical contexts, the actual decision to make a
grant to Johns Hopkins for this purpose was based on much more immediate
and, to a certain extent, purely bureaucratic considerations. High on the list
certainly was the very general respect and affection for Popsy Welch. . . ."

The Rockefellers, in other words, not only did not value the history of
medicine but did not even pretend to; the usual justification memo could
be forgotten. It was obvious that the grant was made very largely, if not entirely, to promote the comfort and dignity of Dr. Welch. But the foundation was confirmed in this by the comparable attitude of Johns Hopkins.
This induced a "slightly irritated feeling" in New York.

Two factors counterbalance the impression we are left with at this point.
One is the clear vision of Welch himself. As noted earlier, if neither the foundation nor the university was very sure what it was doing, Welch knew what
he intended. "The proposal to the General Education Board, which he must
have supervised, if not actually written, reads as if it had been prepared in the
1960s, when other medical educators finally awoke to the constricting effects
of the so-called Flexnerian Revolution." The other factor came into play with
the man Welch chose to be his successor. "As far as the foundation was concerned, the appointment of Henry Sigerist in 1932 marked the beginning of
a new era. . . . Alan Gregg, who became director of Medical Education about
the time the original grant was made, was himself deeply interested in the
broader social and historical relationships of medicine, which Sigerist was so
clearly identified with."

It is evident that Dr. Morison, a Harvard man, began his research for his
presentation at the fiftieth anniversary of the Welch Library and the Institute of the History of Medicine with the feeling that Welch had long been
somewhat overrated. He finished not only with high respect for Welch but

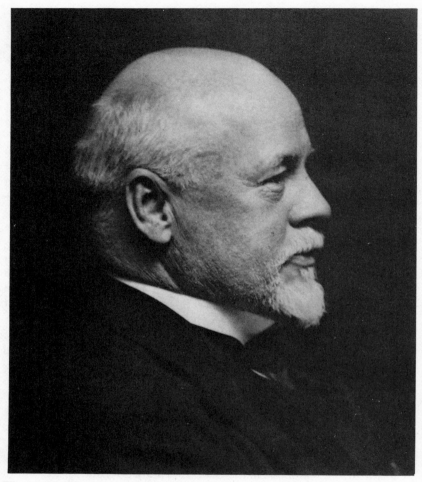

WILLIAM H. WELCH

with a glow of admiration. Matching this was warm appreciation of Sigerist and of the subsequent development of the Institute. Best of all, perhaps, he displayed a lively understanding of what history might mean and might accomplish in some sectors of its concern. The history of the relationship between medical care and health and the origins of the social obligation to provide health services for everyone: both of these appealed to him as insufficiently explored and as well worth further scrutiny. If the story begins on the one side, in New York, in a faint mist of benevolence and sentiment, and on the other, in Baltimore, with a combination of sentiment and opportunism — both sides being ever so slightly befogged — the air was cleared first of all by Welch, then by Sigerist and Alan Gregg and their successors.

Even if there is a good deal more than this to be said about the potential of medical history, this address illustrates (as well as relates) the Institute's message and the Institute's story, forming a suitable climax for its fiftieth anniversary.

In addition to the ten papers that make up this volume—seven of them augmented by a discussant—there were two films and a videotape, which, with the presentation of the Larkey memorial volume already referred to, made up a rewarding evening. The films, which brought Dr. Welch and Dr. Shryock vividly before us, were unfortunately not matched by a similar record of Dr. Sigerist. It is an enduring pity that no film of Sigerist, who was probably nearer to being an actor than were any of his colleagues, was ever made. Industrious research among the recordings preserved by Baltimore radio stations failed to discover an echo of his voice—and he was a splendid talker, several times heard by radio listeners. Welch, Shryock, and Temkin, however, are cherished in recoverable sight and sound, for in addition to the old but excellent films of the first two, the Institute was able to present a new videotape of an interview granted by Temkin at the National Audiovisual Center; better still, Professor Temkin himself was present at the showing and afterwards fielded questions. The frontispiece of the present volume represents him as he appeared in the studio immediately after the making of the videotape.

Two very brief quotations, chosen from the Temkin replies to the questions asked on the evening of 17 October 1979, follow. Both are characteristic—in thoughtfulness, in clarity, and in caution. It is perhaps a paradox to say, but although both quotations exhibit caution, they are at the same time forthright, even blunt.[2]

After he had made a comment about "specialism" the professor was asked if one should aim to be a generalist or a specialist or both, and he replied:

> Now let me tell you first of all I have absolutely no intention to develop here a curriculum of how graduate students and others should behave. That is not my job. What I meant was something different. When I said that personally I'm not much in favor of specialists, I had in mind something which amongst historians is quite natural today. You are not a historian, you are an eighteenth-century man or woman; you are, well, *are* you a nineteenth-century man or are you an *early* nineteenth-century man or a *late* nineteenth-century man? If you are a medievalist I'm very much afraid that very soon you won't remain a whole medievalist, you will become a partitioned medievalist. And so it goes with practically every sphere...that's what I mean by a specialist, and that's what I like to avoid. However, if you have never studied anything in depth—that is to say, acquired the tools to answer the questions which that particular period presents and then tried to go into these questions as far as seems necessary—if you do not possess *that*, then you probably will be bad in every period....But there's a great difference between that and being a specialist in the sense in which many of our recent historians are specialists. I beg their pardon.

Soon afterwards someone in the hall asked Professor Temkin about change in his teaching over the years, inferring "that you are now less concerned with teaching facts, and more concerned with how they [the protagonists] think and their thinking process." To the use of the present tense Temkin reacted at once: "I'm retired. I'm now not concerned with anything at all any more, thank God." But when the laughter died he dealt with the question seriously and succinctly, speaking of a good balance between facts and ideas and also about "unnecessary facts." This taken care of, he added:

> On the other hand, and here I would almost like to raise my voice. . . I would say that you must resist the temptation, which is very strong today, to think and to let your students think, and get away with it, that you can deal with thoughts without knowing facts. And that is particularly dangerous in the history of medicine, because there is a tendency—or perhaps there *was* a tendency, I hope there *was* a tendency. . . [toward the view] that the history of medicine is something which is most fruitful for the student not if he has a *course*, not if he has to *study*, but if he sits with others around a table and has historians and theologians and jurists—and I don't know [who else]—talk about something, and he then participates intelligently in the discussion. He can't participate *intelligently* in the discussion!

Never given to *obiter dicta*, or to resounding declarations *ex cathedra* either, the professor has always been capable of a pithy, compendious sentence. He speaks his mind. The genial manner in which he speaks it may be gathered from a glance at the frontispiece.[3]

NOTES

[1]Charles Webster, ed., *Health, Medicine, and Mortality in the Sixteenth Century* (Cambridge: At the University Press, 1972). In his introduction to this volume, which is dedicated "To the memory of Sanford Vincent Larkey," Dr. Webster gives a brief survey of Larkey's work and writes that Larkey "inherited Osler's conviction that the creation of collections of historical sources, and the compilation of professionally competent bibliographies, were essential prerequisites for the development of the history of medicine. . . .Larkey's conception of humanism differed significantly from that of Osler. . . .Larkey subtly changed the emphasis of medical humanism, in accordance with what he regarded as the intellectual needs of the medical profession and the public, during a period of rapid advance in medical science coinciding with the upheavals caused by the Second World War" (pp. 1–2). Dr. Larkey's valued service as director of the Medical Indexing Research Project is set forth below (p. 79) by Dr. Frank B. Rogers among the origins of MEDLARS.

[2]Two or three unimportant interjections have been cut; a few words not clearly recorded have been supplied, together with appropriate punctuation throughout.

[3]The Rockefeller Foundation, in conjunction with the Johns Hopkins University, created the Institute of the History of Medicine fifty years ago; liberal subvention from the same source made possible the anniversary meeting and helped bring this book to publication.

GREETINGS FROM THE AMERICAN ASSOCIATION FOR THE HISTORY OF MEDICINE

Genevieve Miller

On Wednesday, 12 December 1934 I first set foot in The Johns Hopkins Institute of the History of Medicine as a Goucher College student in Dean Dorothy Stimson's course on the history of science. We had heard an exciting lecture by Dr. Henry Sigerist the preceding Monday at Goucher, and in his absence we were welcomed in the Welch Library by Dr. Fielding H. Garrison at the head of the marble staircase and by Dr. Temkin in the Institute. We were shown, among other treasures, the first edition of Vesalius, which fascinated and stimulated me because it was the first time that I had either seen or handled a really old book. Little did I dream then that forty-five years later I would be president of the American Association for the History of Medicine, retired, and newly resettled in my academic homeland, and extending fiftieth birthday greetings to the Institute!

The Association has been closely associated with the Institute throughout nearly its entire history, beginning in 1927 when Dr. William H. Welch, the first Institute director, was elected president of what was then called the American Section of the International Society for the History of Medicine founded by Dr. E. B. Krumbhaar two years earlier. Under Welch's aegis the Association acquired its present name and its first Constitution. All the subsequent Institute directors have served as president either before or during their Hopkins tenure. In 1938 Sigerist, the Association's energetic secretary, enlarged its scope by establishing Constituent Societies, creating an honorary lectureship, establishing two award medals, and publishing the transactions of the annual meetings in the *Bulletin of the Institute of the History of Medicine*, the new medical history journal which he had founded. Beginning in 1929 the journal became the official organ of both the Institute and the Association with the new name, *Bulletin of the History of Medicine*.

As the first center for graduate instruction in medical history in the United States, the Institute has trained students who have spread throughout the country and generated further interest in the subject. From 360 members in 1927 (of whom 131 had not paid their dues!), the Association grew to 507 in 1945, and has nearly doubled in the following years.

One of the Institute's goals from the very beginning was to raise the standards of American medical historiography, and the annual meeting programs of the Association reflect the gradual improvement of quality that resulted from this and the other graduate teaching centers created in this country since World War II.

On this happy occasion the American Association for the History of Medicine salutes the gifted leaders of the Johns Hopkins Institute—Welch, Sigerist, Shryock, Temkin, Stevenson, and their staffs—who have improved and strengthened medical history in this country, and whose teachings continue to be extended by their disciples. May the good work and inspiration of the Institute continue to flourish!

CAUSES AND PSEUDOCAUSES IN THE HISTORY
OF DISEASES

Erwin H. Ackerknecht

Before discussing some aspects of the history of diseases, I take the liberty of surveying the work done during the last fifty years in a discipline that is about two hundred years old. I know I will not be able to be exhaustive, even in limiting myself to books, and I know that surveys are dull. But they are also useful.

Since the publication of the great classics of Hirsch (1881) and Haeser (1882), no histories of that size have appeared.[1] The field has grown too large for one author. Some have tried shorter books: Colnat, Bett, Henschen, Ackerknecht.[2] Bett, whose excellent book is a cooperative effort, has concentrated on our most common Western diseases. This is quite reasonable; but leaves out such historically relevant diseases as malaria, typhus, cholera, and plague. Another attempt—the book by the historian W. H. McNeill—reads rather like science fiction. The works of eminent bacteriologists-epidemiologists like Charles Nicolle, M. Greenwood, Charles E. Winslow, Cockburn, or M. F. Burnet, though only partly historical, contain many ideas and facts of great importance to the historian of diseases.[3]

As in the beginnings of the historiography of diseases, numerous monographs on single diseases have appeared, mostly on infectious diseases and above all on *plague*—perhaps because plague was the most murderous epidemic disease in history. It is also one of the few that are identifiable with relative ease. The plague has been the favorite of two well-known trends: the one explaining history in terms of diseases; the other explaining diseases in terms of history. Hirst's portrait of the plague has profited from the author's long personal experience with the subject in the East.[4] There are valuable summaries by Pollitzer and Ziegler, and Bowsky's anthology.[5] Mullett is particularly good on old plague "theories"; Shrewsbury enjoys debunking them.[6] Le Roy Ladurie in 1973 dubbed him "the head of the rat school" as opposed to Biraben, "the head of the flea school." Biraben's two volumes on men and the plague in France and in the European and Mediterranean countries are truly monumental.[7] All aspects are discussed. At last somebody has used the more than three thousand studies of local historians on plague. Though one might disagree with the one or the other of Biraben's conclusions, it is probably the most important book of these fifty years in our field. Dols's work on Islam and plague opens new vistas, and Zaddach's study on the plague mortality of the Continental clergy is a very valuable addition to our knowledge.[8]

More of a local character are studies like those by two "classic" authors, J. Guiard and R. Jorge, still working during our period, or those by Rodenwaldt, Cipolla, Charpentier and Bennassar.[9] Charpentier emphasizes the deleterious influence of the repetition of the epidemics, a point made before her by Russell, Lütge, Kelter, and Mullett.[10] According to Charpentier, the enormous loss of human lives during the years 1348 to 1349 worsened a pre-existing economic and moral decline.

Compared to this hypertrophy of plague studies, occupation with the history of other infectious diseases has been sparse. *Cholera* has still done relatively well with the work of Delaunay, Chevalier, Pollitzer, McGrew, and Rosenberg.[11] Charles Rosenberg has followed the course of cholera in the United States from a problem of sin to one of sanitation, from moral dilemma to social problem. But diseases of the importance of *tuberculosis, malaria,* or *influenza* have only found the respective interest of Bochalli and Löffler, Celli and Ackerknecht, and Hoehling.[12] Celli's is the last and most radical formulation of the "malariological" theory of history. *Syphilis,* together with other venereal diseases, has profited from a late work of the famous G. Sticker appearing simultaneously with a book by Jeanselme.[13] Hackett brought important new points into the discussion of treponematoses.[14] The important book by Carter on the African origin of *yellow fever* came out in 1931, Powell's excellent book on the Philadelphia epidemic, in 1949.[15] *Leprosy* has been discussed from different angles by Möller-Christensen and Brody.[16] One of our most eminent polio researchers, J. R. Paul, has given us a history of *poliomyelitis.*[17] The parasitologist Hoeppli wrote an excellent history of *parasitic diseases.*[18] Less successful was the great *typhus* specialist Zinsser, with a history of his main field of interest.[19] There is still no history of *infectious hepatitis,* and we are waiting with impatience for one of *rabies* from Jean Théodoridès.

Still important among regional histories of infectious diseases is Scott's work on tropical diseases.[20] Another Scott has provided us with a history of epidemics in Ghana.[21] D. Cooper traces the history of epidemics in Mexico, a subject also treated in the remarkable studies of Cook and Borah.[22] And there is a whole cluster of books on epidemics in colonial America: Stearns and Stearns, Ashburn, Duffy, and Keehn.[23]

It is surprising that so little effort has been spent on the noninfectious diseases, though they constitute now our main problems. There are but three rather small books on heart disease, and no serious history of cancer has appeared since Jacob Wolff's publication of 1907.[24]

Fortunately one of the foremost *beri-beri* researchers, R. R. Williams, wrote a book on the history of this avitaminosis. And Roe wrote one on *pellagra.* The history of *goiter* was thoroughly studied by Merke. A book on *diabetes* by Papaspyros also exists.[25] Schadewaldt has unfortunately still not brought together in a book his numerous papers on *allergies.* In 1939

W. Grothand published a Düsseldorf thesis on the history of diseases of the *vertebral column*. In Berkeley in 1964 Copeman brought out a short history of *gout*. George Rosen was not only a pioneer in the history of *miner's diseases* but also of *psychopathology*[26] in doing what he called historical sociology. Temkin provided us with a classic work on *epilepsy*. There is also a remarkable study by Norman Cohn.[27] *Ergotism* has been dealt with by Chaumartin, Barger, and Bove.[28] The history of catastrophies overlaps with the history of diseases. An interesting new departure in Wise's book.[29]

Paleopathology, a close relative of our subject, has not developed as it was hoped in the 1920s. But it seems that the efforts of D. R. Brothwell in Britain and S. Jarcho in the United States have had a salutary effect on the situation. J. L. Angel, who since the 1940s has probably made the most numerous valuable contributions to the subject, has regrettably never published a book.[30]

Pathologists and clinicians have increasingly become aware of the existence of historical changes in diseases through the experiences of just the last fifty years.[31] Certain medical sociologists have used materials from the history of diseases, and certain geographers, like André Siegfried, have made important contributions.[32] A number of bibliographies are very helpful, although they cannot, of course, replace true histories.[33]

Two trends have developed more recently in the examination of the history of diseases: "quantohistory" and "psychohistory." They are mainly promoted by historians and are far from being as new as some of their prophets seem to think. As to "quantohistory," Gasquet in 1893 had after all derived much of his evidence from the study of ecclesiastic records. There are, for example, publications of Peller and Kisskalt, in 1920 and 1921 respectively, based on such material, and a Zürich M.S. thesis of 1926 by Baer.[34] In Germany the method had been used rather widely, but was so much misused during the Third Reich for "racial" research that Germans have been very cautious in touching it up to this day. Its only two prominent practitioners in the German language area are two Swiss scholars Imhof and Mattmüller.[35]

The new trend originated rather in France, and to a minor degree in Great Britain after World War II, and was of course reinforced by the rapid ascent of the computer. In France demography had been an early foundation of sociology, as Chevalier correctly states. Demographic historians also went into research in the history of diseases in the early 1950s, among them Yves Renouard, P. Goubert, and L. Henry.[36] The tendency crystallized around Emanuel Le Roy Ladurie, a demographic historian, who became particularly sensitized to the problem of diseases through his interest in climate. Typical of the tendency is a 1972 publication by J. B. Desaive and others.[37] There is no doubt that this trend has often stimulated good work, especially in economic problems, disputed now for decades, but some of its representatives might also do well to exchange their admiration of M. Foucault or psychoanalysis for some knowledge in medical history and medicine.[38]

Of course, the other trend, psychohistory, had antecedents as well: not

only early, with Hecker and Le Bon, but rather recent, with the work of Lu-
cien Febvre, and Baehrel.[39] The gates were opened, however, with William
L. Langer's presidential address to the American Historical Association on
December 29, "The New Assignment."[40] Here Langer, obviously indoctri-
nated by his younger brother, Walter C. Langer, a professional psychoana-
lyst, suggested that future research be based on a psychoanalysis of "long
range psychological repercussions" of diseases. In spite of a great number of
footnotes and references, an aura of dilettantism surrounds this paper. Not
much needs to be said about it, as this has been done so well by Barzun,
Trevor Roper, M. Shepherd, and others.[41] Langer probably dreamt of analyses of history through analysis of diseases. What came out of his manifesto
was something else: a flood of psycho-pathographies (nothing particularly
new) of Hitler, Mao, Stalin, Wilson, Kennedy, Kissinger, Nixon, etc.,
etc.—which, of course, all are based on the mythological Oedipus complex.
Langer himself had called the flood of the psychoanalysis-inspired psychobi-
ographies of the 1920s of "a low order." But most of those of the 1960s and
1970s, following his appeal, resemble qualitatively their predecessors. Is this
perhaps a question of the scientific foundation?

I am convinced that fashions in the history of diseases will come and go
as they do everywhere; the studies themselves will go on. A hundred years
ago Daremberg wrote—not accidentally: "Dans l'histoire de la médecine les
véritables personnages ce sont les maladies." The history of diseases is an
ideal meeting ground for historians and medical historians. The old diseases
are not dead (did a disease ever die?) and it will be a challenge to the researcher to find out, for example, to what extent the "new" virus diseases,
which seem to menace us now, have antecedents.

It is possible that somebody will regard the following discussion of medical theories as not making part of the history of diseases. I feel, on the contrary, that they are inseparable. Certain theories reflect clearly the history of
diseases, certain theories have had a strong influence on the further evolution of diseases. While plague, for example, disappeared from the western
Mediterranean in the beginning of the eighteenth century, it did so only one
and a half centuries later in the eastern Mediterranean as a consequence of
the Turks at last abandoning that great Islamic tradition of passivity towards
God's decisions, like plague, and adopting Western attitudes (last plague in
Constantinople 1841, Asiatic Turkey 1843, Egypt 1840).[42] Biraben has
rightly emphasized the connection between disappearance of plague in the
West and the basing of public health measures there on contagiosity
theories.[43]

The main causal theories for epidemic diseases, the group of diseases we
will mainly discuss here—the influence of gods, devils, and the stars, mi-
asma, and contagion—have been discussed thoroughly elsewhere.[44] But
there are a number of other causal theories—often pseudocausal from our

present-day point of view—which it is perhaps worthwhile to recall to memory: psychological causes, heredity, parasites, sleep, crimes, poverty, wealth, and so on.

What J. Schneck has so aptly called "iatropsychology" comes in waves. We are—or have just been—living through one. Not that any thinking clinician, not even the extreme Greek somaticists or the much-maligned nineteenth-century men, have ever totally failed to consider psychological influences, as some naive and ignorant psychosomaticists have pretended recently. But emphasis on this point has changed repeatedly; so has the list of diseases regarded as psychologically caused. And a psychological explanation has often served to mask plain etiological ignorance.[45]

As an example, to regard *plague* as psychogenic seems to us today rather extreme, and it is not surprising that this opinion is not found in either the Hippocratic corpus or in the writings of Galen. It is, on the other hand, not surprising either that in the "spiritualist" Middle Ages this idea became by no means rare.[46] And that the strange mixture of medieval mysticism and modern observation, Paracelsus, characterizes fear or fright as one of the three main causes of plague epidemics (the other two are natural causes, like spoiled food, or "supernatural," such as God's punishment or the stars). He has also, of course, an infallible preventative to offer: red corals, dissolved in wine, taken twice a day.[47] Nor are such ideas surprising with his follower and the developer of his archeus doctrine, J. B. van Helmont (1577–1644). With van Helmont plague originates through the archeus being frightened.[48]

And it is understandable that later, with Stahl's (1660–1734) animism, a new wave of iatropsychology starts. Not all of Stahl's pupils followed him in the assumption of psychogenic plague. Among them, J. Kanold (1679–1729) and J. Storck (1681–1751) said no.[49] Coschwitz (1679–1729) (developed by Finger) tried a compromise.[50] Psychogenic plague had also been admitted by Chirac (1650–1732) in Montpellier: P. Hecquet in Paris (1661–1737) and Ettmüller (1644–1683) in Leipzig. And a climax was reached by the statement of Ettmüller's disciple, Rivinus (1652–1723), that regards fear and fright as the only cause of plague.[51]

Psychogenic explanations of plague persisted throughout the eighteenth century. The Boerhaave pupils, Gaub (1703–1780) and van Swieten (1700–1772), as well as a Timoni (fl. 1720), or British authors like Manningham (fl. 1750) or Henderson (fl. 1760) recognized them.[52] There is no doubt that these theories interfered with prophylactic measures to isolate cases.

Even the nineteenth century still saw psychogenic explanations for such diseases as typhus,[53] cholera,[54] typhoid,[55] rabies,[56] and general paresis.[57] The famous anticontagionist, Maclean, blamed fearsome quarantining, not contagion, for killing people.[58] For Morton (1689), as well as Auenbrugger (1761), the main causes of consumption were "affections of the soul," especially, nostalgia. Actually, as J. Starobinski has shown, tuberculosis was the main cause of death in "nostalgia."[59] No less a man than Laennec declared tuberculosis noncontagious and (together with cancer) often psychogenic, while his great teacher and friend, G. L. Bayle, opposed this idea for cancer.[60] As late as 1916, Schwarzwald gave a psychogenic explanation of the epidemic of (infectious) hepatitis during World War I![61] Again the practical consequences of these theories are obvious. With increasing knowledge the above-mentioned diseases have ceased to be psychogenic. The principle has been shifted to other conditions.

The second traditionally used causal explanation for diseases that are otherwise not explainable is *heredity*. As Virchow wrote in 1896:

> If one surveys the almost immeasurable number of diseases which have been held as hereditary it soon becomes obvious that the habit of doctors of recognizing the hereditary character of certain diseases has changed almost according to fashion. An inclination in this direction has always existed, as the assumption of heredity protects against any further mental efforts concerning the cause of the condition.[62]

Probably the first conditions regarded as hereditary (in ancient Greece and India) were pulmonary tuberculosis and epilepsy.[63] Hereditary explanations have been present uninterruptedly ever since. The Salernitan regimen, for instance, recognizes six hereditary diseases: sleeping disease, leprosy, favus, phthisis, gout, and stone. Van Helmont mentions that fright and fury produce hereditary pulmonary tuberculosis, lunacy, and epilepsy.

In 1960, Dr. Helmut Semadeni published a very thorough study of the notion of hereditary diseases around 1850.[64] These years must have been the apex of a "hereditary" disease wave. The great Piorry claimed that basically all diseases are hereditary (contradicted by the equally great Louis). Of the over sixty "hereditary" diseases Semadeni dug out from the literature, of which we regard only some as hereditary today, we mention here only asthma (also a typical hereditary disease during the eighteenth century), gout, several eye diseases (here quite a few have been confirmed), and the tendency to hemorrhages. The medieval belief in the heredity of leprosy was still so strong in the nineteenth century that such eminent specialists as Danielson and Boeck asked for sterilization of leprotics. Scabies and favus were still regarded as hereditary in spite of the discoveries of Linné and Schoenlein. Cancer as well as goiter, epilepsy, and mental diseases were explained on the basis of heredity. Rickets and polyarthritis, pulmonary tuberculosis, scrofulosis, and also intestinal worms were hereditary diseases! So too were pellagra and, last but not least, general paresis.[65] Due to the discoveries of bacteriology and biochemistry and the application of better statistics, the hereditary explanations became much rarer after 1900, in spite of German efforts in the 1920s and 1930s to revive them. The growth of experimental genetics after 1900 has, on the other hand, opened a new chapter in this field.

Hoeppli's history of *parasites* in early medicine has revealed—besides early knowledge of pathogenic parasites—an amazing number of nonexisting parasites and pseudoparasites, which were supposedly causing a variety of diseases: heartworm, teethworm, earworm, umbilical worm, hellworm, tongue worm, etc.[66] While a number of *animals* have been rightly accused as carriers of disease (dogs and foxes in rabies, for instance), others have either been overlooked as carriers (rats, vermin) or, although innocent, accused and combated (like dogs, mentioned as carriers of plague, as early as in Homer, Thucydides and Ovid) and persecuted in times of epidemics.[67] A well-known explanation for the spread of epidemics is the "pestis manufacta," employed especially when the extermination of Jews and lepers during the Black Death was to be "justified." But the scapegoat vice is, of course, much older, even in Christendom, and has lasted much longer, whereas the groups (for example, Gypsies, Tartars) and individuals persecuted have changed during the period from the fifteenth to nineteenth centuries.[68] And not so long ago, during the Korean War (1950–1953), the North Korean and Chinese governments, and their sympathizers, accused the United States of spreading plague and other infections in Korea.

It is probably remembered that onanism was for centuries often blamed for producing numerous diseases, all with dire consequences. More of a curiosity is the millenary campaign carried into the eighteenth century from Susruta (by way of Soranus, Salerno, and Avicenna) against the postprandial nap as a pathogenic factor.[69]

When J. P. Frank in 1790 gave his famous lecture, "The People's Misery, Mother of Diseases,"[70] he only expressed an idea that had been alive in the analyses of epidemics by laymen as well as doctors for many centuries: "die Zurückführung der epidemischen Krankheiten auf das soziale Elend," as Emil Behring called it disapprovingly.[71] It struck many contemporaries and historians alike that in epidemics the poor were the ones to suffer first and worst.[72] It is impossible to discuss in detail within the framework of this paper this far-reaching causal theory, which, if analyzed in its elements, was valid in many cases. It, also, has found a lot of attention in recent years. Yet I have brought it in for another reason: to suggest research on the opposite proposition, the *diseases of wealth*. No longer do most of us disappear dramatically in an epidemic or infection (the dramatic remains in the form of accidents, which are also partly a result of our wealth), but we are decaying slowly, largely as a result of our own affluence. One of its consequences, overeating, has been regarded as a source of ill health ever since the time of the ancient Egyptians and Greeks.[73] It was of relatively minor importance in the time of small, overfed elites and hungry majorities. But the twentieth century has allowed large parts of the Western population to overeat. Indirect proof has been given by the decrease of coronary heart disease, diabetes, and other conditions thanks to the enforced moderation in food intake during the two world wars.

As a matter of fact, the idea of diseases of misery is, according to Tissot, somewhat older than that of diseases of wealth, but the latter idea, too, was extant around 1700.[74] It is no accident that this is the time, when acute "fevers" began to recede as well as climatological explanations, and when chronic diseases found more attention. Laws against overeating existed in ancient Rome. Medieval preachers fought it with all their rich vocabulary in explaining that it was not only sinful but unhealthy. Medieval fasting seems to have played a hygienic as well as a religious role. The Salernitan regimen recommends "modest meals." The famous Cornaro (1467–1566) characterizes overeating as "the worst plague."[75]

The medicine of the Enlightenment takes up the problem with new vigor. J. P. Frank quotes Rousseau: "The poor die from want, the rich from plenty."[76] He says: "Most diseases spring from intemperance."[77] Similar opinions are found in Hufeland and B. Faust.[78] Frank claims that gluttony always becomes widespread before the fall of empires. He discusses antigluttony laws in Rome, Athens, Sweden, and Saxony. He also reviews laws against alcoholism, a disease causing addiction among the poor and the rich.[79]

In his *Diseases of Men of the World* Tissot recommends exercise and fresh air to the latter.[80] He sees the devaluation by the wealthy of walking in favor of using carriages as a disease-producing factor, an opinion taken up by Frank.[81] Both observe "degeneration" in the nonworking population.[82] Tissot feels that "passions" form one of the disease-producing elements in these groups, via the nervous system. He comes fairly close to the concept of a "manager's disease," which is, by the way, adumbrated as far back as Galen.[83]

These remarks on the diseases of wealth are only a few glimpses into a field of research that can, I am convinced, eventually yield results relevant to our present-day medical and social problems.

NOTES

[1]A. Hirsch, *Handbuch der historisch-geographischen Pathologie* (Stuttgart, 1881–86); H. Haeser, *Geschichte der epidemischen Krankheiten* (Jena, 1882).

[2]A. Colnat, *Les epidémies et l'histoire* (Paris: Editions Hippocrate, 1937; W. R. Bett, *The History and Conquest of Common Diseases* (Norman: University of Oklahoma Press, 1954); F. Henschen, *The History and Geography of Disease* (New York: Delacorte Press, 1966); and E. H. Ackerknecht, *History and Geography of the Most Important Diseases* (New York: Hafner, 1965).

[3]W. H. McNeill, *Plagues and People* (New York: Anchor/Doubleday, 1976); C. Nicolle, *Destin des maladies infectieuses* (Paris: F. Alcan, 1933); M. Greenwood, *Epidemics and Crowd Diseases* (New York: Macmillan, 1937); C. E. Winslow, *The Conquest of Epidemic Disease* (Princeton: Princeton University Press, 1944); A. Cockburn, *Infectious Diseases* (Springfield, Ill.: Charles C Thomas, 1967); and F. M. Burnet, *Natural History of Infectious Disease*, 3d ed. (Cambridge: At the University Press, 1962).

[4]L. F. Hirst, *The Conquest of Plague* (Oxford: Clarendon Press, 1953).

[5]R. Pollitzer, *Plague*, World Health Organization, Monograph Series, no. 22 (Geneva, 1954); P. Ziegler, *Black Death* (London: Collins, 1969); and W. M. Bowsky, *The Black Death: A Turning Point in History* (New York: Holt, Rinehart, & Winston, 1971).

[6]C. F. Mullett, *The Bubonic Plague and England* (Lexington: University of Kentucky Press, 1956); J.F.D. Shrewsbury, *A History of Plague in the British Isles* (Cambridge: At the University Press, 1971).

[7]J. N. Biraben, *Les Hommes et la peste en France et dans les pays européens et méditeranéens*, 2 vols. (Paris: Mouton, 1975–1976).

[8]M. W. Dols, *The Black Death in the Middle East* (Princeton: Princeton University Press, 1977); B. J. Zaddach, *Die Folgen des schwarzen Todes für den Klerus Mittel-europas* (Stuttgart: G. Fischer, 1971).

[9]J. Guiard, "Histoire de la peste en France au 16ᵉ et 17ᵉ siècles," *Rev. Univ. Lyon* 1 (1933): 53–91. R. Jorge, "La Peste Africaine," *Bull. Off. Intern. d'Hyg. Publ.*, 29 (1935): 1–67; E. Rodenwaldt, *Pest in Venedig 1575–1577* (Heidelberg: Springer-Verlag, 1953); C. M. Cipolla, *Cristofano and the Plague* (London: Collins, 1973); E. Charpentier, *Une Ville devant la Peste: Orvieto et la peste noire de 1348* (Paris: SEVPEN, 1962); and B. Bennassar, *Recherche sur les grandes épidémies dans le nord de l'Espagne à la fin du 16ᵉ siècle* (Paris: SEVPEN, 1969). Much important local information is also contained in E. Olivier, *Médecine et santé dans le pays de Vaud* (Lausanne: Librarie Payot, 1962); vols. 1–2; *Des Origines à la fin du XVIIᵉ siècle: 1675–1798*, vols. 3–4: *Au XVIIIᵉ siècle: 1675–1798*.

[10]J. C. Russell, *British Medieval Population* (Albuquerque: University of New Mexico Press, 1948); F. Lütge, *Jahrb. f. Nationalökonomie u. Statistik*, 162 (1950): 161–213; E. Kelter, ibid., *Jahrb. f. Nationalökonomie u. Statistik*, 165 (1953): 161–208; Mullett, *Bubonic Plague and England.* Wilhelm Abel has studied the disappearance of villages, the so-called "Wüstung," since 1935.

[11]P. Delaunay, *Le Corps médical et le choléra en 1832* (Tours: Impr. Tour angelle, 1933); L. Chevalier, *Le Choléra: La première épidémie du XIXᵉ siècle* (La Roche sur Yon: Impr. Central de l'Ouest, 1958); R. Pollitzer, *Cholera* (Geneva: World Health Organization, 1959); R. E. McGrew, *Russia and the Cholera: 1823–1832* (Madison: University of Wisconsin Press, 1965); and C. Rosenberg, *The Cholera Years: The U.S. in 1832, 1849, 1866* (Chicago: University of Chicago Press, 1962).

[12]R. Bochalli, *Geschichte der Schwindsucht* (Leipzig: G. Thieme, 1940). W. Löffler, "Geschichte der Tuberkulose," in *Handbuch der Tuberkulose*, eds. J. Hein et al. (Stuttgart: Thieme, 1958), 1:1–96. See also C. Coury, *La Tuberculose au cours des ages: Grandeur et déclin d'une maladie* (Suresnes: Lepetit, 1972); A. Celli, *The History of Malaria in the Roman Campagna from Ancient Times* (London: John Bale, 1933). E. H. Ackerknecht, *Malaria in the Upper Mississippi Valley: 1760–1900* (Baltimore: The Johns Hopkins Press, 1945), *Suppl. Bull. Hist. Med.*, no. 4. See also J.W.W. Stephenson, *Blackwater Fever* (Liverpool: Liverpool University Press, 1937); and A. A. Hoehling, *The Great Epidemic* (Boston: Little, Brown, 1961).

[13]G. Sticker, "Entwurf einer Geschichte der ansteckenden Geschlechtskrankheiten," in *Handbuch der Haut- und Geschlechtskrankheiten*, ed. J. Jadassohn, vol. *23 (Berlin: J. Springer, 1931); and E. Jeanselme, Histoire de la syphilis* (Paris: G. Doin, 1931).

[14]C. H. Hackett, "On the Origin of Human Treponematoses," *Bull. Wld. Hlth. Org.*, 29 (1963): 7–44.

[15]H. R. Carter, *Yellow Fever: An Epidemiological and Historical Study of Its Place of Origin* (Baltimore: Williams & Wilkins, 1931); J. H. Powell, *Bring Out Your Dead* (Philadelphia: University of Pennsylvania Press, 1949).

[16]V. Möller-Christensen, "Osteo-Archeology as an Auxiliary Medico-Historical Sci-

ence," *Med. Hist.*, 17 (1973): 411–18; and S. N. Brody, *Disease of the Soul: Leprosy in Medieval Literature* (Ithaca, N.Y.: Cornell University Press, 1974). See also A. Weymouth, *Through the Leper-Squint: A Study of Leprosy from Pre-Christian Times to the Present Day* (London: Selwyn & Blount, 1938).

[17]J. R. Paul, *History of Poliomyelitis* (New Haven: Yale University Press, 1971).

[18]R. Hoeppli, *Parasites and Parasitic Infections in Early Medicine and Science* (Singapore: University of Malaya Press, 1959).

[19]H. Zinsser, *Rats, Lice, and History* (Boston: Little, Brown, 1935).

[20]H. H. Scott, *A History of Tropical Medicine* (London: E. Arnold, 1939).

[21]D. Scott, *Epidemic Disease in Ghana: 1901–60* (London: Oxford University Press, 1965). See also G. W. Hartung and K. D. Patterson, eds., *Disease in African History* (Durham, N.C.: Duke University Press, 1978).

[22]Donald Cooper, *Epidemic Diseases in Mexico City: 1761–1813* (Austin: University of Texas Press, 1965). See also G. M. Foster, *Culture and Conquest: America's Spanish Heritage* (New York: Wenner-Gren, 1960); S. F. Cook and W. Borah, *Essays in Population History*, vol. 1, *Mexico* (Berkeley and Los Angeles: University of California Press, 1971). Cook has been active in this field since 1937, Borah since 1951.

[23]E. Stearns and A. E. Stearns, *The Effect of Smallpox on the Destiny of the Amerindian* (Boston: B. Humphries, 1945); P. M. Ashburn, *The Ranks of Death* (New York: Coward-McCann, 1947); J. Duffy, *Epidemics in Colonial America* (Baton Rouge: Louisiana State University Press, 1953); and P. A. Keehn, *The Effect of Epidemic Diseases on the Natives of North America* (London: Survival International, 1978).

[24]F. A. Willius and T. J. Dry, *A History of the Heart and Circulation* (Philadelphia: W. B. Saunders, 1948); T. East, *The Story of Heart Disease* (London: William Dawson, 1958); J. O. Leibowitz, *History of Coronary Heart Disease*, Wellcome Inst. Hist. Med. Publ., n.s., vol. 18 (London, 1970); and J. Wolff, *Die Lehre von der Krebskrankheit von den ältesten Zeiten bis zur Gegenwart*, vol. 1 (Jena: G. Fischer, 1907).

[25]R. R. Williams, *Toward the Conquest of Beri-Beri* (Cambridge: Harvard University Press, 1961); D. A. Roe, *A Plague of Corn* (Ithaca, N.Y.: Cornell University Press, 1973). For avitaminoses see also E. V. McCollum, *A History of Nutrition* (Boston: Houghton Mifflin, 1957); F. Merke, *Geschichte und Ikonographie des endemischen Kropfes und Kretinismus* (Bern: Hans Huber, 1971); and N. S. Papaspyros, *History of Diabetes Mellitus* (London: Robert Stockwell, 1952).

[26]George Rosen, *The History of Miners' Diseases* (New York: Schuman, 1943); idem, *Madness in Society* (Chicago: University of Chicago Press, 1968). See also I. Veith, *Hysteria: The History of a Disease* (Chicago: University of Chicago Press, 1965); and E. Fischer-Homberger, *Hypochondrie* (Bern: Hans Huber, 1970).

[27]O. Temkin, *The Falling Sickness* (Baltimore: Johns Hopkins Press, 1945); N. Cohn, *The Pursuit of the Millennium* (London: Secker & Warburg, 1957).

[28]H. Chaumartin, *Le Mal des ardents et le feu Saint-Antoine* (Vienne La Romaine: Ternet Martin, 1946); G. Barger, *Ergot and Ergotism* (London: Gurney & Jackson, 1931); F. J. Bove, *The Story of Ergot* (Basel-New York: Karger, 1970).

[29]See for example M. Wolfenstein, *Disaster: A Psychological Essay* (Glencoe, Ill.: Free Press, 1957); J. G. Leithäuser, *Katastrophen: Der Mensch im Kampf mit Naturgewalten* (Berlin: Safari-Verlag, 1956); and W. Wise, *Killer Smog: The World's Worst Air Pollution Disaster* (Chicago: Rand McNally, 1968).

[30]D. R. Brothwell and T. A. Sandison, eds., *Diseases in Antiquity* (Springfield, Ill.: Charles C Thomas, 1967); S. Jarcho, ed., *Human Paleopathology* (New Haven: Yale University Press, 1966): see the survey article of M. Goldstein, "Human Paleopathology and Some Diseases in Living Primitive Societies: A Review of the Recent Literature," *Amer. J. Phys. Anthropol.*, 31 (1969): 285–94.

[31]For example see H. Rolleston, "Changes in the Character of Diseases," *Brit.*

Med. J. 1 (1933) 499–500; W. Doerr, ed., *Gestaltwandel klassischer Krankheitsbilder* (Berlin: Springer-Verlag, 1957).

[32]J. Siegrist, *Medizinische Soziologie* (Munich: Urban & Schwarzenberg, 1974); C. v. Ferber, *Soziologie für Mediziner: eine Einführung* (Berlin: Springer-Verlag, 1975); H. E. Freeman, ed., *Handbook of Medical Sociology* (Englewood Cliffs, N.J.: Prentice-Hall, 1975); E. B. McKinley, *A Geography of Disease* (Washington: George Washington University Press, 1935); J. M. May, *The Ecology of Human Disease* (New York: M.D. Publicationa, 1958); E. Rodenwaldt et al., *Weltseuchenatlas* (Hamburg: Falk-Verlag, 1956); A. Siegfried, *Itinéraire des contagions: épidémies et idéologies* (Paris: Colin, 1960).

[33]A. L. Bloomfield, *A Bibliography of Internal Medicine* (Chicago: University of Chicago Press, 1958–60); M. Fishbein et al., *A Bibliography of Infantile Paralysis: 1789–1949*, 2d ed. (Philadelphia: Lippincott, 1951); J. Schumacher, *Index zum Diabetes mellitus* (Munich: Urban & Schwarzenberg, 1961).

[34]F. A. Gasquet, *The Great Plague* (London, 1893); K. Kisskalt, "Sterblichkeit im 18. Jahrhundert," *Ztschr. f. Hyg. u. Infek. Krank.*, 93 (1921): 438–511; S. Peller, "Zur Kenntnis der städtischen Mortalität," ibid., 90 (1920): 227; M. Baer, *Medizinisch-statistische Ergebnisse aus Zürcher Kirchenbüchern des 17, und 18. Jahrhunderts* (Zürich: H. A. Gutzwiller, 1926).

[35]Erich Keyser, "Neue deutsche Forschungen über die Geschichte der Pest," *Vierteljahresschrift für Sozial- und Wirtschaftsgeschichte*, 44 (1957): 243–53; A. E. Imhof and O. Larson, *Sozialgeschichte und Medizin* (Stuttgart: Fischer, 1976); vol. 12 of *Medizin in Geschichte und Kultur*; M. Mattmüller, *Einführung in Bevölkerungsstatistik der Schweiz* (Basel: 1973). Mattmüller has also formed a group for research in plague history with H. Koelbing, director of the History of Medicine Institute of Zürich.

[36]Y. Renouard, "Conséquences et intérêt demographiques de la peste noire de 1348," *Population* 3 (1948): 459–66; P. Goubert, "En Beauvoisis," *Annales E.S.C.* 7 (1952): 453; L. Henry and E. Gautier, *La Population de Crulai paroisse Normande* (Paris: Presses Universitaires de France, 1958).

[37]E. Le Roy Ladurie, *Histoire du climat depuis l'an mil* (Paris: Flammarion, 1967); idem, "La menorrhoe de la femme," *Annales E.S.C.* 24 (1969): 1589–1601; idem, "Du coté de l'ordinateur," in his *Le Territoire de l'historien* (Paris: Gallimard, 1973); idem, "Un Concept: L'unification microbienne du monde," *Schw. Ztschr. f. Gesch.* 23 (1973): 627–96 (based on Cook and Borah, *Essays in Population History*); and J. P. Desaive et al., *Médecine, climats et épidémies à la fin du 18ᵉ siècle*, Civilisations et Sociétés, no. 29 (Paris: Mouton, 1972).

[38]The fashionable structuralist philosopher M. Foucault has characterized himself well in declaring: "I think in order to forget. What I have written doesn't interest me." N. Meienberg, *Das Schmettern des gallischen Hahns* (Neuwied: Luchterhand, 1966), p. 133. Declarations like that of Peter in Desaive et al., *Médecine, climats et épidémies*, p. 165: "La Tendance hysteroide disparait par l'exécution du père le 21 janvier 1793," are hardly fruits of true quantitative analysis.

[39]L. Febvre, *Le Problème de l'incroyance au XVIᵉ siècle* (Paris: A. Michel, 1947); idem, *Histoire psychologique*; R. Baehrel, "La Haine des classes en temps d'épidémie," *Annales E.S.C.* (1952): 351.

[40]*Amer. Hist. Rev.* 63 (1958): 283–304.

[41]Langer has recently published interesting memoirs of his training in Vienna in 1938 in *J. Hist. Behav. Sci.* 14 (1978): 37–55; J. Barzun, *Clio and the Doctors: Psycho-history, Quanto-history and History* (Chicago: University of Chicago Press, 1974); M. Shepherd, "Clio and Psyche," *J. Roy. Soc. Med.* 72 (1978): 406–12.

[42]W. Griesinger, *Infectionskrankheiten* (Erlangen, 1864), p. 295.

[43]Biraben, *Les Hommes et la peste en France*, 2:183.

[44]See for example E. H. Ackerknecht, "Anticontagionism between 1821 and 1867," *Bull. Hist. Med.* 22 (1948): 562–93; see also H. Ribbert, *Die Lehre vom Wesen der Krankheit* (Bonn, 1899); F. Troels-Lund, *Gesundheit und Krankheit* (Leipzig: B. G. Teubner, 1901); E. Berghoff, *Entwicklungsgeschichte der Krankheitsbegriff* (Vienna: Maudrich, 1947); and K. E. Rothschuh, *Konzepte der Medizin in Vergangenheit und Gegenwart* (Stuttgart: Hippokrates Verlag, 1978).

[45]J. M. Schneck, "Iatrochemistry, iatrophysics and iatropsychology," *Dis. Nerv. Syst.* 22 (August, 1961); E. H. Ackerknecht, "Das Märchen vom verlorenen Psychosomatismus," *Gesnerus* 25 (1968): 113–15; D. Schneider, *Psychosomatik in der Pariser Klinik von Pinel bis Trousseau* (Zurich: Juris Verlag, 1964); and M. Egli, *Psychosomatik bei den deutschen Klinikern des 19. Jahrhunderts* Zürcher medizingeschichtliche Abhandlungen, n.s., no. 23 (Zurich: Juris Verlag, 1964).

[46]Biraben, *Les Hommes et la peste en France*, 2:37–38.

[47]Paracelsus, *Sämtliche Werke*, ed. B. Aschner (Jena: Gustav Fischer, 1926), 1:684, 726.

[48]"Tumulus pestis" quoted in C. Daremberg, *Histoire des sciences médicales*, 2 vols. (Paris, 1870), 1:480–81.

[49]J. Storck, ed. and comment., *Praxis Stahliana* (Leipzig, 1732), pp. 773, 781.

[50]C. S. Finger, *Über den schädlichen Einfluss von Furcht und Schreck bei der Pest* (Diss. Halle, 1722), trans. and ed. H. Koelbing (Aarau: Sauerländer, 1979). See also H. Koelbing, U. B. Hirchler, and P. Arnold, "Die Auswirkungen von Angst und Schreck auf Pest und Pestbekämpfung nach zwei Pestschriften des 18. Jahrhunderts," *Gesnerus* 36 (1979): 116–26.

[51]Quoted by Finger, *Über den schädlichen Einfluss von Furcht und Schreck bei der Pest*, p. 40. Finger also agrees that fear and fright can produce smallpox, measles, typhus, and scabies. No elaborate proof is needed in this respect concerning epilepsy or apoplexy, "as we encounter daily such cases," p. 13.

[52]Ribbert, *Die Lehre vom Wesen der Krankheit*, p. 195; G. van Swieten, *Erläuterungen der Boerhaave'schen Lehrsätze* (Vienna, 1755), 1:298; Mullett, *Bubonic Plague and England*, pp. 265, 311, 322.

[53]Maclean in Ackerknecht, "Anticontagionism," p. 584; Colnat, *Les Epidémies et l'histoire*, p. 160.

[54]Chevalier, *Le Choléra*, pp. 16, 1141.

[55]Chomel in E. H. Ackerknecht, *Medicine at the Paris Hospitals: 1794–1848* (Baltimore: The Johns Hopkins Press, 1966), pp. 101–2.

[56]C. W. Hufeland, *Encheiridion medicum* (St. Gallen, 1839), p. 70. Rabies was generated in dogs by excitement.

[57]T. J. Austin, "Clinical picture of general paralysis of the insane," reprinted in *Three Hundred Years of Psychiatry: 1535–1860*; ed. R. A. Hunter and I. MacAlpine, (London: Oxford University Press, 1963), pp. 1052–57.

[58]Maclean in Ackerknecht, "Anticontagionism," p. 584.

[59]Löffler, *Geschichte der Tuberculose*, p. 25; J. Starobinski, "Le Nostalgie: Théories médicales et expression littéraire," *Studies on Voltaire and the Eighteenth Century* 27 (1963):1505–18.

[60]In Ackerknecht, *Medicine at the Paris Hospital*, p. 95; G. L. Bayle, "Cancer" in *Dict. des sci. méd.* (Paris, 1812), 3:668.

[61]See also E. H. Ackerknecht, "The Vagaries of the Notion of Epidemic Hepatitis" in *Medicine, Science, and Culture: Essays in Honor of Owsei Temkin*, ed. L. G. Stevenson and E. P. Multhauf (Baltimore: The Johns Hopkins Press, 1968) pp. 3–16.

[62]Idem, *Rudolf Virchow* (Madison: University of Wisconsin Press, 1953), p. 206.

[63]Löffler, "Geschichte der Tuberculose," pp. 6, 9; Temkin, *The Falling Sickness*.

[64]Ribbert, *Die Lehre vom Wesen der Krankheit*, p. 120.

[65]H. Semadeni, *Die Erbkrankheiten um 1850* (Zurich: Julius Verlag, 1960); C. Anglada, *Etude des maladies éteintes et les maladies nouvelles, pour servir à l'histoire des évolutions séculaires de la pathologie* (Paris, 1869), p.29.

[66]Hoeppli, *Parasites and Parasitic Infections*, pp. 58, 69, 70, 71.

[67]E. Leclainche, *Histoire illustrée de la médecine vetérinaire* (Monaco: Albin Michel, 1955); Shrewsbury, *History of Plague in the British Isles,* p. 194; Mullett, *Bubonic Plague and England* gives numerous examples of preventative dog killing from the sixteenth and seventeenth centuries (for example, p. 46). Only Petty remarked, in 1667, upon its ineffectiveness. Occasionally also swine and cats were accused as plague carriers. See also Biraben, *Les Hommes et la peste en France,* 2:25.

[68]E. Fröhner, *Kulturgeschichte der Tierheilkunde* (Konstanz: Terra Verlag, 1952–68), 2:176; Biraben, *Les Hommes et la peste en France,* 2:23–25; Colnat, *Les Épidémies et l'histoire,* p. 119; and Ackerknecht, *History and Geography of the Most Important Diseases,* p. 22.

[69]E. H. Hare, "Masturbatory Insanity," *J. Mental Sci.* 108: (1962) 1–25; W. Gubser, "Ist der Mittagsschlaf schädlich?" *Schweiz. Med. Wschr.* 97 (1967): 213–16.

[70]Henry E. Sigerist, trans. and comment., *Bull. Hist. Med.* 9 (1941):81–100.

[71]Quoted in G. Rosen, *From Medical Police to Social Medicine* (New York: Science History Publications, 1974), p. 61.

[72]See Biraben, *Les Hommes et la peste en France,* 2:31; Colnat, *Les Épidémies et l'histoire,* p. 172; Ackerknecht, *History and Geography of the Most Important Diseases,* p. 22.

[73]Ribbert, *Die Lehre vom Wesen der Krankheit,* p. 190.

[74]S. A. Tissot, *Les Maladies des gens du monde* (Lausanne, 1770), p. x.

[75]L. Kotelmann, *Gesundheitspflege im Mittelalter* (Hamburg, 1890); H. Schipperges, *Lebendige Heilkunde von grossen Aerzten und Philosophen aus der drei Jahrtausenden* (Freiburg: Walter, 1962), p. 110; *L'Ecole de Salerno,* trans. C. Méux St. Marc (Paris, 1880), p. 56; and L. Cornaro, *Discourse on a Sober and Temperate Life* (London, 1768), p. 2.

[76]J. P. Frank, *System einer vollständigen medizinischen Polizey,* 9 vols. (Mannheim-Vienna, 1779–1827), 1:19.

[77]Ibid., 3:616.

[78]C. W. Hufeland, *Makrobiotik* (Jena, 1798), p. 55: B. C. Faust, *Gesundheitscatechismus* (Hannover, 1794), p. 1.

[79]Frank, *System einer vollständigen medizinischen Polizey,* 3:621.

[80]Tissot, *Les Maladies des gens,* p.105.

[81]Ibid, p. 30; Frank, *System einer vollständigen medizinischen Polizey,* 1:26.

[82]Tissot, *Les Maladies des gens,* p. 57; Frank, *System einer vollständigen medizinischen Polizey,* 1:39.

[83]Tissot, *Les Maladies des gens,* p. 31; Galen, *Hygiene,* trans. R. M. Green (Springfield, Ill., Charles C Thomas, 1951), p. 51.

Commentary The History of Disease: Now and in the Future

Charles E. Rosenberg

Professor Ackerknecht has evaluated a half century of research and publication. I would like to do something rather different: to describe not what has happened in the past, but to evaluate what is taking place now and will be taking place in the next generation.

Any discussion of the art's present state must begin with the observation that the history of disease is becoming increasingly relevant to historians generally; it is no longer an almost exclusive concern of medical men and medical historians. There are some past exceptions of course; plague, for example, has long occupied a prominent place in the canon of accepted historical subject matter. But the Black Death is atypical. It is only in recent years that disease has come to seem an appropriate subject for historical investigation, and not the occasion for random ancedote.

This increased interest is closely associated with the rise in the past generation of what has come to be called the new social history. For a number of reasons disease has become a natural if not necessary part of that ill-defined but vigorous enterprise. One central element in contemporary social history is demography; the findings, and to some extent, the methods of demography have already become part of our generation's accepted historical canon. Although historians of population agree that there was something they call a demographic revolution, and have demostrated it in local studies and in the aggregate analyses of larger units, they are still unsure of the configuration of factors that brought this change about. Nutrition, birth control, medical skills, and of course sickness and mortality are all relevant candidates for study. Another important element, both motivational and substantive, found in the new social history is an emphasis on what has been called history from below—the study, that is, of ordinary men and women as opposed to the traditional emphasis on the powerful and successful. Most "ordinary" people don't write books or rule countries—or even keep diaries—but they do live and die. Insofar as one hopes to study the quality of their lives, one must of necessity evaluate such factors as diet, agricultural practice, family and household structure, work and religious belief, and of course morbidity and mortality.[1] And no kind of data can be ignored in attempting to reconstruct such everyday realities.

In a few areas such interests have already become prominent. One is the history of Asia, Africa, and the non-West generally. Historians of Africa and Latin America, for example, have become increasingly concerned with the use of mortality data and disease conditions as they seek to understand the texture of life in pre-colonial and post-colonial societies; indeed one fundamental aspect of early contact with the West lies in the impact of disease itself and its consequent relationship to political, economic, military, and even ideological change. Whereas older historians of colonialism — though they would probably not have employed that term — tended to write from the perspective of European capitals and archives and concern themselves with political and administrative questions, their more recent successors have often explored the experience and perceptions of the colonized, not the colonizers. Scholarly interests have shifted to cultural and behavioral questions, and sickness and healing have inevitably played a prominent role among them.[2]

Similarly, social historians of Europe and Anglo-America have turned not only to the behaviors latent in the demographer's aggregate figures, but also — increasingly — to the specific ideas and world-views of ordinary men and women. They have turned, that is, to what French social historians have come to call *mentalité*, for the moment, at least, an indispensable, if neither definable nor entirely translatable, term. Such work brings many of the concerns of the cultural anthropologist into the historian's ken. In particular, that field's interest in world-view necessarily encompasses a long-standing concern with ideas of disease causation and the way in which such concepts reflect fundamental aspects of social structure and social organization. That last half-dozen years have already brought substantial indications that this is going to be a very influential approach in the next decade or two. Such interest in the relation of medical ideas to world-views generally relates, of course, to the movement for writing history from below, inasmuch as this work will deal not so much with high culture, the debates and treatises of professors, as with the ideas of ordinary people.[3] And with a growing sophistication it is becoming clear that this very relationship between high and popular culture is in itself of central importance to an understanding of social structure and social change — while ideas concerning the body and its state of health provide an ideal test case for studying the distribution and uses of knowledge.

In addition to the growing interest in social history, contemporary debate over the place and prerogatives of the medical profession will almost certainly continue to stimulate interest in the history of disease. The most extreme critics of the profession have sought to destroy the moral legitimacy often accorded to medicine as both scientific and efficacious. In many ways the most extreme and widely discussed statement of this position was made a half-dozen years ago by Ivan Illich; yet his views are in some ways consistent with the strictures of such revisionist evaluators of medical history as René

Dubos and Thomas McKeown.[4] Without venturing into the substantive aspects of the debate over the possible role of medicine in lengthening lives and reducing infectious ills, it is certainly apparent at this juncture that the argument has still to be decided. Critics have dismissed the more extreme and ahistorical claims of medical *therapeutics*, but have thus far failed to explain adequately what did cause the vital changes that we have so long and so casually associated with conscious medical policy. (In many ways, of course, this position has a much older lineage. Erwin Ackerknecht's classic monograph on *Malaria in the Upper Mississippi Valley*, for example, published almost four decades ago, is an elegant reminder of the well-established nature of ecological approaches, and of the tenacity of an older social medicine.)[5] But whether we agree or disagree with particular evaluations of the medical profession's historical role, this area of contention has both defined and motivated a renewed concern with disease and its social and economic determinants.

And there are a host of other politically resonant questions that will help keep disease in the foreground of historical concern. One applies with particular force to the United States. This is the growing interest in black history, and with it the way in which disease conditions have shaped one dimension of the collective experience of a group that has left a comparatively small body of traditional literary sources. Studies of slavery and the slave trade in Africa, in the West Indies, and in the United States routinely include materials on medicine, sickness, and mortality.[6] A parallel observation can be made in regard to women's history, where the study of past interactions among doctors, women, and women's health has become an active, if not agitated, field of historical investigation.

All these aspects of the new social history cannot well be separated, for they relate to one another in a number of significant ways. But there is another contemporary trend that has origins and implications quite different from those we have seen as mingling in the new social history. This is an emphasis on the biological history of disease and especially the impact of that natural history on man's social evolution. Biology approximates destiny in this revival of nineteenth-century interpretive styles. Perhaps the most widely discussed example of this genre is William McNeill's *Plagues and Peoples*, which ministers to our natural desire for mechanistic models with which to explain historical change.[7] Such deterministic arguments neatly parallel the current revival of interest in what has come to call itself "sociobiology." Obviously a part of the reason for this revival of biological reductionism lies in the explanatory promise of new scientific information; but much of the motivation must be sought in areas unrelated to the specific content of these ideas. In the case of both sociobiology and "disease as destiny" the hard biological data invoked serve as an egregiously narrow base for an inverted pyramid of speculation. But the very allure of such speculation and continued addition to our store of scientific information—and thus plausible materials for speculation—guarantees that the biological impact of disease will continue to be studied and at times exaggerated.

I would like to conclude with a theme also explored at the conclusion of Professor Ackerknecht's paper. This is a growing interest in the environmental and social dimensions of disease—in seeing disease in relation to its victims' social situation. Partially because of a comparative lack of interest in the infectious ills, and partially because of the contemporary impact of a more general concern for the environment as provoker of disease, our generation has seen an increasing interest in what the nineteenth century would have called "constitutional" ailments. One need only refer to cancer, for example, and the way it has encouraged an interest in questions of environment, of social policy and regional difference, of diet and life-style and their relationship to the economy—all variables commonplace in nineteenth-century medical speculation, but still uncomfortable factors for many clinicians today. Such relationships constitute fertile areas for historical investigation and at the same time mirror many of those interests that have helped make the new social history so important to historical practice in the past generation. These interests should also encourage a renewed empathy with past medical thought; historians at the end of the twentieth century will approach the holistic and environment-oriented conjectures of earlier centuries with far more sympathy than some of their medico-historical predecessors, who had often little patience for the seemingly misguided speculations of past centuries.

A parallel point can be made in regard to heredity. We know a great deal more about it, and the more we know, the more provisional the knowledge of our immediate past appears; the balance between heredity and environment seems once again a central question for the student of disease. Our knowledge of modern genetics has certain other implications as well, for it underlines a much older debate concerning the biological idiosyncrasies of race. Here too disease will constitute a relevant area of investigation—as it has already in regard to black history; immunology and gene distributions may never be the royal road to historical understanding, but they will certainly constitute a path followed by at least some adepts.

I have hoped to be brief and informal and would like to conclude with an appropriate homily. Disease will continue to be a fruitful subject for gaining an understanding of the relationship between biological event and society; there has always been a dialectic between disease as experience, and the social forms and ideas of the society in which that illness occurs and is defined. There is a relationship as well between the economic and social organization of that society and the diseases that arise within it. Such relationships are intrinsically complex and significant and will always constitute an appropriate subject for historical investigation—even if the particular influences and motivations we have seen as influential today fade into the dustbin of historical motivations.

NOTES

[1]Particularly influential in this development has been the example of the so-called *Annales* school; for a representative sample of their work in English, see Robert Forster and Orest Ranum, *Biology of Man in History, Selections from the Annales: Economies, Sociétés, Civilisations*, trans. Elborg Forster and Patricia M. Ranum (Baltimore: The Johns Hopkins University Press, 1975); see also Peter Burke, ed., *A New Kind of History from the Writings of Febvre*, trans. K. Folca (New York: Harper & Row, 1973).

[2]See, for example, Alfred W. Crosby, Jr., *The Columbian Exchange: Biological and Cultural Consequences of 1492* (Westport, Conn.: Greenwood Press, 1972); idem, "Virgin Soil Epidemics as a Factor in the Aboriginal Depopulation in America," *William and Mary Quart.*, 3d. ser. 33 (1976):289–99; Sherburne F. Cook, "The Significance of Disease in the Extinction of the New England Indians," *Human Biology*, 45 (1973):485–508; Gerald W. Hartwig and K. David Patterson, eds., *Disease in African History: An Introductory Survey and Case Studies* (Durham, N.C.: Duke University Press, 1978), and especially K. David Patterson's useful "Bibliographical Essay," pp. 238–50. The work of Philip Curtin on the demography and epidemiology of the slave trade has been particularly influential: " 'The White Man's Grave': Image and Reality, 1780–1850," *J. British Studies* 1 (1961):94–110; "Epidemiology and the Slave Trade," *Political Sci. Quart.*, 83 (1968):190–216.

[3]See, for example, the widely cited study by Keith Thomas, *Religion and the Decline of Magic* (New York: Charles Scribner's, 1971), and Bernard Capp, *English Almanacs, 1500–1800: Astrology and the Popular Press* (Ithaca, N.Y.: Cornell University Press, 1979), pp. 180–214.

[4]Ivan Illich, *Medical Nemesis* (London: Calder & Boyars, 1975); René Dubos, *Mirage of Health: Utopias, Progress, and Biological Change* (Garden City, N.Y.: Doubleday, 1961); Thomas McKeown and R. G. Brown, "Medical Evidence Related to English Population Changes in the Eighteenth Century," *Population Studies* 9 (1955):119–41; McKeown and R. G. Record, "Reasons for the Decline of Mortality in England and Wales during the Nineteenth Century," *Population Studies* 16 (1962): 94–122; McKeown, *The Modern Rise of Population* (New York: Academic Press, 1976); idem, *The Role of Medicine: Dream, Mirage, or Nemesis?* (Princeton: Princeton University Press, 1979). Criticism of medical overemphasis on therapeutics and underestimation of preventive (and especially economic and environmental) variables is, of course, a much older theme in the history of public health and social medicine.

[5]Ackerknecht, *Malaria in the Upper Mississippi Valley: 1760–1900* (Baltimore: The Johns Hopkins Press, 1945); reprint ed., New York, N.Y.: Arno Press, 1977, *Suppl. Bull. Hist. Med.*, no. 4.

[6]See, among many such examples: Richard S. Dunn, *Sugar and Slaves: The Rise of the Planter Class in the English West Indies, 1624–1713* (Chapel Hill: University of North Carolina Press, 1972); Peter H. Wood, *Black Majority: Negroes in Colonial South Carolina from 1670 through the Stono Rebellion* (New York: Knopf, 1974); Todd Savitt, *Medicine and Slavery: The Diseases and Health Care of Blacks in Antebellum Virginia* (Urbana: University of Illinois Press, 1978); Michael Craton, *Searching for the Invisible Man: Slaves and Plantation Life in Jamaica* (Cambridge: Harvard University Press, 1978); Kenneth and Virginia Kiple, "Slave Child Mortality: Some Nutritional Answers to a Perennial Puzzle," *J. Social Hist.* 10 (1977):284–309; Kenneth and Virginia Kiple, "Black Tongue and Black Men: Pellagra and Slavery in the Antebellum South," *J. Southern Hist.* 43 (1977):411–28; B. W. Higman, *Slave Population and Economy in Jamaica, 1807–1834* (Cambridge: At the University Press, 1976).

[7]William H. McNeill, *Plagues and Peoples* (Garden City, N.Y.: Doubleday/ Anchor, 1976).

BIOMEDICAL THOUGHT IN GLISSON'S HEPATOLOGY AND IN WEPFER'S WORK ON APOPLEXY

Nikolaus Mani

Glisson's work on the anatomy of the liver and Wepfer's study on apoplexy were published in the middle of the seventeenth century.[1] The two books have one thing in common: the anatomical description and physiological interpretation of an organ and the physiopathological explanation of a disease-process in the light of Harvey's discovery of the circular motion of the blood.

FRANCIS GLISSON'S HEPATOLOGY

NEW INTERPRETATIONS

Research methods and biomedical thought characteristic of the last twenty years of Glisson's life and work have been the subject of careful examination. R. Milnes Walker presented biographical accounts of Glisson based on archival sources and examined the early research endeavors of Glisson, including the original work leading to his classic study on the anatomy of the liver.[2] In a thorough comparative study, Edwin Clarke analyzed the treatises of Daniel Whistler and of Francis Glisson on rickets, and disclosed the important and independent contribution Whistler made to the study five years prior to the publication of Glisson's book *De Rachitide*.[3] Francis J. Cole published a manuscript of Henry Power on the circulation of the blood that reflected the experimental endeavor of the Glissonian circle at Cambridge.[4] It was Charles Webster who emphasized the influence of Glisson at Cambridge as an early advocate of Harvey's discovery of the circulation of the blood; and he pointed to the importance of the Royal College of Physicians as an early nexus of experimental and medical research in England, and to the role of Glisson in that context.[5] Audrey B. Davis showed Glisson's endeavor to present a "chemical anatomy" of the blood,[6] suggesting that this new interest in "blood chemistry" was enforced by the conviction of the vital primacy of the blood advocated by Harvey, and shared and developed by Glisson. Theodore M. Brown made evident Glisson's vitalistic and nonmechanical concept of secretory processes.[7]

Two major contributions to Glisson's biological thought have substantially widened and deepened our understanding of Glisson as a medical philosopher. Regarding the first, Owsei Temkin uncovered the Galenic roots of Glisson's concept of irritation developed in the *Anatomia Hepatis*.[8] He pointed to the similarity of Glisson's *irritatio* to Galen's concept of *dexis*.[9]

According to Galen, *dexis* (biting, irritation), *achthos* (burdening), and *diatasis* (distention) excite and awaken the uterus, stomach, gut, and bladder to contraction and evacuation of their contents.[10] Temkin traced the long and complex history of the idea of irritation from antiquity to the seventeenth century — from Galen to Harvey and Glisson — identifying the anthropomorphic components of this idea, which was to find its first real focus in Glisson's *Anatomia Hepatis*. Another important contribution to Glissonian thought was that of Walter Pagel, who dealt with the Aristotelian streams of thought in Harvey's and Glisson's biological ideas. He examined the monistic view of life as immanent in matter, a concept shared by Harvey and Glisson and rooted in Peripatetic philosophy. He also showed the similarity of Harvey's belief in a basic reactivity inherent in living matter and Glisson's concept of "perception" as a quality pervading all levels of nature.[11] On the basis of these new interpretations I shall take a fresh look at Glisson's *Anatomia Hepatis*. Four areas of Glissonian work and thought will be examined: (1) anatomy and physiology; (2) chemical views; (3) natural philosophy; and (4) experimental findings.

ANATOMY AND PHYSIOLOGY OF THE LIVER

Glisson's Anatomical and Physiological Research

Glisson's *Anatomia Hepatis* is an investigation of the structure and function of the liver.[12] It is one of the major works in the history of hepatology and it stands as a lasting achievement between Galen on the one hand, and Haller, Kiernan, and Claude Bernard on the other hand. Glisson's *Anatomia Hepatis* represents the first detailed examination of the liver under the aspect of the decisive systemic discoveries of the circulation of the blood and the lymphatic vessels. Glisson described the vascular architecture of the liver: the extra- and intrahepatic distribution of the portal vein; the hepatic veins; the hepatic artery and the bile ducts. He formulated the concept of the portal trias; that is, the common entry and ramification of the hepatic artery, the bile ducts, and the portal vein, all enveloped by a common fibrous capsule. He recognized the peculiar significance of the portal vein as an afferent vessel branching like an artery into the liver parenchyma. Glisson postulated an equal supply of all portions of the parenchyma with capillaries of the portal vein and of the hepatic veins. He envisaged bile formation as a secretion of preformed bile matter from the blood into the bile ducts by the vital action of the liver parenchyma. He believed in a regulation of the bile flow through irritation of the bile ducts and gallbladder by their contents. He characterized the liver as an essentially excretory organ whose function consisted in depurating the blood by elimination of the bile matter from the blood into the bile ducts. Glisson abandoned once and for all the traditional doctrine of hepatic blood generation.

What was the framework of Glisson's biomedical thought and his methods of research? Without any doubt he was a skillful anatomist deeply engaged in morphological research. Moreover, he adopted the methods of experimental physiology that were coming to the fore in the mid-century. On the other hand, Glisson's biological thought was pervaded and essentially shaped by natural philosophy. In the history of philosophy Glisson is known as a representative of hylozoism and a precursor of Leibniz's monadology.[13] His work, *On the Energetic Nature of Substance*, was rooted in neoscholastic thought, and even Glisson's anatomical works were composed in strict logical order, bearing witness to his scholastic formation and inclination.[14] In the history of biology Glisson's name is connected with the concept of irritability as a basic property of living matter.[15]

Methodological Elements

Anatomical Techniques. The *Anatomia Hepatis* emerged from Glisson's "Goulstonian Lecture" for the College of Physicians of London delivered in 1641. Glisson stated: "I was appointed [in 1640] by the physicians of the Coll. of London to read a publick anatomical lecture in the theatre belonging to the Coll. to be performed in the year 1641, thus was allowed about a twelvemonth time for my preparation, so I applied myself to the study of the liver." His main interest at that time was devoted to the vascular tree of the liver; the vascular ramification was demonstrated in the "liver denuded of its flesh" ("hepar carne sou exutum").[16]

The last touch to the *Anatomia Hepatis* was given shortly before it was published. This is particularly true for the last section describing the lymphatic vessels in which reference was made to literature published up to 1653.[17] Glisson was thoroughly acquainted with contemporary anatomical and physiological research. He adopted Harvey's discovery of the circular motion of the blood; he was perfectly familiar with the discovery of the intestinal lacteals by Gaspare Aselli, of the thoracic duct by Jean Pecquet and Thomas Bartholin, and was probably acquainted with the recent description of the lymphatic vessels by Thomas Bartholin and Olof Rudbeck. Terms used by Glisson, *lymphae-ductus* and *canales aquosi*, point to his acquaintance with the treatises of these two authors on the lymphatic system published in 1653.[18] Glisson was personally associated with Wharton's important investigation of the glands and his discovery of the submaxillary duct, which Glisson claims to have found in common with Wharton. Glisson was also deeply impressed by Harvey's embryological opus.[19]

Glisson's anatomical methods and techniques were dissection with the knife; the artificial injection and inflation of vascular structures; the perfusion of organs with the syringe; and the measuring and weighing of organs and ligature of vessels. The goal of anatomy, Glisson stated, was to explore the topography, the structure, the connections, and the anomalies of the organs, and to reveal the faculties, actions, and sympathies of the whole dynamic and purposeful fabric of the human body.[20] Glisson also advocated the use of the microscope ("tubi optici sive microscopia") as a means to reveal little ducts, vessels, and tissue-pores. He cautioned against fallacious interpretation of microscopic observations.[21] Glisson also recommended perfusion techniques with pure water, diluted milk, or water tinged with saffron. If a parenchymatous organ perfused with a colored liquid acquired a homogeneous tinge, this was proof that the liquid permeated the whole parenchyma in a diffuse way and was not confined to a vascular transition.[22]

Vivisection. A further important methodological element was vivisection, which had to be restricted to animal experimentation. Glisson demonstrated the existence of the Asellian chyle vessels and the hepatic lymphatics by means of vivisection, and he excised the heart of living animals in order to ascertain the blood-forming capacity of the cardiac flesh.[23] Henry Power's excellent experimental study of the circulation of the blood was probably due to the stimulating influence of Glisson.

Glisson believed that the anatomist oriented toward research should specialize: that he should devote his efforts to the examination of a circumscribed part of the body. Only in this way could he hope to make new observations and to increase anatomical knowledge.[24] Thus Glisson relied on the whole range of morphological observations and experimental investigations available to a mid-century physician, and he drew important conclusions from these data by reasoning a posteriori. We shall see however that Glisson attributed equal (or perhaps even greater) weight to a priori reasoning: reasoning by a sequence of logical deductions.

VITAL CHEMISTRY

The Elements

Glisson differentiated ultimate from intermediate elements. He adopted without reservation the doctrine of the recent chemists (*chymici*) who distinguished five ultimate elements or principles; namely, spirit, oil, salt, water or phlegm, and *caput mortuum* or *terra damnata* (dead earth). According to the chemists these elements were the ultimate parts into which any substance could be divided by human industry and ingenuity.[25] The doctrine of five elements was very common in the seventeenth century, and the division used by Glisson can be found in the writings of various chemical authors of the early seventeenth century: writers such as Jean Beguin, Sebastian Basso, or Etienne de Clave.[26] The intermediate elements were obtained by incomplete separation of mixed bodies. The most diverse intermediate elements were isolated according to the nature of the chemical operations employed.

These operations consisted of filtration, precipitation, flotation, distillation, extraction, fermentation (separation of foamy matter from sediments with formation of an intermediate liquor), and the making of new combinations of matter by the action of peculiar affinities (as occurred in the "granulation" of salts and crystallization of sugar).[27] This property of specific affinity was seen as pervading the whole of nature—mineral, vegetable, and animal. The four Galenic humors belonged to the intermediate elements, and practical medicine endeavored to evacuate these humors. This last was the legitimate goal of traditional dogmatic medicine, while elementary analysis into the ultimate elements belonged to the theoretical part of medicine.[28]

Application of Chemistry to Biology and Medicine

Chemistry described the material and elementary composition of the humors of the body. Analysis of bile, for example, yielded evidence of a small amount of spirits, some sulphur, and much salt, water, and earthy element. Chemistry also explained fundamental physiological phenomena as the formation of chyle and blood, the origin of vital heat, and the process of secretion.[29]

The Spirits

The most powerful chemical and vital agents were the spirits. Spirits, in a wider sense, were defined as substances of a subtle, active, penetrating, and volatile nature such as the spirit of vitriol, the spirit of vinegar, and the spirit of salt. More appropriately and specifically, the term spirit designated an element that spontaneously acquired a state of volatility in a fermenting process, as did the spirit of wine.[30] The spirit called (among other things) mercury by the chemists occurred in two forms: as a fatty or sulphurous spirit; and as a meagre or saline spirit.[31] The fatty spirit was obtained in the form of oil (e.g., chemical oils, the spirit of roses), while the meagre, or saline, spirit was represented, for instance, by the spirit of wine and other ardent waters.[32] Both the saline and sulphurous spirit were highly volatile and prevailed in activity over all other elements, even if the spirit was present in minimal quantity. This is also the reason why the highly exalted spirits formed the substratum of vital heat and would then be called vital spirits.[33] The spirits occurred in three states: first, a state of fixation to thick matter; second, a state of fusion or half-way liberation from the thick principle; and third, a state of volatility which was produced by the most intense exaltation of the spirits.[34] The spirits had a strong proclivity to dissipate: to evade lest they be coerced and restrained.[35] The gradual acquisition of volatility occurred in a struggle aroused between the spirits and thick matter (lucta excitate, concertatio). The fermenting process and the production of vital heat resulted from such a fight.[36]

Although fermentation and vital heat shared with the spirits an intense propensity towards expansion and volatility there still existed specific differences between fermentation, putrefaction, and the formation of vital heat.

The blood contained a large quantity of spirits together with a considerable amount of sulphur or fatty substances. The vital heat excited the spirits to become volatile and to dissipate; after dissipation of the sweet and agreeable spirits the gross sulphur was burnt to the bitter substance of bile. The formation of chyle and blood consisted in a gradual transition of food into blood. Three stages of maturation could be distinguished as follows: (1) the solid food ingested containing fixed spirits; (2) the spirits reaching a state of fusion in the stomach, by means of fermentation and addition of aqueous matter, to produce a milky juice termed chyle; (3) the chyle, being full of mild spirits, infusing into the venous bloodstream until it reached the heart, where the spirits would acquire a volatile state and form the substratum of vital heat. The vital spirits resided potentially in the food; they lacked only due preparation towards exaltation.[37]

This was a remarkably *chemical view* of the vital process of assimilation. One has to bear in mind, however, that for Glisson, the spirits were of a dynamic, active, and reactive nature, and in no way mere dead matter. Fermentation, putrefaction, chylification, and sanguification all expressed an inner fight, a dynamic interaction between gross and spiritual matter. These views were support for Glisson's belief in a unity of nature, and for his presentation of vital phenomena in terms of "vital chemistry."

From the material composition of the blood containing a rich amount of spirits and boiling in vital heat, a dissipation of volatile matter could be deduced a priori. Loss of volatile matter by evaporation and transudation could also be demonstrated a posteriori, by empirical investigation. Santorio Santorio measured the insensible transpiration (*transpiratio insensibilis*), which he computed to be half of the solids and liquids ingested.[38] Not all of these "exhalations" consisted of evaporated spirits, but the cause of insensible transpiration of subtle matter was the expanding tendency of the spirits (*nisus expansivus spirituum*).

NATURAL PHILOSOPHY

The Elements

In the *Anatomia Hepatis* Aristotelian and Galenic thought pervaded Glisson's biological ideas. Glisson reconciled the four elements of the Peripatetics with the five elementary principles of the "chemists." Fire corresponded to spirit, the air to the oily element, the water to phlegm, and the earth to the salt and to the earthy element.[39]

Matter and Form

The concept of matter and form was a general and all-embracing theme in Glisson's morphology and physiology. Matter was a body apt to be formed and shaped according to the design and purpose of an agent. Form was a modification of matter to serve a specific purpose designed by an agent. Nature herself selected with perfect discretion the matter that was most apt to receive an appropriate and optimal form.[40]

Similar and Organic Parts

The concept of matter and form was Glisson's leading criterion to distinguish and differentiate the parts of the body. Glisson adopted the ancient division into similar and dissimilar parts: in particular, the form of similar parts, on the one hand, and organic parts on the other.[41] The similar parts, Glisson stated, were characterized by their material essence (e.g., blood, bone-substance, liver parenchyma). The organic or instrumental parts were defined by their form, their instrumental structure (e.g., the vascular ramifications of the liver, the structure of the heart).[42] The actions of the similar parts consisted in material change (e.g., assimilation of chyle to blood) or in vital attraction ([attractio similaris] e.g., attraction of bile particles from the blood into the liver parenchyma). The functions of the organic parts were mechanical in nature (e.g., the filtration of urine by the kidneys, the elimination of the glandular juices through the excretory ducts [salivation, lacrimation], or the transportation of blood to the various organs).[43] There were likewise similar and organic diseases; that is, pathological alterations of the material composition of the parts or lesions of the structure (form) of the organs.[44]

The Causes

Glisson's doctrine of causes was intimately connected to the concept of matter and form. The distinction of matter and form presupposed a material and formal cause. In addition, Glisson adhered to the concept of final causes at a time when atomists and mechanists began to concentrate their interest and research on the working of the efficient causes. Any action, Glisson stated, had an efficient cause by which it was performed; but every action had also a final cause that determined the useful and significant result of an action.[45]

Action and Use

The final cause determined the usefulness, the use, of an action. A given organ had both a private and public use: the private use concerned the action of an organ for its own and proper benefit; the public use designated the usefulness of this action for the whole organism. Given that the body formed a harmonious federation of parts (*foedus sociale*), it was inconceivable that a private action should be meaningful and useful to the whole by sheer accident.[46]

Similar Attraction

Similar attraction—also called, by Glisson, magnetic attraction—was perhaps just the common expression of ancient wisdom that like enjoys like (*simile simili gaudet*). Glisson rejected the corpuscular doctrines of magnetic attraction just as Galen had denied the mechanical and atomistic explanations of Epicurean philosophy. According to Glisson, the conditions of similar attraction were threefold:[47] (1) two bodies were to possess similarity, affinity, familiarity; (2) at least one of these bodies had to excite in the other a desire for union; (3) to make this excitation effective there had to be an actual endeavor (*actualis conatus*) and mutual appetite for congregation (*nixus coeundi*).[48]

In Glisson's explanation of similar or magnetic attraction we recognize basic elements of his theory of irritation: The excitation corresponded to the "irritation," and the *nisus coeundi* to the *appetitus* which was followed by motion. Similar attraction meant an enticement (*allectatio*) or incitation (*incitamentum*) whereby similar bodies would strive to congregate.[49] The term attraction, according to Glisson, was somewhat misleading; it pointed to a mechanical pulling that was not operative in similar attraction. Similar attraction thus differed from organic or mechanical attraction, similar attraction being based on familiarity, similarity, and affinity between the attracted and the attracting body.[50] Similar attraction was widespread in nature. It produced magnetic attraction and crystallization, and was present in those plants which attracted the appropriate food by means of their roots. Similar attraction was particularly conspicuous in animals whose organs attracted the useful and rejected the useless (e.g., in those where fecal matter was segregated from the chyle and bile matter was attracted from the blood into the hepatic parenchyma).[51]

In Glisson's concept of similar attraction we recognize the Galenic doctrine of natural faculties. We see Glisson's view of a general dynamic unity of nature throughout the animal, vegetable, and mineral realms. There is an almost anthropomorphic presentation of similar attraction in which similar matter was mutually excited to fuse with a drive of common appetite.

EXPERIMENTAL FINDINGS

The Problem of Blood Generation

Glisson made reference to the age-old controversy between Aristotelians and Galenists on the blood-producing organ of the body. The Peripatetics attributed the power of sanguification to the heart, the Galenists to the liver. Glisson states that recent findings in his time had led to the rejection of both the Galenic and Aristotelian views on sanguification.[52]

Generation of Primitive Blood

The formation of blood in the embryo was due to a natural cause. By necessity, this cause acted uniformly and in the shortest and most economical way. If the natural agent producing embryonic blood persisted in adult life, blood generation had to follow by necessity the same pattern.[53] Primitive blood was formed in the ovum long before heart, liver, or blood vessels were shaped; therefore these organs could not be the source of embryonic blood. Primitive blood, rather, was generated by the vital spirit residing in the first seminal matter of the ovum.[54] The vital spirits expanded the vital liquor of seminal matter, excavated channels, and established a circular flow: the dance of life began before the blood reddened.[55] This same vital spirit was also present in the adult body and continued its blood-forming function.[56]

Role of Heart and Liver in Sanguification

A further reason to assume that neither heart nor liver produced blood was the fact that their substance was very different from blood; this excluded consideration of that assimilative process in which the two organs were thought to change chyle into blood.[57] A posteriori reasoning based on clinical experience and experimental evidence led to the same conclusion. Severe hemorrhages were followed by a rapid loss of blood generation, although heart and liver were in perfect health.[58] The heart, vitalized by the blood of the coronary arteries, depended on this blood supply to maintain its vitality and was unlikely to produce blood. The experiment demonstrated an excised heart cleansed of its blood was not able to convert milk or chyle into blood. Vivisection also showed that the cardiac flesh of a living animal was less hot than the blood contained in the ventricles. Henry Power, a student of Glisson, described in more detail this experiment in a manuscript dated 1652.[59]

The Lymphatic System and Sanguification

Sanguification in Glisson's time meant conversion of chyle into blood. The discovery of the thoracic duct by Jean Pecquet had shown that the chyle was infused into the blood stream of the vena cava superior. The first chyle-receiving organ was the heart; therefore the heart, and not the liver, had to be the instrument of sanguification. For Jean Pecquet, Thomas Bartholin, Johannes van Horne, and Olof Rudbeck,[60] experimental evidence was the main reason to overthrow the traditional doctrine of hepatic sanguification. For Glisson, these experimental data were certainly strong arguments against the Galenic theory of blood generation by the liver, but in contrast to these authors, he thought it not the only argument. It rather corroborated his own conclusion obtained by reasoning a priori. This involved: (1) the thinking in terms of analogy (heat generally reddens substances, and as the most intense heat resides in the vital spirits of the blood, the blood must be the source of a continuous generation of new blood).[61] (2) The conviction that natural actions were consistent, uniform, and strictly determined by the same causes throughout embryonic and adult life (in the embryo the vital spirits residing in the seminal matter produced blood; in the adult body the same vital spirits operated in the blood and assimilated chyle to blood). (3) The division of physiological functions into similar and organic actions (sanguification was a similar action [assimilation] performed by a similar part — the blood — which converted, or assimilated chyle into blood in a process of material change).[62]

Bile Secretion

In the process of bile secretion similar and organic actions took place. The similar actions were as follows: (1) the generation of bile in the blood by combustion of thick sulphur into bile matter;[63] (2) the bile matter of the aortic blood channelled into the mesenteric and coeliac arteries and conveyed from there to the liver to be excreted (the mass of bile accumulated in the gall-bladder would attract by specific affinity the bile particles of the aortic blood into the coeliac and mesenteric arteries); and (3) the mucous portion of the blood being in the stomach and gut is attracted by the mucus lining of the gastric and intestinal cavities. This last arrangement was for Glisson the expression of nature's perfect working. It showed the adaptive integration of physiological functions and the harmonious cooperation of private and public use. The private action of the stomach and gut was the extraction of mucus from the blood to the inner surface of the intestinal tube for the purpose of protection and lubrication. At the same time this action prevented a mucous obstruction of the portal blood and of the liver, that being the public use of mucus secretion.[64] The intestinal bypass had an additional effect: that the fermenting power of stomach and gut assist the separation of bile and blood.[65]

A special case was found in the liver parenchyma. According to Glisson, it was composed of two portions: a substance similar to blood and a substance similar to bile. The biliary portion attracted the bile from the portal capillaries and conveyed it to the bile ducts while the sanguineous portion of the parenchyma attracted the blood, which was then infused into the roots of the hepatic veins.[66] Blood and bile had almost the same consistence, and a mechanical separation (as, for example, in urinary filtration) was therefore impossible; specific affinity was required. This property of specific affinity was immanent in the liver parenchyma and it imparted to the liver the highest functional dignity of all abdominal viscera.[67]

Organic Apparatus of the Liver

The organic apparatus of the liver was represented by the network of blood vessels and bile ducts and of the fibrous capsule. Although this apparatus was of admirable architecture, it was only auxiliary to the basic function of "similar secretion." The organic part of the liver carried the portal to the liver, conveyed the bile to the gallbladder and duodenum, and stopped or allowed the bile flow by the operation of sphincter mechanisms.[68] The bile flow was performed mechanically and regulated vitally through irritation.

As regards the portal trias, the pulse imparted to the portal vein by the hepatic artery and the coercion of the spirits in the portal vein by the com-

mon capsule produce a revival of the portal blood (*revivescentia*), an igni-
tion of the sparks of life, and a mechanical activation of the portal blood
stream.[69]

CONCLUSION

In the introductory chapters of Glisson's study—considered to be superflu-
ous scholastic exercises by enlightened anatomists of the eighteenth century
—Glisson set the stage for his *Anatomia Hepatis*.[70]

1. The ancient concepts of matter and form—of similar and organic
parts—determined his presentation of the structure and function of the
liver. The similar parts induced material change and specific attraction. The
main similar part of the liver was the parenchyma, which separated bile from
blood. The organic parts of the liver exerted mechanical effects: transportation of blood and bile through vessels and ducts. The bile flow was performed
mechanically and controlled vitally by periodic irritation and consecutive
contraction of the bile ducts and gall bladder discharging their bile content.

2. Vital chemistry explained the processes of material change. Sanguification consisted in a mutual reaction between spiritual and thick elements.

3. Magnetic attraction, the specific selection of food by the plant roots
and by the animal organs, bore witness to the basic unity of nature where
specific affinities were to be found at all levels. After Glisson, the similar
part of the liver, the hepatic parenchyma, was neglected and sank almost
into oblivion. It became a passive, rigid, and lifeless part functioning strictly
as dead mechanical filter. Xavier Bichat and Johannes Müller vitalized the
glandular parenchyma again into an active and elaborating substance, and
Claude Bernard revealed the chemical working of Glisson's similar substance.[71]

JOHANN JACOB WEPFER'S WORK ON APOPLEXY

HISTORICAL STUDIES

In 1658 Johann Jacob Wepfer (1620–1695), town physician of Schaffhausen,
published a book on apoplexy.[72] Wepfer's study of apoplexy presented a
fundamentally new interpretation of a cerebral disease; it was based on the
concept of blood circulation, on the anatomical study of the cerebral blood
vessels, and on morbid anatomy of the brain. The core of Wepfer's contribution was the explanation of apoplexy in terms of physiopathology. Apoplexy
became a vascular disease affecting the cerebral circulation.

Conrad Brunner and Wilhelm von Muralt inaugurated the modern historical studies on Wepfer and his school. They published letters of Swiss
physicians of the seventeenth century and gave an all-around and well-docu-

mented picture of Swiss medicine of that epoch. A chapter was devoted to
Wepfer and his achievements as head of the unchartered Schaffhausen
school of medicine.[73] Hans Fischer gave an enlightening interpretation of
Wepfer's place in seventeenth-century medicine, with particular emphasis
on Wepfer's contribution to clinical and experimental toxicology. An accurate study of Wepfer's anatomical work was done by Henry Nigst; this study
shows Wepfer's technical skill and power of observation in the realm of morphology. Heinrich Buess and his students made substantial contributions to
the life and work of Wepfer. Buess pointed to Wepfer's description of em-
bolic processes, and together with S. Joos-Renfer and M. L. Portmann he
studied the achievement of Swiss physicians in morbid anatomy between
1670 and 1720. Buess also showed the prominent part played by Wepfer as
senior head of the Schaffhausen medical school. The most extensive and accurate biographic study of Wepfer was published by Pietro Eichenberger, a
student of Buess. Eichenberger based his work on important manuscript
sources and added much documentary evidence on Wepfer's medical training,
private practice (which covered a wide area of Switzerland and southwestern
Germany), and public duties as town physician. He devoted particular attention to Wepfer's clinical pathology. Eichenberger also published an important autobiographical sketch of Wepfer which provided new information
on Wepfer's student life, medical thought, and academic connections.[74]

WEPFER AND THE CIRCULATION OF THE BLOOD

Harvey's discovery of the circular motion of the blood was praised by Wepfer
as the great and sagacious discovery of the century.[75] For about fifteen years,
from 1643 to 1658, the circulation of the blood remained the pivotal point,
the main and central problem of Wepfer's student years and of the first
decade of his medical practice. In a letter written in 1656 to the physician
and polyhistor Johann Conrad Brotbeck of Tübingen, Wepfer dealt with the
early reception of Harvey's circulation theories in Strassburg, Basel, Italy,
and German lands. When Wepfer studied at Strassburg from 1639 to 1643,
nobody mentioned Harvey's discovery.[76] At that time Wepfer read the epis-
tolary treatise of Johannes Walaeus (Jan de Wale) to Thomas Bartholinus,
"On the Motion of the Blood," which made him acquainted with Harvey's
discovery and impressed him deeply.[77] When he continued his studies in
Basel he checked that problem experimentally together with Felix Platter II
(1605–1671), at that time professor of physics at the University of Basel.
This removed practically every doubt, but Wepfer remained silent about it
for fear of displeasing his professors.[78] A true revelation occurred in Padua
where he went in 1644 to study for three years. In particular, it was Johann
Vesling, professor of anatomy, and his student circle (which included
Thomas Bartholin) who convinced Wepfer conclusively of the truth of
Harvey's discovery: both by arguments and by visual demonstration. When

Wepfer returned to Basel in 1647 the climate had changed and the circulation doctrine was widely known.[79]

WEPFER'S THESIS *DE PALPITATIONE CORDIS*

In 1647 Wepfer took his medical degree in Basel; his inaugural dissertation was "On the Palpitation of the Heart."[80] In his thesis the circular concept formed an essential element of clinical pathology, although Wepfer did not use the term of circulation to point only to the mode of cardiac revolution as described by Realdo Colombo, William Harvey, and Hermann Conring.[81] Palpitation of the heart, Wepfer stated, was not a distention of the heart by thick vapors or spirits. It was, on the contrary, an active, vehement, frequent, and faulty motion of the heart whose pulsific faculty was irritated by molesting conditions (*facultas cordis irritata a re molesta*) and by adverse stimuli (*stimulus adversus*).[82] The fibers of the heart were the very substratum of cardiac contraction. If the heart was removed from living animals (fish and quadrupeds) and cleansed of its blood, it continued to beat for a shorter or longer time, provided the fibers maintained their integrity and some heat was conserved.[83] The heart had the faculty (*potentia*) to perceive (*agnoscere*) harmful things, probably by means of its nerves. In any case, experiments on living animals demonstrated that a heart stung with a needle jumped, which proved that it was endowed with sensation.[84] Thus, for Wepfer, palpitation was an intense cardiac contraction caused by continuous irritant conditions. These conditions could have been an excess of blood burdening the heart, or obstacles resisting the ejection of blood from the heart (e.g., blood coagula or carneous excrescences at the basis of the heart); the same irritant effect could also be produced by acrimonious humors.[85] These conditions formed the proximate causes of palpitation. The palpitation of the heart was easily perceived by putting the hand under the left nipple.[86]

In Wepfer's thesis we recognize the following elements: (1) explanation of clinical pathology on the basis of morbid anatomy and experimental physiology; (2) the endeavor to ascertain the immediate, proximate causes of disease-processes, in this case the various pathological conditions leading to irritation of the cardiac fibers; and (3) the assumption that the cardiac fibers responded to irritations, this being the clue to the understanding of palpitation. In this last, however, the notion of irritation was applied specifically to heart pathology and was not presented in terms of a generalized biological concept, as Glisson was to do later.[87]

WEPFER AND MODERN MEDICINE OF HIS TIME

After graduation in 1647 Wepfer was appointed town physician in Schaffhausen. He built up a large private practice, engaged in medical research and established a veritable though unchartered medical school. Of overall importance was the fact that he received permission from the magistrate to perform post-mortem examinations on patients who died in the hospitals of his home town.[88]

In his "Apoplexia" Wepfer hailed the emergence of a new medicine. After the "instauration of anatomy" in the preceding century,[89] an acceleration of research occurred and a series of new discoveries were made in his own time: the discovery of the chyle vessels, of the circulation of the blood, of the thoracic duct, and the lymphatic vessels, each bringing considerable confusion and turmoil to pathology.[90] On the other hand, medicine has become so narrow-minded that the physicians who professed new opinions based on observed facts were considered quacks by dogmatic tyrants who boasted of the authority of Galen.[91] The dogmatic Galenists, nurtured exclusively in traditional views, were reluctant to deviate a finger's breadth from the doctrines of their master.[92] But those open to new ideas knew that the actions and uses of the organs had to be rechecked and reinterpreted in the light of the new discoveries. When Wepfer became acquainted with the circular motion of the blood he grasped the significance of this revolutionary discovery for the whole of medicine and he began a systematic reinterpretation of pathology under the aspect of circulation. He opened the bodies of numerous patients who had died from most diverse diseases.[93]

EMPIRICAL RESEARCH

From the beginning of his medical career Wepfer stated that he had refused to rely exclusively on the wisdom of books, and that he had consulted Nature herself whenever he had the opportunity.[94] Knowledge of physiology and pathology had to be obtained through the testimony of the senses (*sensuum testimonio*), combined with substantial and pertinent arguments.[95] The existence of visible and palpable structures could only be demonstrated with the eye and the skillful hand of a master in dissection.[96]

PHYSIOPATHOLOGICAL MECHANISMS

Wepfer was deeply convinced that the circular concept had changed the very foundation of physiology and pathology. Those who had observed in living animals the perpetual flow of blood from the heart to the arteries, and the continuous reflux of blood through the veins to the heart, could no longer share the traditional dogma of blood flow. According to the traditional doctrine, the blood moved intermittently towards the periphery, either by attraction of the various organs for the purpose of nutrition or by being pushed from the back by the blood, which was continuously generated in the liver.[97] For a given disease, not only the affected part (Galen's *topos*) had to be known, but also the proximate causes (*causae proximae*) and the mode of generation (*modus generationis*).[98] Thus the anatomical localization and physiopathological mechanisms of disease had to be assessed. Wepfer himself acknowledged that he was particularly indebted to Thomas Bartholin.

By personal and most agreeable conversations at Padua in their student days, and from the study of Bartholin's writings subsequently, he became convinced of two things required in medical research: the need to register day after day the course of rare diseases, and the effects of remedies; and the need to investigate the morphological features of these diseases by morbid anatomy.[99]

APOPLEXY: WEPFER'S CLINICAL PATHOLOGY

Wepfer's medical research emerged from clinical problems. The point of departure of his work on apoplexy were four cases of stroke which he observed clinically and then submitted to post-mortem examination.[100] The clinical picture was characterized by loss of consciousness and paralysis of motor and sensory functions. It appeared suddenly as total apoplexy or developed gradually with headache, speech disorders, loss of language, and hemiplegia turning to complete apoplexy.[101] The anatomical lesions of the brain were massive ventricular and meningeal hemorrhages, and rupture of cerebral arteries.

Up to Wepfer's time the main cause believed to produce apoplexy had been obstruction of the ventricles of the brain by viscid and cold matter.[102] This traditional doctrine, Wepfer stated, became untenable once one correlated anatomical and pathological data with the circular motion of the blood. The brain belonged to the organs with the largest blood supply.[103] Large arteries ramified to arterioles and capillary vessels and conveyed an incessant stream of blood to all regions of the brain. The functional portions of the brain were not the ventricles but the cerebral substance, particularly the medullary portion. Here the spirits were filtered from the blood and generated motion and sensation.[104]

For Wepfer the main pathogenetic process of apoplexy consisted of cerebral ischemia: an interruption of blood flow to, and through, the brain. This occurred by ruptures of cerebral arteries, obstruction of the carotid arteries with muco-fibrous coagula, and by repletion of the small arteries of the brain with viscid blood particles.[105] Rupture of cerebral arteries stopped the formation of the animal spirits and the functional portions of the brain suffered additional damage by compression with extravasated blood.[106] The obstruction of the internal carotid or of the arteria basilaris led also to cerebral ischemia; the obstruction was caused by muco-fibrous blood coagula originated *in loco* or carried from the left ventricle to the carotid.[107] In apoplexy the animal actions (sensation and motor functions) were paralyzed while respiration and cardiac activity continued.[108] Therapeutic success or failure depended on the extent and nature of the morbid process. Ruptures of large arteries were irreparable, and obstruction of the carotid arteries did not respond to bloodletting or cauterization.[109] In both cases the anatomical lesion was too profound to be influenced by any therapeutic measure. The best chances of healing were present in the cases of obstruction of the small cerebral arteries by viscid blood particles. Spontaneous recovery or therapeutic success indicated a reversible process.[110] According to the extent and to the localization of the vascular lesions and circular alterations, the psychic, sensory, and motor functions were impaired differently. Some patients were only deprived of language; others suffered from hemiplegia if one side of the brain was affected, and true apoplexy if the whole brain was involved.[111]

Wepfer's work on apoplexy was the first example of modern research into that disease. From a process of humoral pathology in the form of obstruction or repletion of the cerebral ventricles, apoplexy became a vascular and circulatory disease of the brain.

CONCLUSION

Wepfer, a powerful clinical observer as well as an accomplished anatomist and morphologist, tried to assess pathogenetic mechanisms — that is, the "proximate causes" and the "mode of generation." But he was of a pragmatic and eclectic turn of mind, free of dogmatic fixation. There was no overall theoretical approach to medicine: no demand of "mechanical explanation" (Walaeus);[112] no physical model to be applied to biology (such as Pecquet's pneumatic physics); no mechanistic reduction of physiology in the Cartesian way.[113] For Wepfer, anatomical facts and experimental results formed the ultimate criteria of biomedical knowledge. In that respect he took approximately the same position as Thomas Bartholin,[114] who stressed the dignity and validity of experimental criteria to gain new knowledge and to decide controversial issues. Wepfer is above all a clinical, morphological, and experimental observer with a remarkable power of integration.

Glisson on the other hand possessed a highly theoretical and scholastic mind. The fabric of his presentation of the structure and function of the liver is Aristotelian and Galenic, entailing the division into similar and organic parts, and into similar and organic actions. While the organic fabric operated mechanically, the similar parts caused material transformation (assimilation) and similar attraction. Thus Glisson's views on motion and assimilation were still largely Aristotelian and Galenic. He adhered firmly to tradition and did not assume corpuscular mechanisms to underlie motion and change in the way of Walter Charleton, who rejected "*Attraction Similarly*; because in Nature there is no Motion by Attraction, but all from Impulsion."[115] Glisson also elaborated a vital chemistry effective in the workshop of nature causing such fundamental biological phenomena as sanguification and nutrition.

Both works — that of Glisson and of Wepfer — represent a rich and complex picture of medical research and thought in the mid-seventeenth century. Both Glisson and Wepfer were accomplished anatomists, relying on physiological observation and experimentation. Both accepted the important physiological discoveries of the first half of the seventeenth century; both rejected central Galenic positions on blood flow and blood formation. But while Wepfer—a generation younger—was essentially an empirical observer of great critical acumen, Glisson's thought was more complex. Glisson was essentially a theoretician, a man entrenched in tradition trying to reconcile moderns and ancients. Already in his *Anatomia Hepatis* he developed, with great imagination and conceptual force, a first draft of his later notion of irritability.[116]

NOTES

[1]Francis Glisson, *Anatomia Hepatis cui praemittuntur quaedam ad rem anatomicam spectantia* (London, 1654) (hereafter cited as *Anat. Hep.*); Johann Jacob Wepfer, *Observationes anatomicae ex cadaveribus eorum, quos sustulit apoplexia, cum exercitatione de eius loco affecto* (Schaffhusii, 1658) (hereafter cited as *Apoplexia*).

[2]R. Milnes Walker, "Francis Glisson and His Capsule," *Annals Roy. Coll. Surg. Engl.* 38 (1966): 71–91; idem, "Francis Glisson," *Cambridge and Its Contribution to Medicine*, ed. A. Rook (London: Wellcome Institute, 1971), pp. 35–47; an excellent biographical sketch is Owsei Temkin's article "Glisson," *Dictionary of Scientific Biography*, ed. Charles C. Gillispie (New York: Charles Scribner's Sons, 1972), 5:425–27.

[3]Edwin Clarke, "Whistler and Glisson on Rickets," *Bull. Hist. Med.* 36 (1962): 45–61.

[4]Francis J. Cole, "Henry Power on the Circulation of the Blood," *J. Hist. Med. and Allied Sci.* 12 (1957): 291–324.

[5]Charles Webster, "Henry Power's Experimental Philosophy," *Ambix* 14 (1967): 150–78; idem, "The College of Physicians: 'Salomon's House' in Commonwealth England," *Bull. Hist. Med.* 41 (1967): 393–412.

[6]Audrey B. Davis, "Some Implications of the Circulation Theory for Disease Theory and Treatment in the Seventeenth Century," *J. Hist. Med. and Allied Sci.* 26 (1971): 28–39; idem, "The Circulation of the Blood and Chemical Anatomy," in *Science, Medicine and Society in the Renaissance: Essays in Honor of Walter Pagel*, ed. A. G. Debus (New York: Science History Publ., 1972), 2:25–37.

[7]Theodore M. Brown, "The Mechanical Philosophy and the 'Animal Oeconomy': A Study in the Development of English Physiology in the Seventeenth and Early Eighteenth Century" (Ph.D. diss., Princeton University, 1968), pp. 54–55.

[8]Owsei Temkin, "The Classical Roots of Glisson's Doctrine of Irritation," *Bull. Hist. Med.* 38 (1964): 297–328.

[9]Ibid., pp. 307–8.

[10]Galen, *On the Natural Faculties*, trans. A. J. Brock (London: Heinemann; Cambridge: Harvard University Press, 1952), p. 288 (b. 3, chap. 12); Temkin, "Classical Roots of Glisson's Doctrine," pp. 307–8.

[11]Walter Pagel, "The Reaction to Aristotle in Seventeenth-Century Biological Thought," in *Science, Medicine and History: Essays in the Evolution of Scientific Thought and Medical Practice Written in Honour of Charles Singer*, ed. E. A. Underwood (London: Oxford University Press, 1953), 1:489–509 (pp. 503–9 fr. *Anat. Hep.*); Walter Pagel, "Harvey and Glisson on Irritability, with a Note on Van Helmont," *Bull. Hist. Med.* 41 (1967): 497–514.

[12]Nikolaus Mani, *Die historischen Grundlagen der Leberforschung*, 2 vols. (Basel: Schwabe, 1967), 2:104–20 (fr. *Anat. Hep.*).

[13]Friedrich Überweg, *Grundriss der Geschichte der Philosophie,* vol. 3, *Die Philosophie der Neuzeit bis zum Ende des XVIII. Jahrhunderts* (Tübingen: E. S. Mittler, 1953), p. 193; Werner Ziegenfuss, ed., *Philosophen-Lexikon. Handwörterbuch der Philosophie nach Personen* (Berlin: De Gruyter, 1949), 1:391 (article: Glisson); Pagel, "Reaction to Aristotle," pp. 489–509; H. Marion, *Franciscus Glissonius quid de natura substantiae, seu vita naturae senserit et utrum Leibnitio de natura substantiae cogitanti quidquam contulerit* (Lutetiae Parisiorum: Baillière, 1880).

[14]Glisson took his medical degree in 1634, at the age of thirty-six. Before that he had been lecturer in Greek and fellow of the Gonville and Caius College from 1624 to 1634, and dean in 1629 (See Walker, "Francis Glisson and his Capsule," p. 36). The scholastic framework of thought is particularly obvious in the prolegomena of the *Anat. Hep.,* pp. 1–46. See also Marion, *Franciscus Glissonius:* "Vir (scil. Glisson) nempe subtilissimus, et indefessus, et scholasticis argutiis mirum in modum eruditus, perplexis itineribus quasi delectatur, per innumeros circuitus lectorem trahit, a proposito centies digreditur, divisa rursus dividit, haeret in distinctionibus, rationes rationibus innectit atque implicat" (pp. 25–26); this qualification of Marion refers to Glisson's work *Tractatus de natura substantiae energetica* (London, 1672). See also Erik Nordenskiöld, *Geschichte der Biologie* (Jena: Fischer, 1926): "Seine Schlussätze formt er nach dem Muster der Scholastik, und die physiologischen Probleme, die er aufstellt, löst er auf rein abstrakte Weise" (p. 150); and Hermann Conring, *In universam artem medicam singulasque eius partes introductio, cura et studio G. Chr. Schelhammeri* (Helmstadii, 1687): "Anglorum plurimi Harvei exemplo inducti, in eo suam operam collocarunt. Numerantur in his Nathanael Highmorus, Gualtherius Charleton, Franciscus Glissonius (qui tamen de pluribus, veterum potius more egerunt) Thomas Wharton, qui de glandulis sollicitus novos salivales ductus inferiores adinvenit, et primus descripsit" (p. 182). And see also note 70 below.

[15]Temkin, "The Classical Roots of Glisson's Doctrine," pp. 297–328; Pagel, "Reaction to Aristotle," pp. 489–509; idem, "Harvey and Glisson on Irritability"; Albrecht Haller, *Bibliotheca Anatomica* (Tiguri, 1774), 1:452: "De irritabilitate nemo ante Glissonium rectius cogitavit, quam equidem paulo liberalius fere omnibus corporis humani partibus tribuit."; Thomas S. Hall, *Ideas of Life and Matter* (Chicago: University of Chicago Press, 1969), 1:396; Karl E. Rothschuh, *History of Physiology,* trans. and ed. Guenter B. Risse (Huntington, N.Y.: R. E. Krieger, 1973), p. 86.

[16]Walker, "Francis Glisson and His Capsule," p. 78; idem, "Francis Glisson," p. 43; *Anat. Hep.,* "Lectori."

[17]*Anat. Hep.*: "in ipso operis exodio, de lymphae-ductibus paulo fusius egimus" "Lectori"; *Anat. Hep.,* chap. 45: "De actione et usu Lymphae-ductuum, sive Canalium aquosorum" (pp. 401–58).

[18]Gaspare Aselli, *De lactibus sive lacteis venis, quarto vasorum mesaraicorum genere novo invento* (Mediolani, 1627). Reference to this treatise is made in *Anat. Hep.,* chap. 35, p. 313; Jean Pecquet, *Experimenta nova anatomica quibus incognitum chyli receptaculum, et ab eo thoracem in ramos usque subclavios vasa lactea deteguntur* (Paris, 1651). Reference to this book is made in *Anat. Hep.,* chap. 35, pp. 315–17; Thomas Bartholin, *De lacteis thoracicis in homine brutisque nuperrime observatis historia anatomica* (Copenhagen, 1652). Reference to this work is found in *Anat. Hep.,* chap. 35, p. 315; idem, *Vasa lymphatica nuper Hafniae in animantibus inventa et hepatis exsequiae* (Copenhagen, 1653); Olof Rudbeck, *Nova experimenta anacomica, exhibens ductus aquosos hepaticos aquosos, et vasa glandularum serosa* (Arosiae, 1653); "A translation of Olof Rudbeck's *Nova Exercitatio Anatomica* announcing the discovery of the lymphatics," trans. A. E. Nielsen with a biographical note by G. Liljestrand, *Bull. Hist. Med.* 11 (1942) 304–39. See also Nikolaus Mani, "Darmresorption und Blubbildung im Lichte der experimentellen Physiologie des

17. Jahrhunderts," *Gesnerus* 18 (1961): 93–121. The terms *canales aquosi* and *lymphae-ductus* used by Glisson in *Anat. Hep.*, chap. 45, p. 401, point to his acquaintance with these two works, although in chap. 35 of *Anat. Hep.*, p. 315, he does not mention the rejection of hepatic blood formation by Bartholin.

[19]*Anat. Hep.*, chap. 45, pp. 438–439: "Vasa excretoria, glandibus maxillaribus propria, a D. Whartonio et me primum (uti arbitror) reperta sunt" (p. 439); ibid., chap. 35, p. 301.

[20]Ibid., "Prolegomena," chap. 1: "Anatomia est ars, quae per artificiales dissectiones, commensurationes, ponderationes, inflatus, injectiones per siphonem, ligaturas, aliasque utiles operationes corporis humani singularium eius partium structuram, proportiones, complementa, defectus, elementa, communitates, differentias, sympathias, antipathias, facultates, actiones atque usus eius luculenter explicat" (p. 5).

[21]Ibid., "Prolegomena," chap. 10, p. 42; Webster, "Henry Power's Experimental Philosophy," pp. 160–61.

[22]*Anat. Hep.*, "Prolegomena," chap. 10, p. 42; ibid., chap. 21, pp. 210–12; ibid., chap. 33, pp. 286–88.

[23]Ibid., "Prolegomena," chap. 1: "Imo vero sola bruta ipsius partis artis, quae vivorum dissectio appellatur, subiecta aestimanda sunt" (p. 4); ibid., chap. 35; "Chylum plus minusve dilutum, in diversis animalibus etiamnum viventibus ad Asellii norman dissectis, facile videre est. In quibus animalibus saepe eum crassum lacteumque sum conspectus" (p. 313). On pp. 315–17 of chap. 35, Glisson describes personal investigations of the lymphatics. See also p. 321.

[24]Webster, "Henry Power's Experimental Philosophy," pp. 153–54; Cole, "Henry Power on the Circulation," pp. 318–19, 323. Here, Power refers to the perfusion of the liver as a fundamental experiment of Glisson; *Anat. Hep.*, "Prolegomena," chap. 1, p. 6.

[25]*Anat. Hep.*, "Prolegomena," chap. 8, pp. 26–34; ibid., chap. 38, 39, pp. 344–77; ibid.: "Horum (scil. elementorum) duo sunt genera, intermedia nempe, et ultima" (p. 27); ibid.: "Quod ad mistorum corporum in elementa ultima divisionem attinet; existimen, sententiam Chymicorum esse verissimam; nempe quinque principia ab iis dicta, puta spiriutum, oleum, salem, aquam sive phlegma, et caput mortuum sive terram (ut vocant) damnatam, esse partes ultimas in quas res ullae vel ingenio vel industria humana dissolvi queant" (p. 32).

[26]Allen G. Debus, *The English Paracelsians* (London: Oldbourne, 1965), p. 39; Robert P. Multhauf, *The Origins of Chemistry* (London: Oldbourne, 1966), pp. 276–77; James R. Partington, *A History of Chemistry* (London: Macmillan, 1962), 3:1–8; Jean Beguin, *Tyrocinium Chymicum autore Johanne Beguino*, ed. Christopher Glückradt, 6th ed. (n.p., 1625), pp. 34–39; see also Multhauf, *Origins of Chemistry*, and Partington, *History of Chemistry*, pp. 2–4. The numerous editions of the *Tyrocinium Chymicum* are discussed by T. S. Patterson, "Jean Beguin and his *Tyrocinium Chymicum*," *Annals of Science*, 2 (1937):243–98; See also P. M. Rattansi's article "Beguin" in *Dictionary of Scientific Biography*, ed. Charles C. Gillispie (New York: Charles Scribner's Sons, 1970), 1:571–72; The five elements of Basso are: spirit (or mercury), oil (or sulphur), salt, earth (faeces, caput mortuum), and phlegm. See Partington, *History of Chemistry*, p. 7. See also P. M. Rattansi's article, "Sebastian Basso," *Dictionary of Scientific Biography*, p. 495; and for Etienne de Clave's elementary doctrine see Heléne Metzger, *Les doctrines chimiques en France du début du XVIIᵉ à la fin du XVIIIᵉ siècle* (Paris: Presses Univ., 1923), p. 57–58.

[27]*Anat. Hep.*, "Prolegomena," chap. 8, pp. 27–29.

[28]See section "similar attraction" of this paper; *Anat. Hep.*, "Prolegomena," chap. 8, p. 30–31.

[29]*Anat. Hep.*, chap. 38, pp. 344–45: "Elementa e quibus (bilis) constat, videntur

esse pauci spiritus, aliquantulum sulphuris, plurimumque salis, aquae et terrae"
(p. 344); Ibid., chap. 39, pp. 347–73; Davis, "Some Implications of the Circulation
Theory," pp. 28–39.

[30]*Anat. Hep.*, chap. 39, pp. 348–54; and ibid.: "Spiritus vocabulo intelligendum
venit elementum illud, quod, post debitam fermentationem, licet haud antea, sua
sponte sursum nititur, et fit volatile" (p. 349).

[31]Ibid.: "Mercurius sive spiritus iste, est duum generum: est enim Mercurius pin-
guis, sive sulphureus, est etiam macer, sive salinus" (p. 349).

[32]Ibid., pp. 349–50.

[33]Ibid., p. 352.

[34]Ibid., pp. 353–54.

[35]Ibid., pp. 353–54, 365–66.

[36]Ibid.: "Fermentatio autem est calor intus exoriens, ob luctam inter spiritus et
partes crassiores; dum illi conantur sese expandere, atque avolare, hae vero illi nisui
adversantur. Similiter, vitalis calor provenit ab interna concertatione, inter spiritus
sanguinis vitales, huiusque elementa crassiora, dum illi id sedulo agunt, ut tum ipsi,
tum sanguis reliquus dilatentur; haec autem isti conatui oppido reluctantur. Adeoque
fermentatio et vitalis calor in hoc conveniunt, quod in utroque spiritus nitantur sese
expandere" (p. 366).

[37]Ibid., pp. 365–68.

[38]Ibid., pp. 369–70. Glisson refers to Santorio Santorio (Sanctorius): *De statica
medicina*, 1st ed. (Venice, 1614).

[39]*Anat. Hep.*, "Prolegomena," chap. 8: "Commodissimum itaque mihi videtur,
elementa Aristotelica, Chymicorum principiis conciliare, inque gratiam mutuo
reducere. Si nempe Aristotelis elementum ignis, proportione respondet Chymicorum
spiritui; aer, oleo; aqua, phlegmati; terra sali simul et capiti mortuo" (p. 33). See also
Davis, "The Circulation of the Blood and Chemical Anatomy," p. 29.

[40]*Anat. Hep.*, "Prolegomena," chap. 4: "Materiae igitur definitio generalis est,
ut sit corpus, aptum fingi et formari ad scopum agentis....Formae autem definitio
generalis est, ut sit modificatio quaedam ab agente in materiam introducta, qua usui
destinato commode inservit." (p. 11). Ibid.: "Natura vero delectu exquisitiore utitur;
ideoque ipsamet sibi materiam parat operi proposito plane accomodam." (p. 12).

[41]Ibid., chaps. 5, 6, 7, pp. 13–26: "Veterum ergo distinctio (in partes similares
et organicas) sola realem usum in Medicina obtinet" (p. 14). Apart from the division
of the parts into similar and dissimilar, Aristotle and Galen also differentiated similar
parts from instrumental or organic parts *Homoiomere Moria* and *Organica Moria*. See
Aristotle, *Generation of Animals*, trans. A. L. Peck (London: Heinemann; Cambridge: Harvard University Press, 1953), bk. 2, chap. 1, p. 152, bk. 2, chap. 4,
p. 190, bk. 2, chap. 6, pp. 212–14; see also Galen, *In Hippocratis de natura hominis
commentaria tria*, ed. J. Mewaldt (Lipsiae et Berolini: Teubner, 1914), "Corpus
Medicorum Graecorum," bk. 5, chap. 9, sec. 1, p. 6 (the same passage is found in
Kühn's edition, bk. 15, p. 7); *Galeni in Hippocratis librum de alimento commen-
tarius*, bk. 3, chap. 1 (in Kühn's edition, bk. 15, p. 252).

[42]*Anat. Hep.*, "Prolegomena," chap. 6: "Quod partes itaque sint similares, id
materiae debent; quod autem organicae, id formae acceptum referunt" (pp. 16–17)

[43]Ibid., chap. 34: "Porro actio atque usus partium distingui possunt in similares et
organicas....Fatemur certe usum semper, sensu iam dicto, vel alii cuipam parti, sive
agenti, vel toti inservire: non tamen id semper facit organice sive mechanice" (pp. 297–
98); chap. 35: "Pro concesso enim habeo sanguificationem esse actionem similarem,
et per modum assimilationis perfici debere" (p. 307); chap. 35: "Assero sanguinem
ipsum qui efficitur, esse corpus simile; chylumque ex quo fit, pariter similarem
esse; et chylum non facessere in sanguinem, separatione ullius eius partis ab alia
(quemadmodum urina et bilis oriuntur) verum exaltatione quadam spiritus illius
naturalis in vitalem; dum spiritus vitales eundem calorem sive motum diffusivum,

atque micationem, quam ipsimet obtinent, in naturalibus exuscitant: quod manifeste assimilando peragitur, estque actio mere similaris" (p. 311); chap. 41: "Quippe bilis est humor crassior multo, quam urina; nec potest eiusmodi colatura separari, quae expressione mechanica potissimum perficitur; qua partes tenuiores premendo eliciuntur, crassioresque per alia vasa remeant. Ipse quoque bilem separandi modus est praestantior, utpote qui attractionem similarem accuratam magis quam urinae segregatio, postulet" (p. 384); chap. 43: "Colaturae, quae ad excretionem spectant, trifariam dividi possunt. Quarum prima est, cum parte tenuiore reiecta, forasque extra corpus educta, parsque crassior retinetur. Atque huius colaturae specimen in renibus evidentissime conspicitur, ubi potulenta materia a sanguine secernitur: idemque etiam in sudatione, lacrymatione, salivatione, etc. videre est. . . . Colaturae artificiales sunt ut plurimum plane mechanicae; naturales autem licet insignem mechanicen semper adminiculantem habeant, pars tamen actionis earum praecipua, videtur esse similaris. Quippe mechanica earum pars est organica sive instrumentalis; similaris vero est, cui organum immediate inservit, quaeque opus perficit" (p. 392); chap. 43: "Partes organicae, quae bili a sanguine secernendae operas suas immediate conferunt, sunt rami portae, et radices cavae, atque pori bilarii. . ." (p. 393).

[44]Ibid., "Prolegomena," chap. 7: "nimirum morbos humano corpori accidentes, ad alterum horum generum referri posse, scil. ad partes similares, vel organicas; sive (quod eodem redit) ad partium materiam vel formam" (p. 23); See also Galen, *De differentiis morborum*, chap. 13, ed. Kühn bk. 6, p. 876, where Galen differentiates diseases of similar and organic parts.

[45]*Anat. Hep.*, chap. 34: "Quaelibet enim actio, ut causam efficientem, sic et finalem obtinet: eademque finalis causa, quamdiu est in intentione agentis, manet etiamnum causa finalis; quamprimum vero ad executionem perducitur, ut rei propositae fructus est, ita ipsiusmet actionis usus dici debet" (pp. 294–95).

[46]Ibid.: De actione atque usu hepatis" (pp. 294–99): "Ususque etiam privatus est, utpote privatae solum partis (a cuius actione profluxit) commodo inserviens" (p. 295); "pars est cum aliis, ad totius salutem, sociali foedere coniuncta" (p. 295); "Quapropter licet organum absolute (ceu agens naturale, nulloque ad totum respectu habito) consideratum, suis tantum rebus consulat, quatenus tamen cum toto foederatum est, debet necessario dare operam illius commodo, publicaeque actioni atque usui, quos producit, incumbere; neutrum vero eorum fortuito consequi" (p. 296).

[47]*Anat. Hep.* "Prolegomena," chap. 8, pp. 29–30; chap. 20, pp. 200–5; chap. 20, pp. 200–2; Galen, *On the Natural Faculties*, trans. Arthur John Brock (London: Heinemamm; Cambridge: Harvard University Press, 1952), bk. I, chap. 14, pp. 71–81.

[48]*Anat. Hep.*, chap. 20: "Tria ad hanc rem (scil. attractio similaris sive magnetica) requiro. 1. Ut sint duo, vel plura corpora, quibuscumque similitudo, affinitas, sive familiaritas mutuo intercedat. 2. Ut ab uno saltem eorum, in alio unionis desiderium excitetur. 3. Ut excitatio haec sit proficua, oportet adsit *nixus coeundi* sive *actualis conatus* quo corpora ad se invicem congregentur. . . corpora hoc pacto excitata, mutuum congressum appetunt" (p. 203).

[49]*Anat. Hep.*, chap. 20, p. 204: "Ex dictis constat, quid per attractionem similarem sive magneticam, intelligam: nempe allectationem, sive incitamentum, quo corpus naturale ad aliud sui simile fertur" (p. 204).

[50]Ibid.: "At vero inquis, vocabulum (scil. attractio) eo sensu acceptum, haud proprie attractionis titulum merebitur; cum toto genere ab eo differat, quod mechanice perficitur. . . . Dixi autem attractionem similarem, ut ab organica sive mechanica distinguerem. Nam licet attractio huiusmodi in corporis organis reperiri possit, illa tamen haud organice perficitur; sed a similitudine, familiaritate, atque affinitate corporis attrahentis cum attracto, promanat; eademque similitudo in constitutione partium *similari*, non *organica*, fundatur" (pp. 204–5).

[51]Ibid.: "Prolegomena," chap. 8: "Separationes quaedam fiunt per congregationem

vel attractionem magneticam, sive similarem....Ita quoque consimilis naturae
partes facile inter se congregantur, relictis aliis, quibuscum illis minus convenit; uti
videre est in salium granulatione; in crystallizatione sacchari....Id certe constat,
qualitatem hanc (sc. attractio similaris) in animalibus maxime conspicuam esse,
eademque etiam habere organa huic usui destinata; quod occultae actionis naturae
maxime convenit...Variae plantae in eadem area consitae, sibi quaeque diversum ac
peculiarem succum eligunt; idque radicum ope, quibus in hunc finem donantur.
Animalium quoque pars quaelibet alimentum sibi congruum attrahit, retinetque;
excrementa vero sive partes inutiles reiicit. Hoc pacto chylus separatur ab excre-
mentis; bilis a sanguine..." (pp. 29–30).

[52]Ibid., chap. 35: "Litigatum est olim inter Peripateticos et Galenicos, cuinam vis-
ceri sanguificandi munus conveniat: dum illi cordi, hi vero hepati officium illud attri-
buunt...Nuper autem facta penitiore illius rei indagatione, clare constitit, nullam
earum (scil. sententiarum) veritati consonam esse" (p. 299).

[53]Ibid., pp. 299–311; see also Howard B. Adelmann, *Marcello Malpighi and the
Evolution of Embryology* (Ithaca, N.Y.: Cornell University Press, 1966), pp. 1350–
52, with Latin text and English translation. The book offers Glisson's views on the
generation of primitive blood and the sequence of the formation of blood, heart, and
liver. *Anat. Hep.*, chap. 35, p. 300: "Causae vero naturales brevissimo optimoque
agendi modo strictius adalligantur; debentque, quamdiu eaedem permanserint, rem
eandem agere, nisi alicunde impeditae fuerint....Quoniam igitur causa sanguinis
primi effectrix, est agens naturale; si in animali usque perstiterit, oportet quoque
idem semper opus instituat..." (p. 300).

[54]Ibid.: "Si vero accurate pensitemus quidnam sanguinem primitivum efficiat;
liquido constabit, non hepar, neque cor, nec etiam venas, sed spiritum vitalem in
prima seminali materia hospitantem, illius auctorem esse. Nam in ovo incubato
sanguinem reperias, antequam cor, hepar, venaeve efformatae fuerint; imo vero
priusquam in ipso puncto saliente vel minimum sanguinis extiterit" (p. 300); "Quae
omnia clare indicant, cuiusnam opera (in sanguineis animalibus) succus vitalis in sanguinem excoquatur, quidque hunc ipsum incolumem conservet: est nempe calor
spiritus vitalis, in ipso saepe redintegratus, absque quo sanguineus illius color subito
evanescit" (p. 304); "Est quidem verissimum, fieri aliquo pacto debere primum sanguinem: non potest autem fabricari a corde aut hepate, aut aliqua solidarum partium, quia post natum sanguinem hae efformantur; ineptumque est credere, partem
aliquam agere posse antequam existat. Quamobrem nihil superest, quod primum
sanguinem effingat, praeter spiritum vitalem, qui in vitali liquore continetur" (p. 306).

[55]Ibid., pp. 301–2; Adelmann, *Marcello Malpighi*, pp. 1350–51.

[56]*Anat. Hep.*, chap. 35: "asserimus porro, debere idem agens in consimili opere
ad ultimum vitae terminum persistere. Nam spiritus hic vitalis non solum in corpore
permanet, verum in dies fit vegetior, calidior, et ad opus promptior, donec animal ad
aetatis florem pervenerit....Neque sane putandum est, agens aliquod naturale
(qualis est spiritus hic vitalis) ab opere omni feriari, actionemque suam suspendere,
aut vires integras non exerere; ideoque quamdiu vita suppetit, oportet eidem muneri
incumbat...(puta) revera, spiritum vitalem, dum vitalem succum in colorem san-
guineum excoquit, primum sanguinem efficere; eundemque spiritum in sanguine
iam facto commorantem, et ab hoc adiutum, maiori semper postea facilitate idem
opus exequi" (pp. 306–7).

[57]Ibid., pp. 307–9: "Ratio aliqua generalis, quae cordi, venis atque hepati pariter
sanguificandi munus adimat, haec statui potest: quia nulla harum partium sanguini
satis assimilis est, ut officio hoc defungantur. Pro concesso enim habeo sanguificationem esse actionem similarem, et per modum assimilationis perfici debere" (p. 307).

[58]Ibid.: "Accedit in sententiae nostrae confirmationem ipsamet experientia: saepe
enim usu venit, ut quorum corda, iecinora, venae aliaeque solidae partes, integrae

illibataeque sanitatis sunt, si tamen casu aliquo ingentem sanguinis iacturam faciant (nempe vel narium haemorrhagia, vel ruptione venarum, vel ab inflictis vulneribus) sanguificatio statim manifeste laedatur" (p. 309); "Cordi particulariter sanguificandi munus denegatur hoc argumento; quod cor ipsum, vitalem omnem calorem atque activitatem a sanguine vitali in ventriculis ipsius contento, inque substantiam eius per arterias coronarias distributo, foeneretur.... Quoniam igitur cor illico a sanguificationis officio cessat, quamprimum sanguis vitalis e ventriculis eius eductus fuerit; fas est concludere, vim sanguinis generatricem haud primario in solida ipsius substantia sitam esse, sed in alio quopiam: debetque adeo in eo posita esse, cuius absentia fit, ut virtus illa elanguescat; nempe in sanguine vitali" (p. 321); "Evelle protinus sani animalis cor, sanguinemque inde omnem elue, ac mox (dum etiamnum calet) chylum aut lac in ventriculos eius infundito, visurus, numnam liquor ille sanguinis faciem aliquam induiturus sit: experieris profecto eundum neutiquam immutatum iri" (p. 321); "Viventium certe dissectionibus compertum habemus, calorem vitalem maiorem esse in cordis ventriculis, quam in ipsius substantia, in quam sanguis e ventriculis derivatur" (p. 322).

[59]Cole, "Henry Power on the Circulation," p. 299.

[60]Mani, "Darmresorption und Blutbildung," pp. 93–121.

[61]*Anat. Hep.*, chap. 35, p. 303–4; see notes 54 and 56 above and the section of this chapter entitled "Application of chemistry to Biology and Medicine."

[62]See notes 53, 54, and 56 above.

[63]*Anat. Hep.*, chap. 39: "Ideoque si suaves eius (scil. sanguinis) spiritus continue disperdantur, necesse est, ut calor (dispendii illius autor) sulphur quoque crassum adurat, atque eidem amarorem conciliet, humoremque adeo felleum progeneret" (p. 366).

[64]*Anat. Hep.*, chap. 40, pp. 374–79; Mani, *Die historischen Grundlagen der Leberforschung*, pp. 113–14.

[65]Ibid., pp. 376–79.

[66]Ibid., chap. 43: "Verisimile equidem est, parenchyma e partibus similaribus diverismodis constitui; aliasque humorum excernendorum uni, alias alteri convenire: quo fit, ut humores illi se partibus iis accomodent, cum quibus similitudo maxima atque affinitas ipsis intercedit: estque istud secretionis eorum initium. Particulae nempe, quibus maxima cum humore felleo est familiaritas, eundem ad sese alliciunt, inque pori bilarii extrema capillaria dirigunt. Similiter, particulae illae, quibus cum sanguine puro potissimum res est, hunc ad se attrahunt, posteaque ad capillares radicum cavae extremitates deducunt" (p. 393).

[67]Ibid., chap. 41, pp. 383–85.

[68]Ibid., pp. 383–85, 390–94; Mani, *Die historischen Grundlagen der Leberforschung*, pp. 111–13, 117–18.

[69]*Anat. Hep.*, chap. 42: "Probabile est sanguinem in hepate ob duplicem portae tunicam, spiritus in ea caeteroquin avolaturos coercentem, obque motum pulsatilem iam dictum, vitalitatis quosdam veluti igniculos recuperare, et micationem aliquantillam acquirere: talem nempe, quae parenchymati hepatis vivificando sufficiat.... Poterit etiam porro huius sanguinis revivescentiae documentum peti a cordibus viperarum, aliorumque consimilis vivacitatis animalium: ea enim e corporibus execta, mensaeque imposita, pulsum diu servant; tandemque, absumpto iam plane calore vitali, si modo calente saliva attigeris, revivescunt protinus, pulsumque denuo ad tempus redintegrant, Talis nempe est haec vitae scintillula, in sanguine intra portam resuscitata..." (pp. 388–89).

[70]Antoine Portal, *Histoire de l'anatomie et de la chirurgie*, (Paris, 1770), 3:47: "Glisson a consacré huit chapitres à des prolegomenes superflus, et totalement étrangers à son objet"; N.F.J. Eloy, *Dictionnaire historique de la Médecine ancienne et moderne* (Mons, 1778), 2:358: "Si l'on pardonne à l'auteur (Glisson) les réflexions

scholastiques dont il a rempli quelques chapitres de cet ouvrage (scil. *Anat. Hep.*), il ne se mêle guere de raisonner; il s'arrête aux faits anatomiques, et se tait lorsqu'ils lui manquent."

[71]Mani, *Die historischen Grundlagen der Leberforschung*, pp. 213–18, 324, 340–69.

[72]See note 1 above.

[73]Conrad Brunner and Wilhelm von Muralt, *Aus den Briefen hervorragender Schweizer Aerzte des 17. Jahrhunderts* (Basel: Schwabe, 1919), pp. 70–106.

[74]Hans Fischer, "Johann Jakob Wepfer (1620–1695)," *Mitteilungen der Naturforschenden Gesellschaft Schaffhausen* (1929–30), 9:93–201 (also published separately, Zürich, 1931); Hans Nigst, "Das anatomische Werk Johann Jakob Wepfers," in *Veröffentlichungen d. Schweiz. Ges.f.Gesch. d. Med. u.d. Naturwiss.* (Aarau: Sauerländer, 1947), Fasc. 16; Heinrich Buess, "Zur Geschichte des Embolie-Begriffs bis auf Virchow," in *Schweiz. Med. Jahrbuch* (1946), pp. 57–60; Susi Joos-Renfer, Marie-Louise Portmann, Heinrich Buess, "Pathologisch-anatomische Beobachtungen bedeutender Schweizer Ärzte 1670–1720" *Basler Veröffent-lichungen z. Gesch. d. Med. u.d. Biol.* (Basel: Schwabe, 1961), fasc. 13; Pietro Eichenberger, "Johann Jakob Wepfer (1620–1695) als klinischer Praktiker" *Basler Veröffentl. z. Gesch. d. Med. u.d. Biol.* (Basel: Schwabe, 1969), fasc. 26; idem, "Autobiographisches von Johann Jakob Wepfer in einem Briefwechsel mit Johann Conrad Brotbeck," *Gesnerus* 24(1967):1–23.

[75]*Apoplexia*, p. 21: "tum ignotus sanguinis circularis motus, qui nostri seculi praeclarissimum omnino, sagacissimi D. Harvaei inventum est...."

[76]Eichenberger, "Autobiographisches von Johann Jakob Wepfer," pp. 8, 13.

[77]Ibid. For Walaeus and Wepfer see J. Schouten, *Johannes Walaeus. Zijn betekenis voor de verbreiding van de leer van de bloedsomloop* (Assen: Van Gorcum Co., 1972), p. 72–73.

[78]Eichenberger, "Autobiographisches von Johann Jacob Wepfer," pp. 8, 13.

[79]Ibid., pp. 9, 14–15: "Incidi tum in doctissimos huius sententiae (schil. circulationis sanguinis) propugnatores Clarum Dominum Veslingium, Johannem Leonicenum, Dominum Thomam Bartholinum ex Sicilia et Malta reducem, Dominum Gilianum Garz Hamburgensem Anatomicum accuratissimum et contubernalem meum, qui omnes quicquid dubii mihi supererat quotidianis colloquis et argumentis ex ipsa rei natura et oculari demonstratione penitus sustulerunt" (pp. 8–9).

[80]Johann Jacob Wepfer, *Disputatio medica inauguralis De palpitatione cordis* (Basileae, 1647). (No pagination: divided into sections 1–13.)

[81]Ibid., section 2.

[82]Ibid.: "Haec de nomine: definiri potest palpitatio cordis quod sit motus pravus, vehemens, velox, creber, authore facultate eius irritata a re molesta, quam excutere conatur" (section 2); "Causa proxima in singulis cordis partibus, et vicinis, subsistere potest, modo adverso stimulo ad cor pertingere valeat" (section 3).

[83]Ibid: "Subjectum huius motus primarium est cor, quod alias indesinenter contrahitur et dilatatur...." (section 3); "Reliquum igitur est, principalem huius mali causam, facultatem cordis, eamque irritatam dicere, cum ad tam impetuosum motum peragendum robur aliquod requiratur. Cordi enim facultas pulsifica indita est....Cor nempe corpore exciso, vacuum sanguine, per aliquod temporis spatium adhuc movetur...non solum piscium cordibus exemptis, quorum cordis motus per integrum etiam diem perdurat: sed et quadrupedum....Peragit (scil. cor) autem motum insito calido, quo copioso perfunditur, et fibris...quamdiu enim cor calet, et fibrae continuantur, etiam corpore exemptum movetur; tenues vero in auras si calidum abiverit, et fibrae dissecentur, statim consueta agitatio cessat" (section 4).

[84]Ibid.: "Potentia praeterea instructum est cor, qua noxia et damnosa agnoscit, quae tactus est....Ut ut sit, certe experientia cordi sensum inesse facile confirmabit,

si cor nudum, vel acu, vel alio instrumento pungatur; tum oculis usurpare licebit quos saltus facturum sit, quos conatus ad rem molestam repellendam adhibeat..." (section 4).

[85]Ibid., sections 5, 6, 7. According to Wepfer the heart can be brought to contraction by irritation and stimulation of many kinds ("irritamentum, incitamentum, stimulus adversus"). In section 5 Wepfer mentions the Galenic concept of burdening, weight, and biting: "Alibi expultricem ad operam Ania Galeni cogit, quae sub se molem, pondus et mordax comprehendit...."

[86]Ibid.: "manum sub mamilla sinistra appositam ictus vehementius et frequentius feriunt..." (section 10).

[87]Temkin, "The Classical Roots of Glisson's Doctrine," pp. 308–9, 323.

[88]Eichenberger, "Johann Jacob Wepfer," pp. 27–28; Brunner and von Muralt, *Aus den Briefen hervorragender Schweizer Aerzte des 17. Jahrhunderts*, p. 85.

[89]*Apoplexia*, p. 172.

[90]Ibid: "Venas lacteas, circulationem sanguinis, ductus chyliferos, vasa lymphatica atque alia huius saeculi inventa, non exiguas in pathologia turbas excitasse, norunt illi, qui veterum dogmatibus innutriti, nova quoque addidicerunt" ("Preface to the Reader").

[91]Ibid.: "Ad eas angustias redacta est medicina, ut si quispiqm ratione et sensuum fide edoctus, aliter sentiat ac plurimi, qui Galeni authoritate gloriantur, statim apud hos ingeniorum tyrannos, novator et sciolus audiat" (p. 162).

[92]Ibid.: "tum denique Galeni authoritas, cui pridem quam plurimi nimium, quam ex re veritatis erat, studebant, adeo ut piaculum duceretur, ab eius sensu vel latum unguem discedere" (p. 21).

[93]Ibid.: "Nam cum de plurimarum partium usu et actionibus necessario aliter quam hactenus sentiendum sit, non pauca immutanda, emendanda, aut aliter explicanda erunt...postquam ante aliquot annos sanguinis motum agnovissem, plurima humana cadavera, tum apud exteros, tum hic in patria, et solus, et comitibus ac huius utilissimi laboris sociis...aperui..." ("Preface to the Reader").

[94]Johann Jacob Wepfer, *Historiae apoplecticorum et exercitatio de loco apoplexia affecto* (Amstelaedami ap. Janssonio-Waesbergios, 1710), p. 310: "Ex quo tempore medicinae operam dedi, nolui totus a libris pendere, ipsemet, quoties occasio offerebatur, Naturam consului, non paenitendo fructu, non enim raro aliter se rem habere, quam vulgo traditur, inveni" (dedicatory letter to Johann Jacob Stokar of 2 Febr. 1675).

[95]*Apoplexia* ("Preface to the Reader").

[96]Ibid.: "At partis enim visibilis et palpabilis existentiam demonstrandam, firmissimum testimonium nonnisi ab oculis et dextra artificis manu petitur: imo solis his fides debetur" (p. 36).

[97]Ibid.: "Neque enim possibile est, ut ille, qui perpetuum sanguinis fluxum e corde per arterias et refluxum eius per venas ad cor in vivis animalibus, intellexerit, idem sentiat, cum illis, qui sanguinem perpetuo intra venas stagnare credunt, et nonnisi a partibus penuria aliqua laborantibus attrahi, aut a nuper generato sanguine, lento gradu, protrudi, aut alias ob causas tardissime ad partes transportari putant" (p. 173).

[98]Ibid.: "Quo autem felicius affectum locum in apoplexia indagare valeam, eius causas proximas et generationis modos simul succincte tradam, cum his neglectis, alias minus commode negotium successurum sit" (p. 173).

[99]Ibid.: "Potius Exc. D. Thomas Bartholinus, in defens. dub. de lact. Thorac. contra Riol. cp. 2. audiendus videtur, ita enim ille: Optarem certe plures in urbe Parisiensi Ballonios, qui in civitate frequentissima, et Nosocomiis instructissima, debita diligentia, per dierum seriem, consignassent, et raros morborum eventus, et remediorum successus, et observata in morbidorum cadaverum dissectione....At-

que haec Cl. D. Bartholini amica invitatio, non parum animi mihi ad harum observationum editionem addidit, cuius scriptis et iucundissimo colloquio, dum Patavii eramus, me plurimum in his adiutum fuisse, ingenue fateor" ("Preface to the Reader"). The passage cited is from Thomas Bartholin, "Defensio dubiorum anatomicorum de lacteis thoracicis a Joanne Riolano," in *Defensio vasorum lacteorum et lymphaticorum adversus Joannem Riolanum* (Hafniae, 1655), chap. 2, p. 113.

    [100]*Apoplexia*, pp. 1–19. See also Joos-Renfer, Portmann, Buess, *Pathologisch-anatomische Beobachtungen bedeutender Schweizer Ärzte*, pp. 70–72.

    [101]*Apoplexia*, "Case I: Sudden Complete Apoplexy" pp. 1–5; "Case II: Speech Disorders, Loss of Language, Then Hemiplegia and Complete Apoplexy" pp. 5–11.

    [102]Ibid., pp. 20–21. Wepfer quotes Galen: *De locis affectis*, bk. 3, chap. 11, ed. Kühn 8, p. 200.

    [103]Ibid.: "De veritate desperassem, nisi mihi constitisset circulationem sanguinis aeque in cerebro atque in aliis partibus, necessario locum habere...(p. 98); "Et quoties animo revolvo magnitudinem et numerum arteriarum, quae partim substantiam eius (scil. cerebri) subeunt, partim superficiem perreptant, immerito cerebrum tanquam frigidum traduci...nullum enim viscus in toto corpore est, si cor, pulmonem et uterum in gravidis excipias, quod cerebrum arteriarum copia et mole non superet...." (p. 82).

    [104]Ibid.: "Atque ita apparet, firmumque et stabile manet, vasa per substantiam cerebri excurrere, eaque plurima, sed parva et capillaria" (p. 94); for further passages on blood supply and filtration of spirits see pp. 72, 173, 304; Nigst, *Das anatomische Werk Johann Jakob Wepfers*, pp. 11–25.

    [105]*Apoplexia*: "Apoplexiam produci ante omnia, ceu in praeloquio ponam, vel propter sanguinis per arterias affluxum ad cerebrum denegatum, vel ob spiritus animalis effluxum ex cerebro et cerebello per nervos et spinalem medullam, prohibitum, vel ob utramque causam" (p. 173). Regarding rupture of cerebral arteries, see pp. 8–9, 235–41. Regarding obstruction of carotids by muco-fibrous coagula, see pp. 196–203; see also Buess, "Zur Geschichte des des Embolie-Begriffs," p. 59. Regarding obstruction of small cerebral arteries, see p. 205–10.

    [106]*Apoplexia*: "Igitur quae apertio vasorum apoplexiam effectura est, potius intra cranium fiet, hac enim ratione medullosa substantia, sanguine, proxime in usum ipsius cessuro, orbatur, quin etiam premitur, aliaque quae ab extravasato sanguine, suam indolem protinus perdente ac noxio evadente, perpetitur" (p. 223).

    [107]Ibid., pp. 196–203.

    [108]Ibid.: "In apoplexia vero abolitis actionibus animalibus, nihilominus respirant, arteriae pulsant, extrema calida ut plurimum deprehenduntur. Et quandoque facies rubicunda conspicitur" (p. 202).

    [109]Ibid.: "Atque ob haec argumenta apoplexiam a sanguine extravasato generatam adhuc immedicabilem existimo" (p. 241).

    [110]Ibid.: "Et ipsa curandi ratio frequenter tales apoplexias, maxime illas, a quibus aegri plenam valetudinem brevi recuperant, a tali obstructione nasci comprobat" (p. 209).

    [111]Ibid.: "Obstructio vero haec (obstruction of arterioles) non una ratione animales actiones prosternit, sed pro eius conditione nunc plures nunc pauciores, prout scilicet paucae vel multae arteriolarum, perfectius vel imbecillius obstruuntur. Hinc quidem tantum loquela privantur; si in uno latere oppilentur, hemiplegia subsequitur: si utrinque, vera apoplexia exoritur, curatu facilior vel pertinacior, prout imbecillior vel validior illa fuerit" (p. 209).

    [112]Mani, "Darmresorption und Blutbildung," pp. 103–4.

    [113]Nikolaus Mani, "Naturwissenschaftlich-biologische Grundlagenforschung in der Medizin des 17. Jahrhunderts," *Med.-Hist. J.* 11: (1976) 181–205; idem, "Jean

Riolan II (1580–1657) and Medical Research," *Bull. Hist. Med.* 42 (1968):121–44 (for Pecquet, see pp. 141–42).

[114]Mani, "Darmresorption und Blutbildung," pp. 132–34.

[115]Walter Charleton, *Natural History of Nutrition of Life and Voluntary Motion* (London, 1659), p. 99.

[116]Temkin, "The Classical Roots of Glisson's Doctrine," pp. 297–328.

Commentary

Robert G. Frank, Jr.

In surveying and analyzing the two very different *oeuvres* of Glisson and Wepfer, Mani's paper suggests a host of fascinating insights into the research enterprise of medicine in the early modern period. I should like to highlight two themes that run through both the present paper and through a recent, more general article by Mani on basic research in seventeenth-century medicine.[1] First, Mani's presentation exemplifies the role of seminal discoveries in shaping subsequent medical research. Second, his treatment illustrates a paradox in the relationship between, on the one hand, the conservative natural philosophy and investigative methods of men such as Glisson and Wepfer, and, on the other, the innovative nature of their results.

SEMINAL DISCOVERIES

Mani's paper brings out both the direct and the indirect ways in which important—one might even say revolutionary—conceptual innovations influence subsequent research. Two such revolutions are discussed here: (1) Harvey's insight into the motion of the heart and resultant circulation of the blood, announced in 1628; and (2) the discoveries, ca. 1650–1653, by Pecquet, Rudbeck, Bartholin, and others concerning the thoracic duct and associated lymphatic system. Both of these have emerged in clear outlines only recently in the historiography of medicine. Our knowledge of the first we owe largely to the investigations of scholars like Keynes, Pagel, Whitteridge, Webster, and Bylebyl.[2] The nature of the second revolution has been established largely by Mani himself.[3] Here I wish to focus most especially on the seminal role of circulation theory, since it is in this respect that the scientific careers of Glisson and Wepfer show the greatest parallelism.

As Mani notes, Wepfer's conversion to a belief in the circulation was both gradual and conditioned by his contacts with his slightly older peers. Although Wepfer was first exposed to the ideas in reading the work of Jan de Wale, it was only at Basel and Padua in the mid 1640s, where the doctrine was the subject of experiments and discussion with an active circle of Wepfer's anatomical confreres, that he came over to "the Harveian side." The circulation then became the basis for Wepfer's doctoral dissertation. It inspired him to conduct dissections and post-mortems whenever possible, which in turn became the starting point for his explanation of apoplexy. Also out of this crucial student period in Wepfer's career arose his commitment to the belief that clinical observations and their associated post-mortem findings should be recorded in detail, as a foundation upon which genuine innovation in medicine could be based. Wepfer was true to his aspirations. Eichenberger has discovered at the University of Leiden over 12,000 pages of Wepfer's clinical notes, and from these has been able to reconstruct that intermingling of science and art which characterized Wepfer's medical career.[4]

The circulation—and the anatomical research it motivated—was similarly a theme of Glisson's life at almost exactly the same time. Glisson knew Harvey at the Royal College of Physicians of London during the 1630s, and by late in the decade had become an intimate friend and anatomical collaborator of George Ent, one of Harvey's earliest and staunchest English defenders. By 1640, Ent had started Glisson on dissections of the liver, with an eye towards redefining that organ's functions in light of the new doctrine of the circulation. In the mid 1640s Glisson and Ent were participants in a London scientific club (a precursor of the Royal Society) that attempted to explore by discussion and experimentation such recent innovations as the circulation of the blood. Other collaborative research in the late 1640s, this time at the College of Physicians, resulted in Glisson's book of 1650 on rickets, in which he fully integrated the circulation into his explanation of the disease's pathology. Finally, the *Anatomia Hepatis* (1654) was nudged into print in response to the revolutionary discoveries of Pecquet et al. during the years 1650 to 1653. Building upon a knowledge of the thoracic duct and lymphatic system, Glisson recast the anatomical results of ten years' research on the liver into a new framework, one in which that organ no longer occupied its Galenic role as the manufactory of blood.[5]

Wepfer and Glisson, although separated by native language, culture, and hundreds of miles, moved in parallel intellectual paths, each responding to scientific innovations that had captured the attention of their respective professional circles during a formative period in each man's life. To complete the parallel, I would note that Glisson, like Wepfer, left behind many thousands of pages of manuscripts that testify to the assiduity with which he also pursued the ideal of scientific methods applied to clinical observations.[6]

It seems then that seminal or "focal" discoveries influence subsequent research in a number of different ways. Allow me to suggest a few that by no means exhaust the possibilities:

1. They permit—and in many cases necessitate—a fresh evaluation of traditional explanations in cognate areas. Glisson's ideas of liver structure and function, as well as Wepfer's reinterpretation of apoplexy, are perfect examples of this.
2. They provide model protocols for conducting investigations. Harvey's careful dissections, his use of comparative evidence, his techniques of

section and ligature, his vivisectional observations—all were imitated and extended by those who accepted his discoveries.

3. Such discoveries validate an investigator's faith in both the possibility and significance of innovation. Thorndike remarked long ago on the profusion of seventeenth-century books with the word "new" in the titles. But a general faith in intellectual progress cannot long be maintained unless shored up by substantive discoveries. The circulation of the blood and the lymphatic system provided concrete, reproducible evidence of scientific progress, and were so construed by seventeenth-century writers.

4. Seminal discoveries provide the practitioner with the scientific underpinnings for reconsidering accepted explanations in pathology, and therefore infuse his daily activities with a new meaning. One may see this very clearly in the clinical investigations of Wepfer and Glisson.

5. In transitional periods, when opinion on an innovation is still divided, focal discoveries may provide the occasion for discussion and collaborative research that is a rallying point and source of identity for the participants who are adherents of a new doctrine.

NATURAL PHILOSOPHY AND INVESTIGATIVE METHODS

A second theme that may be extracted from Mani's paper is the paradox that, in seventeenth-century biomedical research, both the natural pholosophy that underlay innovation and the investigative methods by which novelty was secured may well be rather conservative and traditional. This is in contrast to the historiography of the physical sciences, where the seventeenth century is commonly interpreted as a period in which substantive innovations were based on concomitantly new natural philosophies and investigative methods. The achievements of men like Kepler, Galileo, Descartes, Boyle, and Newton are placed in the context of a rejection of Aristolelian philosophy because of its verbal and qualitative nature. Innovation in the physical sciences is seen as being intimately connected with matter-and-motion explanations, mathematical analysis, and the use of experiment rather than ratiocination as an arbiter of truth.

Mani's paper suggests that, at least in the case of Glisson and Wepfer, there was no such chasm between ancients and moderns with regard to matter-theory and methodology—a point that recent scholarship has also emphasized with respect to Harvey. Glisson, like Harvey, worked happily and fruitfully within the accepted Aristotelian/Galenic natural philosophy; both accepted goal-directed processes, the philosophical distinction between matter and form, the four causes, similar attraction, and many of other explanatory entities that the seventeenth century had inherited from antiquity. Both also used the largely traditional investigative methods to be found in the works of Galen or Vesalius: exposure and careful description of an organ; comparison of the organ's appearance in different animals; limited use of injection and inflation to expose the vascularity of tissues; section of vessels to expose contents; ligature of vessels to trace the flow of fluids; and vivisection to expose dynamic interactions. None of these methods could be called truly new to the seventeenth century. Rather, investigators in the early modern period took the techniques of observation and experimentation that had constituted only a part of biological reasoning in traditional medicine and elevated them to a place of great prominence (or in the case of Wepfer, preeminence) as sources of medical knowledge.

By way of contrast, only three areas of seventeenth-century biomedical research come to mind in which new methods played a significant part: (1) the respiratory and metabolic investigations of Boyle, Lower, Mayow, and their circle; (2) the microscopic anatomy of the lungs, kidneys, glands, and body fluids as carried out by men such as Malpighi and Leeuwenhoek; and (3) iatrochemical analyses of processes such as gastric digestion by Sylvius and his friends. But even the results in these three areas cannot be characterized as depending wholly on new methods. Lower and De Graaf had to do traditional vivisectional experiments to confirm or refute the conclusions drawn from, respectively, pneumatic and chemical investigations. Microscopy, an undeniably new technique fell out of favor for medical research in the late seventeenth century and was not revived until its optical shortcomings were remedied in the early nineteenth century. Chemistry also proved to be insufficiently developed in the seventeenth century to provide the basis for new research methods. Even the mechanical physiologies that had such a great vogue in the late seventeenth and early eighteenth centuries, although they profoundly reshaped both the physiologist's explanations and assumptions about the material substrate of life, were much less successful in enriching the armamentarium of the experimental investigator.

Indeed, when one considers many of the major accomplishments of biomedical research in the seventeenth century—Harvey on the circulation of the blood; Aselli, Pecquet, Rudbeck, Bartholin, and De Graaf on digestion; Wirsung, Steno, Malpighi, Glisson, Wepfer, Brunner, and Peyer on glands—one realizes that most of these advances were secured through the traditional methods of anatomical observation, vivisection, extirpation, section, ligature, and injection. Advance, at least in these cases, came through old methods prosecuted with skill and ingenuity.

If one were to combine my two themes—the role of focal discoveries and the conservative posture of natural philosophies and investigative techniques—one might state the whole in an exaggerated form. Traditional methods, pursued with vigor, proved capable of producing concrete and seminal discoveries that overthrew some old explanations, called others into doubt, and in turn incited more research to be carried forward with an increased expectation of novelty. Unfortunately, abbreviation often leads to caricature. Even I, with the commentator's license to speculate, would not be happy with so complacently Hegelian a conclusion. But it does emphasize the still unresolved tensions in our interpretations of the medical sciences of the seventeenth century. It is only through scholarship such as Mani's, which attempts simultaneously to analyze the metaphysical, physiological, pathological, and clinical dimensions of medical thought, that we have any hope of understanding such a crucial period in the history of medicine as the seventeenth century. I wish to thank him for providing us the occasion to consider these important issues.

NOTES

[1] Nikolaus Mani, "Naturwissenschaftlich-biologische Grundlagenforschung in der Medizin des 17. Jahrhunderts," *Med.-Hist. J.* 11 (1976): 181–205.

[2] See especially: Geoffrey Keynes, *The Life of William Harvey* (Oxford: Clarendon Press, 1966); Walter Pagel, *William Harvey's Biological Ideas: Selected Aspects and Historical Background* (Basel and New York: Karger, 1967); Walter Pagel, *New Light on William Harvey* (Basel and New York: Karger, 1976); Gweneth Whitteridge, *William Harvey and the Circulation of the Blood* (London: MacDonald, 1971); Charles Webster, "William Harvey's Conception of the Heart as a Pump," *Bull. Hist. Med.* 39 (1965), 508–17; Charles Webster, "Harvey's *De generatione*: Its Origins and Relevance to the Theory of Circulation," *Brit. J. Hist. Sci.* 3 (1967): 262–74; Jerome J. Bylebyl, "The Growth of Harvey's *De motu cordis*," *Bull. Hist. Med.* 47 (1973): 427–70.

[3] Nikolaus Mani, "Darmresorption und Blutbildung im Lichte der experimentellen Physiologie des 17. Jahrhunderts," *Gesnerus* 18 (1961): 85–146; Nikolaus Mani, *Die historischen Grundlagen der Leberforschung*, vol. 2, *Die Geschichte der Leberforschung von Galen bis Claude Bernard* (Basel: Schwabe, 1967), esp. pp. 80–103.

[4] Pietro Eichenberger, *Johann Jakob Wepfer (1620–1695) als klinischer Praktiker* (Basel: Schwabe, 1969).

[5] In addition to the references on Glisson cited by Mani, see Robert G. Frank, Jr., "The Physician as Virtuoso in Seventeenth-Century England," in Barbara Shapiro and Robert G. Frank, Jr., *English Scientific Virtuosi in the 16th and 17th Centuries* (Los Angeles: William Andrews Clark Memorial Library, 1979), pp. 57–114.

[6] British Library, London, MSS. Sloane 574B, 681, 2251, 2326, 3258, and 3306–3315.

THE GENESIS OF THE WILLIAM H. WELCH MEDICAL LIBRARY AND THE JOHNS HOPKINS INSTITUTE OF THE HISTORY OF MEDICINE

Janet B. Koudelka

In celebrating the fiftieth anniversary of the dedication of the William H. Welch Medical Library and the inauguration of the Institute of the History of Medicine, we might recall that these institutions did not materialize overnight. The beginnings of the library and the Institute can really be said to date back much earlier than 1929. Lectures in the history of medicine were given at the Johns Hopkins University a century ago, before the Hospital and Medical School were built, and the need for a central medical library was recognized very early in the life of the medical institutions.

The plans for The Johns Hopkins Hospital provided only limited space in the administration building for a library—the preliminary plans had provided none at all. This is remarkable because the planner was Dr. John Shaw Billings who, in 1865, along with his other important activities, had become librarian of the Surgeon General's Library in Washington. At the time the library contained about 1800 books. Under Billings's direction the collection increased to more than 100,000 volumes by 1891, making it by far the largest medical library in the United States.[1]

While some medical societies—such as the Boston Medical Association, the College of Physicians of Philadelphia, and the New York Academy of Medicine—had impressive book collections, medical schools in the 1890s did not include large libraries. For example, in 1895 Yale had 185,000 volumes in its general library compared to 3,000 in its medical library. At Harvard the disparity was even greater—292,000 volumes to 1,500.[2] In Baltimore at the time of the opening of The Johns Hopkins University, medical library facilities were rather meager. While the Medical and Chirurgical Faculty of Maryland, the state medical society, had 5,882 volumes in 1877, the medical school of the University of Maryland, founded in 1807, had about 1,000 by 1890.[3]

Billings wrote in 1876: "It may be said that almost all attempts to establish medical libraries in connection with medical schools have been failures. Commenced with enthusiasm, they soon become antiquated, are rarely consulted...are never properly catalogued or cared for.... Students and teachers want the recent books and journals only."[4] Many teachers recognized the

69

value of books and encouraged their use by students. But there were also those "practical" men, themselves possessors of fine libraries, who thought otherwise.[5] Their attitude was voiced by Dr. Abraham Jacobi, eminent New York pediatrician, in his discussion of a paper in which William Osler told of his custom of instructing students in medical literature. Dr. Jacobi said that his experience had made him regard the drawing of the students' attention to medical literature a very dangerous practice in most cases. He thought that the students who read were the ones who neglected the clinics and left college ill-equipped for the practical side of the professional life ahead of them.[6]

This perhaps suggests why Billings, who, in addition to real clinical teaching, advocated small classes, laboratories in the basic sciences, and other sound teaching reforms, seemed to pay so little attention to providing a medical library in a hospital that was to be regarded as a teaching institution and would be associated with a medical school.[7] But Billings also had something else in mind. Under his direction the Surgeon General's Library had not only grown steadily but was well organized. In 1879, in collaboration with Dr. Robert Fletcher, Billings had begun to issue the *Index Medicus*, and in 1880 the first volumes of the *Index Catalogue of the Surgeon General's Library* appeared. These important medical reference tools could be used by researchers outside Washington. Baltimore physicians were particularly fortunate because, as Billings said, "Washington is but an hour's ride away, and thus there is no difficulty in using the collections there."[8]

In fact Billings made an arrangement with The Johns Hopkins Hospital to send books requested by members of the medical staff. But the hospital had to assume responsibility for their safe return. In addition, Hopkins physicians often made the trip to Washington to use the Surgeon General's Library and Billings even granted direct borrowing privileges to a favored few, among them Dr. William Osler. Osler related that on returning from Washington one day, he left a library book on the train. It was never recovered and, despite their close friendship, Billings punished Osler by suspending his borrowing privileges for a year—the friendship endured nevertheless. The book in question was Thomas Peacock's *On Malformations of the Human Heart*.[9] It is reassuring to see that the book is not listed in the *Bibliotheca Osleriana*.

For medical researchers the Surgeon General's Library, like its present-day successor, the National Library of Medicine, was a great resource, but the need to have at Hopkins a working library that would include current periodicals was undeniable. The space provided in the hospital soon began to fill up. The collection grew through transfer of pertinent volumes from the university library, exchanges with the *Bulletin of the Johns Hopkins Hospital*, purchases, and particularly through gifts. By the time the medical school opened in 1893 the hospital library contained more than 2,500 volumes and received regularly 127 periodicals. In that year a full-time librarian was engaged. Two years later it was decided to keep the library open from nine in the morning until nine at night, as the library committee minutes record, "by employing a young woman at a moderate price, say $10.00 or $12.00 per month."[10]

The start of classes in The Johns Hopkins Medical School in 1893 brought an increased demand on the facilities of the hospital library, which was accessible to the medical students. Then, in 1899, a new medical school building was completed. In addition to housing the departments of physiology and pharmacology and the administration offices, it provided space for a library in which were shelved books on preclinical subjects, chiefly for the use of first- and second-year students. This library grew rapidly, a library attendant was in charge, and in 1908 the collection contained some 5,000 volumes.[11] The policy of depositing preclinical books in the Medical School had a geographical advantage since the Medical School library was in the midst of laboratories and classrooms, while the hospital library, two blocks away, was in the building where the housestaff had living quarters.

Both libraries were recipients of gifts of books. Many of the early medical staff were bibliophiles—Welch, Osler, Hurd, Halsted, Kelly, and others were frequent donors. Dr. Howard Kelly had been very generous in his gifts of books since the hospital had opened. Then, in 1914, he presented most of his private medical library to the hospital. The collection numbered upwards of 4,000 books, many on Dr. Kelly's own specialty, gynecology, but included were rare works on other branches of medicine. Dr. Kelly continued to collect rare books—he even had his own cable address to speed communication with European booksellers—and in all gave some 9,000 volumes to Hopkins.[12]

William Osler also made many gifts of books during his tenure at Hopkins, and he did not forget the Hopkins medical libraries after he left for Oxford. In 1907 he learned that a London dealer had for sale a whole medical library, from the dispensary of the Warrington Academy in England. The collection numbered about a thousand books published between 1531 and 1800. Osler engaged the interest of Mrs. William Marburg, a Hopkins trustee, who generously purchased the collection for the Medical School library.[13]

The bulk of Osler's own considerable collection was left to his alma mater, McGill University. But Hopkins received his books on cardiology and his son's collection on English literature.

Dr. William Halsted bequeathed to the Medical School library his collection of surgical books numbering nearly 4,000 volumes, including rare books.[14]

In 1916, the General Education Board of the Rockefeller Foundation established, as a branch of The Johns Hopkins University, a School of Public Health and Hygiene with Dr. Welch as director. Construction of a planned new building was delayed by the war, and the school was housed temporarily in buildings formerly used by the faculty of Arts and Sciences. Active preparations for gathering a library were made immediately. One of the early acquisitions was a collection of 1,600 journals given by Dr. Welch. The school moved into its Wolfe Street building in 1925. By 1928 the library contained about 11,000 volumes.[15]

In an address delivered in the Medical School in 1907, Dr. Osler said: "When the plans for the medical school were under discussion, I drew in outline what I should like to see on this plot of land. . . . On the Monument Street front was a beautiful structure in stone devoted to the library. As year by year the books increase in number such a building will be a necessity."[16]

And Dr. Henry Hurd, in his report as superintendent of the hospital, wrote: "The medical library. . . is much too crowded. A new and distinct building for the exclusive use of the library is urgently needed."[17] At the time of the gift of the Kelly collection the need was reiterated by Osler for a building large enough to house the several collections safely and also include space for instruction in the history of medicine.[18]

Formulation of a plan to deal with the problem of a central library began in 1916, when Dr. Halsted presented a proposal to the Advisory Board of the Medical Faculty for raising money for a library building.[19] The proposal was regarded favorably by the Board of Trustees and one of the trustees, Mr. George McGaw, offered $100,000 to help finance the building. As chairman of a committee to survey the features to be embodied in a library building, Dr. Llewellys Barker sent out a letter asking for suggestions.[20] Recipients included professors of the Hopkins medical faculty, some librarians including Fielding H. Garrison of the Surgeon General's Library, and also Drs. Harvey Cushing and Arnold Klebs. For the most part detailed answers were received, some with sketches. There was general agreement that the libraries should be combined and provisions made for rare books and a department of the history of medicine: also that an auditorium should be included. All suggestions were put into the hands of an architect, and tentative plans were drawn up. Unfortunately, Mr. McGaw died in 1919, before the additional funds to complete a library building were raised. However, with the support of Mr. McGaw's gift, a building containing an auditorium as well as offices for the visiting clergy was eventually erected. In compliance with Mr. McGaw's original desire, the building, dedicated in 1932, was named the Henry M. Hurd Memorial Hall in honor of the first superintendent of The Johns Hopkins Hospital.[21]

During the early 1920s, a survey of the needs of the ever-growing Johns Hopkins Medical Institutions was made, along with the resolution to approach the General Education Board of the Rockefeller Foundation.[22] Funds were granted for various new buildings and services. And in 1925, the dean of the Medical School, Dr. Lewis H. Weed, was encouraged to draft a proposal for submission to Dr. Abraham Flexner of the General Education Board. In it he emphasized the value of the medical library collection of over 50,000 volumes, the lack of adequate housing and accessibility of the books and journals, and the dispersement of the collection.[23] A New York architect, Edward L. Tilton, was consulted and tentative plans made. In February 1926 the General Education Board agreed to provide $1 million to support the building of the library and to provide endowment funds. However, Hopkins was to raise an additional $500,000.[24] It took little more than a year to complete the library building, but the university had been unable to raise the additional funds. The problem was solved in 1929 when Mr. Edward Harkness, long a generous friend of Hopkins, gave the entire amount still needed.

The William H. Welch Medical Library was dedicated on 17 October 1929. It provided adequate stack space, a large reading room, offices, and study carrels, and on the top floor a department of the history of medicine, the realization of a goal long sought by many members of the medical faculty.[25] Teaching of medical history had begun at Hopkins with a course of lectures given by John Shaw Billings at the University in 1877. In 1891–92 he gave a course for graduate students, and in 1893 he was appointed lecturer in the History and Literature of Medicine in the Medical School.[26] In speaking of Billings's lectures, Harvey Cushing said that they were badly attended and boring. William H. Howell, who was to become professor of physiology at Hopkins and dean of the Medical School, viewed Billings's lectures quite differently. On the advice of Isaiah Bowman, president of the university, he attended the course as an entering student. Later he recalled that "this survey of the history of medicine was very stimulating and made him gladder than ever that he was going into medicine."[27] At first only for graduate students, Billings's course appeared in the curriculum of the Medical School in 1895. He continued to teach until 1905, when he moved to New York and there became director of the New York Public Library.

After Billings's departure, the course in medical history was dropped from the curriculum. But instruction in the history of medicine and interest in its pursuit did not abate at Hopkins. Many of the professors introduced historical discussions in their lectures, in the laboratory, and at the demonstration of cases. William Osler was one who especially favored this treatment of the subject. In the everyday work of the wards and the outpatient department he tried to instill in the students the habit of looking at a subject from the historical standpoint. Osler also had regular informal meetings with his clinical clerks — over "beer and baccy," as he called it. He would give a short talk on one of the masters of medicine, when possible demonstrating with original works.[28]

The Johns Hopkins Hospital Historical Club was organized in 1890, largely through the efforts of Osler, Welch, and Kelly. At its first meeting Welch was elected president, and Osler and Kelly presented papers. In the early years the club held monthly meetings throughout the winter session in the hospital library. The meetings were well attended and often featured invited speakers from outside. This club still exists today as The Johns Hopkins Medical History Club.[29]

During the first decades of the twentieth century, formal teaching in medical history was introduced into some medical schools in the United States. And in Baltimore, the University of Maryland Medical School had in 1903 appointed Eugene Cordell to conduct courses.[30] With the planning of the new central medical library at Hopkins, the desirability of creating a department of the history of medicine came to the fore. When approached, the General Education Board made it clear that funds would be appropriated for such a department if Dr. Welch would accept the chair. He was at first reluctant on the score of age and the fear of emphasizing a spirit of dilettantism. But on the urging of Abraham Flexner he finally gave in, saying that "the time is ripe and the opportunity splendid for getting the subject of medical history well established and properly recognized both on the research and the teaching sides in our medical schools." In 1926, then aged 75, Welch retired as active head of the School of Hygiene and assumed the newly created chair.[31]

With characteristic vigor, Welch immediately began making plans, leaving for an extensive trip to Europe to visit libraries, to buy books, and to meet medical historians, especially at the Institute of the History of Medicine of the University of Leipzig, which was the prototype of what he wished to see at Hopkins. He did not want just a *Lehrstuhl*, which he said would be like a chair in physiology or pathology without laboratory, assistants, or budget. He talked to Karl Sudhoff and his successor as director of the Leipzig Institute, Henry E. Sigerist, as well as with other members of the staff. In his diary he wrote of meeting a young assistant, Dr. Temkin, and discussing Sydenham and Hippocrates with him. The entry goes on: "Temkin seems a capable, industrious worker—perhaps worth thinking about him for Baltimore." A cogent remark, one might say!

Welch returned to Baltimore in the fall of 1929 and set about finding staff for the library and the Institute. It had long been the wish of Welch and others to offer the directorship of the library to Col. Fielding H. Garrison, librarian of the Army Medical Library, editor of *Index Medicus*, and author of a comprehensive text on medical history. In 1929 Garrison arranged for army retirement and accepted the Hopkins post. The personnel of the original Hopkins medical libraries were transferred to the central library. Garrison was also appointed lecturer in the history of medicine. Other appointments in the Institute included Stephen D'Irsay, physiologist and medical historian, who had been working at the Leipzig Institute, and John Rathbone Oliver, Anglican priest and psychiatrist, who had successfully given courses in medical history at the University of Maryland Medical School.

It had been universally agreed that the medical library at Hopkins be named the William H. Welch Medical Library, and the director of the Institute of the History of Medicine bear the title, William H. Welch Professor of the History of Medicine. Besides honoring Welch, these designations are reminders of the role he played in the creation of the two institutions.

Under Garrison's successors as director of the Welch Library, Sanford V. Larkey, Alfred N. Brandon, and Richard A. Polacsek, the library has increased its collections, expanded its services, introduced new equipment and techniques, conducted training programs, and kept abreast of new developments in the medical library field. The Institute, under the direction of Henry E. Sigerist, Richard H. Shryock, Owsei Temkin, and Lloyd G. Stevenson, has provided regular courses for undergraduates and sponsored research and the publication of works on medical history. Through its graduate and fellowship programs, it has provided medical historians for universities around North America and abroad — as far away as South Africa and Korea. It is to be hoped that the achievements of the library and the Institute fulfill the dreams of Dr. Welch and the other supporters and sponsors who made these two institutions possible.

NOTES

[1]Fielding H. Garrison, S. V. "Libraries, Medical," *Reference Handbook of the Medical Sciences*, 3rd ed. (New York: W. Wood, 1915), 5:904.

[2]Bayard Holmes, "The Medical Library for the Medical School in a Small Community," *Bull. Amer. Acad. Med.* 2 (1895–1897): 247–48.

[3]Eugene F. Cordell, *The Medical Annals of Maryland: 1799–1899* (Baltimore: Williams & Wilkins, 1903), pp. 69–70; Archibald Malloch, "A Century of American Medical Libraries, 1830–1930," in *Celebration of the Centennial of the Library of the Medical and Chirurgical Faculty of the State of Maryland: 1830–1930* (Baltimore, 1931), pp. 3–11.

[4]John S. Billings, "Literature and Institutions," *A Century of American Medicine: 1776–1876*, by Edward H. Clarke et al. (Philadelphia: Henry C. Lea, 1876), p. 351.

[5]Malloch, "Century of American Medical Libraries," p. 8.

[6]James MacFarlane Winfield, "The Medical Library as a Factor in Medical Education," *Med. Libr. and Hist. J.* 2 (1904): 185–86.

[7]Richard H. Shryock, *The Unique Influence of the Johns Hopkins University on American Medicine* (Copenhagen: Ejnar Munksgaard, 1953), p. 14.

[8]Alan M. Chesney, ed., "Two papers by John Shaw Billings on American Medical Education," *Bull. Hist. Med.* 6 (1938): 358.

[9]Edgar Erskine Hume, "John Shaw Billings as an Army Medical Officer," *Bull. Hist. Med.* 6 (1938): 264.

[10]*Fifth Report of the Superintendent of the Johns Hopkins Hospital for the Year Ending January 31, 1894* (Baltimore: The Johns Hopkins Press, 1894), p. 19; The Johns Hopkins Hospital, Minutes of the Executive Committee, Board of Trustees, meeting of 23 April 1895.

[11]"Report of the Librarian," *Johns Hopkins University Circulars*, 25, no. 183 (1906): 113.

[12]"Valuable Additions to the Library of the Johns Hopkins Hospital by Dr. Howard A. Kelly," *Bull. Johns Hopkins Hosp.* 26 (1915): 415–17; Audrey W. Davis, *Dr. Howard A. Kelly: Surgeon, Scientist, Christian* (Baltimore: The Johns Hopkins Press, 1959), pp. 97–98.

[13]William Osler, "On the Library of a Medical School," *Bull. Johns Hopkins Hosp. 18 (1907): 109*–11.

[14]"Report of the Librarian," *Johns Hopkins University Circulars*, 42, no. 348, (1923): 118–19.

[15]*The School of Hygiene and Public Health of the Johns Hopkins University*, American Journal of Hygiene, Monograph Series, no. 6 (Baltimore, September 1926) pp. 1–10.

[16]Osler, "On the Library of a Medical School," p. 11.

[17]*Twenty-second Report of the Superintendent of the Johns Hopkins Hospital for the Year Ending Jan. 31, 1911* (Baltimore: The Johns Hopkins Press, 1911), p. 19.

[18]Osler, "On the Library of a Medical School," p. 111.

[19]Minute adopted by the Advisory Board of the Medical Faculty at its meeting on 26 May 1916 and referred to the president and Board of Trustees. The Johns Hopkins University, Minutes, vol. E, p. 170.

[20]A copy of this letter and the replies to it are in the Alan M. Chesney Archives of The Johns Hopkins Medical Institutions.

[21]W. H. Smith, "The Henry M. Hurd Memorial Hall," *Bull. Johns Hopkins Hosp.* 52 (1933): 267–70.

[22]*The Johns Hopkins Hospital, Baltimore* (a 32-page pamphlet issued in 1921 for a campaign to raise funds), p. 18; Minutes of the Medical Faculty, vol. F, 306th meeting, 29 April 1921, pp. 9–10.

[23]Lewis H. Weed, "Proposal for a Medical Library at The Johns Hopkins Medical Schools." The probable date of this document is 9 October 1923.

[24]W. W. Brierly, General Education Board, to Hopkins president Frank J. Goodenow, March 1, 1927; also "Report of the President, 1926–27," *Johns Hopkins University Circulars* 48, no. 314 (1927): 754.

[25]"The William H. Welch Medical Library of The Johns Hopkins University," *Bull. Johns Hopkins Hosp.* 46 (1930): 3–153.

[26]Fielding H. Garrison, *John Shaw Billings: A Memoir* (New York: G. P. Putnam, 1915), p. 202.

[27]Sanford V. Larkey, "John Shaw Billings and the History of Medicine," *Bull. Hist. Med.* 6 (1938): 362.

[28]William Osler, "A Note on the Teaching of Medical History," *Brit. Med. J.* 12 July 1902, p. 93.

[29]W. G. MacCallum "The Early Days of the Johns Hopkins Historical Club," *Bull. Hist. Med.* 10 (1941): 513–19; Victor A. McKusick, "The Minutes of the Johns Hopkins Medical History Club: 1890–1894," ibid. 26 (1953): 177–81.

[30]Eugene F. Cordell, "The Importance of the Study of the History of Medicine," *Med. Libr. and Hist. J.* 2 (1904): 268–82; Arnold C. Klebs, "The History of Medicine as a Subject of Teaching and Research," *Bull. Johns Hopkins Hosp.* 25 (1914): 1.

[31]Simon Flexner and James T. Flexner, *William Henry Welch and the Heroic Age of American Medicine* (New York: Viking Press, 1941), p. 419. For Welch's role in the realization of the central library and Institute of the History of Medicine, see Thomas B. Turner, *Heritage of Excellence: The Johns Hopkins Medical Institutions: 1914–1947* (Baltimore: The Johns Hopkins University Press, 1974), pp. 187–99.

THE ORIGINS OF MEDLARS

Frank B. Rogers

In the beginning, John Shaw Billings was acting as adviser to President Gilman and to the trustees of The Johns Hopkins Hospital. As early as the spring of 1876, Billings was writing to Gilman proffering suggestions and admonishing him "to condemn or object without the slightest hesitation; it will be to me as if you said that you do not think I shall ever be able to write a great epic, or that I shall ever be seven feet high."[1] At the time, Billings was developing the Surgeon General's Library in Washington, which even then he was calling the National Medical Library. In 1877 Billings was delivering a series of lectures on the history of medicine at Hopkins; in 1879 he drew up plans for The Johns Hopkins Hospital, and before and after he was instrumental in establishing the curriculum of the new School of Medicine.

In 1930, having just brought out the fourth edition of his *Introduction to the History of Medicine* in the previous year, Fielding Garrison became the first librarian of the Welch Medical Library. Garrison had received his undergraduate degree from the Hopkins forty years earlier, and all of the intervening time he had spent in bibliographic work at the Surgeon General's Library: his first years under Billings, his later years as editor of the *Index Medicus*. During most of 1930, Garrison was shuttling between Baltimore and Washington, at first spending his Sundays in Baltimore, trying to get moving in his new tasks, and later spending his Saturdays at the library in Washington, trying to tie up loose ends. He gave lectures and seminars in the history and bibliography of medicine at the new Hopkins Institute until his death in 1935.

I speak of Billings and Garrison because they are heroic figures from our recent medical past, and because they exemplify the long-standing bonds between the National Library of Medicine, the Welch Medical Library, and the Institute of the History of Medicine, and also because these ties account for my being here today.

From 1949 to 1963 I was director of the National Library of Medicine, in Washington and in Bethesda, and during the early years, as it happened, I found myself spending many hours, and indeed days, here at the Welch Medical Library. Thereon hangs a tale. That tale involves vast periodical indexes, punch cards, computers, the semantics of medical terminology, and the genesis of MEDLARS—the Medical Literature Analysis and Retrieval System—operated by the National Library of Medicine. It also involves Sanford Larkey, who was Garrison's successor here at the Welch Medical Library. But first, as in so many things, to set the scene we must go back to Billings's day.

The burgeoning periodical literature of science and medicine during the nineteenth century posed problems of unprecedented magnitude for those concerned with bibliographic control. Whereas in 1847, at the time of the founding of the American Medical Association, there were only 33 American medical periodicals being published, thirty years later Billings counted 262 American titles among 864 medical periodicals world-wide. And whereas in 1779 Albrecht von Haller was bringing out, single-handedly, his *Bibliotheca medicinae practicae* — in four volumes and 52,000 annotated entries — in 1879 Billings had to organize a team endeavor to produce the *Index Medicus,* a classified index to the current periodical literature of medicine. He capitalized on division of labor according to skills, and standardized procedures, varying the manner in which parts were assembled in order to achieve multiple aims. His *Index Medicus* was a bibliography of current materials for purposes of current awareness. When these same materials were placed in a different arrangement and embedded among other materials of different periods, they were metamorphased into the *Index Catalogue of the Library of the Surgeon General's Office.* The *Index Medicus* appeared monthly; the *Index Catalogue* came out in one volume per year, typically requiring about twenty years to complete each alphabetical cycle and get on to the next. In 1879 the *Index Medicus* listed 18,000 articles; within fifty years its annual coverage had trebled.

Billings was of course very much aware of the problems attendant upon sheer volume. In an address in 1881 he asked:

> What is to be the result of this steadily increasing production of books? What will the libraries and catalogues and bibliographies of a thousand or even a hundred years hence be like, if we are thus to go on in the ratio of geometric progression, which has governed the press for the last few decades? The mathematical formula which would express this, based on the data of the past century, gives an absurd and impossible conclusion, for it shows that if we go on as we have been going there is coming a time when our libraries will become large cities, and when it will require the services of every one in the world, not engaged in writing, to catalogue and care for the annual product.[2]

By 1929, Garrison was glumly stating that "there are too many medical periodicals in the modern world." By the late 1940s, the *Index Medicus* which by this time had become the *Quarterly Cumulative Index Medicus,* under the auspices of the American Medical Association, was experiencing printing slowdowns, rising costs, and the accumulation of massive backlogs. The library in Washington was struggling to bring out a weekly index called the *Current List of Medical Literature,* as well as the *Index Catalogue.* In 1948, the fifty-seventh volume of the *Index Catalogue,* by that time in the middle of its fourth series, was published. In those fifty-seven volumes, subject references to three million monographs and periodical articles had been

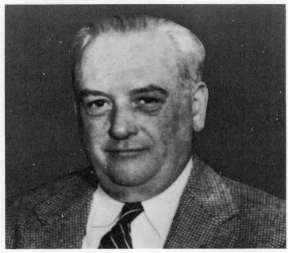

SANFORD V. LARKEY

presented; the shocking thing was that in the same period references to two million additional articles had had to be withheld in backlogs.

In that year of 1948, during the directorship of Colonel Joseph H. McNinch, a Committee of Consultants for the Study of the Indexes to Medical Literature Published by the Army Medical Library was established. This Committee on Indexes, as it came to be called, had as its first chairman Dr. Lewis H. Weed of Johns Hopkins and the National Research Council, and the membership represented some of the best minds in American medicine and bibliography. The major question before the committee was that of continuance of the *Index Catalogue*, and the eventual recommendation was to close it out. To serve as the research arm of the committee and to assist in its deliberations, the Medical Indexing Research Project was established at the Welch Medical Library under the direction of Sanford Larkey. The principal members of Dr. Larkey's project staff were Helen Field, Williamina Himwich, and Eugene Garfield.

Over a period of five years, the Welch Project sorted out issues, brooded over alternatives, made elaborate tabulations of data, and published reports of findings. It listed the titles of current medical periodicals throughout the world, tabulating them by language and by subject field, and calculating the annual yield of indexable articles. It reported on the coverage, and the overlap of coverage, of the biomedical literature among the several indexing and abstracting publications available. It studied the problems of subject headings — the indexing vocabulary — and devised a method of study (which Dr. Larkey called "categorization") to get at the issues more intimately and to be able to derive more readily the actual authority listings that came to be used in the daily work of the *Current List*. This area — the study of subject headings and the elaboration of the concept of categorization — to my mind represents the greatest achievement of the Larkey group, and their most important contribution to the development of medical bibliographic practice and the subsequent emergence of powerful new systems.[3]

In all of the project's work, the use of punch cards and their supporting apparatus of sorters, collators, and tabulators figured prominently. The project even produced a paper describing step-by-step a method of constructing a large medical index from a machine-manipulated punch card base. This was a stunning tour de force, but, as I see it, merely a tour de force. Still, it pointed up some useful notions; anyone who works with machines must quickly learn the importance of having accurate and detailed quantitative data on every aspect of the operation: from the average number of authors per article to the average number of typographic characters per entry. The project identified and tackled questions of this sort.

The Welch Project is but one example of that ferment of ideas in bibliography and bibliographic methods during the 1950s that suggested new approaches and provided promising new concepts. Calvin Mooers came up with his notion of the "descriptor" as a kind of subject heading with special characteristics, and it threw a whole new light on the problems of subject analysis. Mortimer Taube described coordinate indexing, and the use of Boolean expressions of symbolic logic to indicate subject relationships, as well as the distinction between direct and inverted files. H. P. Luhn published papers on sophisticated coding techniques, automatic abstracting, and the development of keyword-in-context indexes. Seymour Lubetzky at the Library of Congress provided a critique of the standard cataloging rules for entry, offering a proposed design for their revision.

In 1956, in the midst of all this activity, the library in Washington was designated the National Library of Medicine, and in the following year plans for a new indexing system began to be drawn up. Seymour Taine of the library staff was the new system's chief architect, and we had the major encouragement and support of Verner Clapp and the Council on Library Resources.

The new system was put into operation in 1960, coinciding with the return of the *Index Medicus* as a monthly publication of the library. In 1960, the system handled 125,000 citations, with multiple entries for each. It employed tape-actuated typewriters for the repetitive printing of the unit entry across the top of a Hollerith card, the keypunching of filing indicia into a reserved area of each card, the employment of sorters and collators to arrange the cards into appropriate author and subject subsets, and the use of a high-speed rotary step-camera. The camera, capable of varying its aperture to fit the number of lines in the entry, would photograph the cards on film strips that could be cut into column length. The decks of cards for the monthly issues were then resorted, refiled, and dumped into the camera once more, for production of the cumulated issues.[4]

The library had hoped to achieve two objectives under this arrangement: a publication system for the *Index Medicus*; and a bibliographic retrieval system for tailor-made responses to single questions. The bibliographic retrieval system was to derive from the publication system: the idea being that the subject codes punched into the cards as filing indicia for publication could also serve as search keys for individual bibliographic searches. As it turned out, while the publication system worked fairly well, and was certainly a great improvement over the predecessor system, the bibliographic retrieval system was not viable. The massive decks of cards could be disturbed before cumulation only at great peril, and sorting and collating times were prohibitive. Early on we came to the realization that if we were ever going to realize both objectives within a single scheme, it would be necessary to reverse the order of priorities with which we had approached the design of the automatic camera system. It would be necessary to start with the design of a retrieval system, and then to proceed with the publication system as the subsequent and derivative problem. That indeed proved to be the crux of the matter. If it appears to be a simple and self-evident idea now, it was far from that twenty years ago.

And so, early in 1959 (and thus even before the automatic camera system had become operational) we began planning a new system, one which Seymour Taine and I dubbed MEDLARS at the very beginning. We knew that a computer would be at the heart of the new system; and with Taine's insistence finally overcoming my initial reluctance, we began to count on developing a special high-speed printing device. About all we knew for certain was that the printer would have to have graphic arts quality — several fonts, upper and lower case — in contrast to the monotonous capitals of the regular computer printers.

We struggled to write down the aims of the proposed system, and after many false starts, we succeeded. We wrote out our requirements in terms of purposes, and not in terms of specific techniques. Indeed, we were only vaguely aware, and in the most general ways, of the techniques that could be used. But we also were certain that bibliography is defined by its purposes, and not by any particular technology.

We received the enthusiastic support of the National Library of Medicine's Board of Regents under its chairman, Dr. Michael DeBakey, and we received the financial backing of the National Heart Council. In February 1961 we sent out our statement of requirements for the new system to seventy-two commercial organizations, inviting them to submit proposals for the study, design, and installation of MEDLARS. We received a total of twenty-five such proposals. I well remember the day in late April 1961 when Taine and I separated the duplicate copies of the twenty-five proposals into two piles, one for him and one for me. I carried my pile home in two big cardboard cartons, and settled down for two weeks of reading.

It was discouraging. Proposal after proposal offered schemes that bore little discernible relationship to the specifications we had issued. Many of the proposals indulged in what I considered to be mere fanciful speculation. Finally, I reached the bottom of the pile, and that last proposal happened to be the one submitted by the General Electric Company. It almost immediately conveyed to me the sense of being on the mark, and when Taine and I carefully reviewed our assessments of the whole lot, we found ourselves in easy agreement on selection of the General Electric proposal.

Some competitor-inspired doubts at the departmental level above us threatened our choice, but after these doubts were disposed of a contract was awarded to General Electric in August 1961 covering the first phase of the project, preliminary design, which comprised study and amplification of system requirements, design of possible system and subsystem configurations, and recommendation of that system configuration which could best meet the library's objectives. In February 1962 the second phase began, involving detailed design, ordering of long term lead items, and planning for system implementation. The overlapping final phase, implementation, began in early 1963 and lasted until shortly after the first issue of the *Index Medicus* to utilize MEDLARS was produced on schedule in January 1964.[5]

The General Electric team responsible for the work included engineers, systems analysts, and computer programmers, and had the able leadership of Richard F. Garrard. Taine and his staff followed the work closely, and many were the discussions, often heated but always friendly, between the library and its contractor. Some idea of the magnitude of the project is gained by noting that it required thirty man-years of programming effort alone to mount the computer operation. Another measure is the total cost of the development; this approached $3 million, including hardware costs, but excluding costs of the in-house library effort.

The hoped-for special output device turned out to be a high-speed photomechanical composing machine, developed for the library by Photon, Inc., which acted as subcontractor. This machine, which we called GRACE for "Graphic Arts Composing Equipment," composed at the rate of 300 characters per second. GRACE accepted input directly from magnetic tape, which had been reworked by the computer into a page-block format. GRACE contained a matrix of 226 characters etched on a glass plate; these characters were in several fonts and sizes, with a complement of diacritical marks. Behind each character on the matrix there was a high-speed flash tube; the circuitry of GRACE timed the flashing of these lights. Between the matrix plate and a 9-inch wide roll of film there was a mirror and reciprocating lens, constantly roving back and forth, photographing one line of characters, character by character, across the entire width of the three-column page, at 1.7 seconds per sweep. In its day, that was thought to be very fast. Still, it may be calculated that to compose the five volumes and 8,900 pages of the 1968 *Cumulated Index Medicus*, for instance, with its 200,000 citations multiplied under author and subject, GRACE had to labor for 150 hours. No doubt the original GRACE was a significant step in computer-controlled typesetting, and this was recognized by her retirement in 1969 to the collection of the Smithsonian Institution.

MEDLARS also served as a comprehensive data base from which two dozen other publications, such as the *Index to Dental Literature* and the *International Nursing Index*, were derived. It provided cross sections of the literature for particular specialty areas, the cross sections being derivative from, and a subset of, the materials in the larger data base.

Besides that, MEDLARS functioned as a mechanized information retrieval system, with the computerized information files being queried directly. In 1965, some 1,800 computer searches, defined according to subject parameters specified by individual users, were performed; six years later this figure had topped 18,000. A whole new dimension of bibliographic service was made manifest.

Within six years of its inception the MEDLARS files contained over a million citations, which were written on forty-eight reels of tape. Since the computer required three minutes to read each reel, it took two and a half hours to read the tape file of a million citations. It is obvious that under such conditions it was not efficient to carry out individual searches, one at a time, through the entire file. Only the placing of a number of searches — say thirty — together in one search batch, and running the batch in a single pass against the file, made serial searching of such magnitude reasonable. The computer, in a final sort, could assign the proper answer to the proper question.

Over the last decade, the old tape-oriented MEDLARS system has been transformed into MEDLINE, an on-line system made possible by the advent of large direct-access storage devices now at the National Library of Medicine which provide a capacity of ten billion characters of bibliographic data, by a communications network of long lines leased under favorable rate structures, and by cheap, fast terminals providing dependable service. Dr. Cummings and his staff at the National Library of Medicine have directed the growth of the MEDLINE system to a flowering that is nothing short of spectacular. There are now more than 800 medical institutions operating terminals in the MEDLINE network, and they are handling annually over 500,000 requests on the *Index Medicus* data base, which is now adding 250,000 articles a year from 2,500 journals. Such figures testify to the real advances that have been made in medical bibliography, just as they speak, as well, to the awesome complexities of contemporary medicine and contemporary society.

Only fifteen years have gone by since the original MEDLARS system began operations, and already that system looks fairly primitive. It is only thirty years ago that the first commercial computer was being readied for shipment to the Bureau of the Census, at about the same time that Dr. Larkey's Welch Medical Library Indexing Project was getting into stride. It is just one hundred years since the beginning of *Index Medicus*; in that same year of 1879, young Herman Hollerith, nineteen years of age and just graduated from Columbia University, was arriving in Washington to begin work at the Census Bureau, where John Shaw Billings was providing consulting services. "And so it happened," Hollerith later wrote, "that one Sunday evening at Dr. Billings's tea table he said to me there ought to be a machine for doing the purely mechanical work of tabulating population and similar statistics. . . . After studying the problem I went back to Dr. Billings and said I thought I could work out a solution for the problem and asked him would he go in with me. The Dr. said no he was not interested any further than to see some solution of the problem worked out."[6]

Such were the modest beginnings of Hollerith's "punched cards" and attendant machines, first used to tabulate the mortality statistics of the city of Baltimore in 1887, then used to tabulate the data of the Eleventh Census in 1890, and eventually forming the nucleus of what is now the IBM corporation. Perhaps it is not too fanciful to think of MEDLARS as being the result of two of Billings's ideas, starting out circling in opposite directions, and finally meeting again eighty years later, to the saving of one and the glory of the other, and to the benefit of all who serve and are served by medicine.

NOTES

[1]Sanford V. Larkey, "John Shaw Billings and the History of Medicine," *Bull. Hist. Med*. 6 (1938): 360–76.

[2]John S. Billings, "Our Medical Literature," *Boston Med. & Surg. J*. 105 (1881): 217–22. Address at the Seventh International Medical Congress, London.

[3]Johns Hopkins University. Welch Medical Library Indexing Project, *Final Report on Subject Headings and Subject Indexing*. 1955. (Mimeographed.)

[4]"The National Library of Medicine Index Mechanization Project," *Bull. Med. Libr. Assoc*. 49, no. 1, pt. 2 (1961): 1–96.

[5]National Library of Medicine, *The MEDLARS Story* (Bethesda, Md: National Library of Medicine, 1963); Charles J. Austin, *MEDLARS: 1963–1967* (Washington, D.C.: GPO, 1968); Scott Adams, "The Way of the Innovator: Notes Toward A Prehistory of MEDLARS," *Bull. Med. Libr. Assoc*. 60 (1972): 523–33; Frank B. Rogers, "Computerized Information Retrieval Services," *Library Trends*, 23 (1974): 73–88. Scott Adams and Davis B. McCarn, "From Fasciculus to On-Line Terminal: One Hundred Years of Medical Indexing," *Communication in the Service of American Health . . . a Bicentennial Report from the National Library of Medicine* (1976) pp. 14–25; Mary E. Corning and Martin M. Cummings, "Biomedical Communications," *Advances in American Medicine: Essays at the Bicentennial* 2 (1976): 722–73; *Medical Informatics*, vol. 3, no. 3. (September, 1978): Entire issue devoted to articles on MEDLINE.

[6]J. Fraser Muirhead, "Doctors Afield: John Shaw Billings," *New England J. Med*. 268 (1963): 778–79; Albert G. Love, "Development and Description of Electrical Accounting Machines," in *Tabulating Equipment and Army Medical Statistics* (Washington, D.C.; Dept. of the Army, Office of the Surgeon General, 1958), pp. 36–51; Leon E. Truesdell, "The Two Men Who Originated the Punch Card System," in *The Development of Punch Card Tabulation at the Bureau of the Census: 1890–1940* (Washington, D.C.: GPO, 1965), pp. 26–34; Frank B. Rogers, "The Index Medicus in the Twentieth Century," in *Centenary of the Index Medicus: 1879–1979* (Bethesda, Md.: National Library of Medicine, 1980), pp. 53–61.

PRIVATE PHYSICIANS AND PUBLIC COLLECTIONS: MEDICAL LIBRARIES IN THE UNITED STATES BEFORE 1900

Whitfield J. Bell, Jr.

Although we are well into the observance of the semicentennial of the Welch Medical Library and the Institute of the History of Medicine, we might profitably recall the time in which the library was dedicated and the Institute inaugurated.[1] The news that October 1929 has a familiar sound to us fifty years later. Disarmament talks were being planned, a revolutionary plot in Cuba had been uncovered, and in Jerusalem shops were closed in anticipation of demonstrations by Arabs. A professor at Johns Hopkins announced he had a solution to the traffic problem, a professional educator expressed his opinion that students must be taught how to live effectively in an urbanized society, and (contriving to get at least one truth and one error in a single statement) a former president of the American College of Surgeons declared that the use of alcohol prolongs life and adds to its joys. One headline informed those gathered in Baltimore on 17 October 1929 that "Favoritism [was] hinted in Power Deal"; another that "Bureaucracy [was] held [a] Danger to Form of U.S. Government"; and a third reported there was hope of a substantial reduction of taxes in Baltimore. Not every report could be repeated half a century later: as Madame Curie, on a visit to New York to receive an ounce of radium, came down the gangplank of her ship, men removed their hats in respectful tribute.

As was natural and proper, there was an air of confidence and satisfaction at the ceremonies in 1929. Several hundred distinguished guests, including the governor of Maryland and the eminent Professor Sudhoff, "crowded" the Great Hall and "overflowed" other parts of the Welch Library. The extent and tone of news coverage evinced the city's pride in its most famous institution; in editorials on three successive days the Baltimore *Sun* commented on the event and its significance. The energy and robustness of Dr. Welch, it declared in a warmly appreciative comment, if applied to other fields, "might have built skyscrapers or merged five hundred power companies."[2]

The opening of the Welch Medical Library, created by consolidating the three separate libraries of the hospital and medical school, was the culmination of one of several movements in the dramatic march of medicine that had begun here within living memory. It may help to explain the mood half a century ago to recall the span in which those present measured time. Many who attended on that occasion could remember when the site of the hospital was a hill and nothing more; they could recall when the first medical class was graduated only thirty-odd years before; and when Osler, dead only ten years, had left Baltimore for Oxford in 1905—no more distant in time from them in 1929 than 1955 is from us. And there on the platform was Dr. Welch, who had played so many founding roles in the institution, alert and vigorous at seventy-nine, about to perform yet another service to medicine and the university. We are fond of saying that we have witnessed rapid changes in the past generation (not a few began the week after the dedication of the Welch Medical Library when the papers reported "Stocks' Wildest Plunge in Worst Selling Scare in 15 Years"); but those changes can hardly have been greater or more beneficent than those that the men of 1929 had seen in the science and practice of medicine in the preceding forty years.

As the metropolis of early America, Philadelphia possessed the first hospital, the first medical school, and the first professional academy in the country. Each of these institutions had, or thought it should have, a library; and the stories of their respective collections, often told and well known, afford an instructive introduction to the history of medical libraries and their founders in the nineteenth century. To the managers of the Pennsylvania Hospital in 1762, Dr. John Fothergill of London presented a copy of William Lewis's *History of the Materia Medica*.[3] Encouraged by that act of generosity and foresight, the hospital physicians recommended the next year that the managers allocate to a medical library fees paid by students attending hospital practice. In 1767 the executors of Dr. Lloyd Zachary presented 43 medical books, and in the same year Deborah Morris gave 55 volumes from the library of her late brother Benjamin Morris, who was a medical graduate of Leyden. A list of the library's holdings was made soon afterwards for Benjamin Franklin in order to guide his solicitations among English friends. One of these was the printer William Strahan, who in 1774 presented books worth £100. Thus were laid the foundations of what became, and for many years remained, the largest medical library in the country.

From the beginning a sufficient room was provided for the books, and when that was filled they were moved to larger quarters. The books were catalogued, regulations for lending were adopted, and close attention was paid thereafter to recovering overdue and lost volumes. From its inception the library appears to have been generally regarded as a valuable adjunct to the lectures, and, because of its proximity to the patients, to clinical observation and practice as well. Surviving records show that students as well as staff borrowed regularly. The combination of lectures, hospital observation, and library constituted the singular attraction that drew medical students to Philadelphia from all parts of the continent, and even from the West Indies and Europe, before the American Civil War.

Dr. John Morgan, sometimes called "the father of medical education in America" because it was he who proposed the first American medical school, appreciated the importance of a medical library both in the instruction of students and as a source of prestige. In his inaugural address on the institution of medical schools in America he suggested that a library might be supported by a small annual fee levied on the students and by gifts of books and money from the practicing physicians of the city. Morgan's appeal to the trustees of the College of Philadelphia and to fellow members of the profession seems to have gone unheeded; yet he did not relinquish his objective. Sent to the West Indies in 1772 to raise money for the college, he so far ignored his instructions as to receive, if not to solicit, gifts for a medical library. The trustees were dismayed when they heard, but did not disavow their agent or return the subscriptions. As it fell out, however, neither the college nor its medical library benefited as expected, for a disastrous hurricane swept the islands soon afterwards and most of the pledges were never paid.[4] The College of Philadelphia (and its successor, the University of Pennsylvania) remained without a respectable medical library for more than a century thereafter.

Like the hospital library, the library of the College of Physicians of Philadelphia began with a gift. No mention of a library or librarian appears in the college's charter and by-laws of 1787. The next year, however, a committee was appointed to draft the plan of a library, and the fellows were asked to contribute to it.[5] Accordingly, Drs. John Jones, Thomas Parke, and Caspar Wistar were asked to prepare a list of books for purchase, not exceeding £50 in value; and Dr. Morgan donated 24 volumes "to be added to the College library." Other gifts followed; a few books were imported; and in 1792 two fellows volunteered to serve as librarians. By 1794 there were enough pamphlets to require binding, and in 1819 a catalogue was compiled. The collection grew slowly — in 1835 there were fewer than 300 volumes, and they had been neglected and had fallen into disrepair. Measures of preservation were ordered; probably they had little effect, for in 1843 it was reported that the library was "rarely, if ever used."

The histories of the libraries of hospitals, medical schools, and medical societies elsewhere are not unlike those of the Philadelphia institutions. The New York Hospital adopted in 1797 a long series of rules for its library, which was open four days a week for an hour a day, was accessible to students, and made special regulations for use of the London and Edinburgh periodicals. The first by-laws of the Massachusetts Medical Society in 1782 mentioned a library; four years later rules were adopted for the loan of books and a purchase order was placed with a bookseller. Dr. James Lloyd gave the society a few books, and other gifts were made by Drs. Cotton Tufts, Aaron Dexter, Edward Holyoke, and others; but in 1788 there were still only 26 titles. The books were kept in the houses of successive secretaries until 1819, when they were placed in the Massachusetts Medical College. No money was available for purchases, and in 1822 the library still numbered only 300 volumes — and many of them could not be found.[6] At the Philadelphia Almshouse the directors recognized the need for a library in 1805, and they began one three years later: some books were purchased, rules were written, and the senior resident student was put in charge.[7]

In 1849 a committee of the newly formed American Medical Association, under the chairmanship of Dr. John P. Harrison of the Medical College of Ohio in Cincinnati, reported on the state of American medical literature and libraries.[8] Ten institutions were listed, the largest, that of the Pennsylvania Hospital with 10,000 volumes, being characterized as a "vast depository of medical literature." The others in the committee's list were Transylvania University (7,000 volumes), New York Hospital (5,345 volumes), University of Louisville (3,000 volumes), the library "connected with the Boston Athenaeum" (3,000 volumes), Medical School of Maine (2,400 volumes), Medical College of Ohio (2,000 volumes), medical library of Harvard College (1,769 volumes), Medical and Chirurgical Faculty of Maryland (1,200 volumes), and Massachusetts Medical College (1,200 volumes).

Whatever these statistics might mean, conditions within the libraries gave scant reason for satisfaction. Few books in any collection were new or current; most were long out-of-date and of little value. The Massachusetts Medical Society claimed 744 volumes in 1850, but 280 were missing; and as late as 1864 its librarian reported that "the library was in its usual condition, and that one member of the Society had, during the year, intimated an intention of taking out books, but had not done so."[9] The library of the College of Physicians of Philadelphia had been reported in 1835 to be "in bad condition and going to decay" — for more than a year not a single volume had been called for — and when it was learned in 1840 that the magnificent library of 15,000 volumes formed by Dr. John Redman Coxe could be had, the college made only half-hearted inquiries to that end. Nothing came of a proposal to form a Medical Hall Association in Philadelphia in 1840 to provide "a commodious, safe, and permanent depository" for the medical books of the city.[10] In Baltimore's Medical and Chirurgical Faculty at midcentury, years of growth and neglect had alternated crazily, and in 1857 the executive committee was authorized to close the library.[11] The library of the Philadelphia Almshouse was housed in the 1830s and 1840s in the lunatics' wing, where little attention was paid it by anyone. "On the contrary," wrote Dr. D. Hayes Agnew in 1852, "it has been plundered by the vandalism, to which it has been exposed, of much valuable matter." Although they were hardly interested in their libraries or able to care for them, the institutions were nonetheless unwilling to release them to others who needed and wanted them: a request from the Navy Department to purchase some volumes for the United States Exploring Expedition was indignantly rejected by the managers of the almshouse.[12]

In the light of these facts the American Medical Association's committee suggested—rather bravely, one thinks—that the profession "in every principal city" should establish a "public medical library," accessible to all qualified persons. In towns where there was a medical school this could be the more readily accomplished if the faculty opened its library to their professional brethren. In every such public collection, the committee recommended in conclusion, periodicals should form a principal part of the collection.

The reference to periodical literature was a recognition of the rapidly changing nature of medical communication at mid century. Knowledge was now increasingly reported and disseminated through short reports in quarterly, monthly, ultimately even weekly, publications. Transactions and proceedings of state societies and academies were now joined, in some instances superseded, by the periodicals of new specialist associations and even by journals established by commercial publishers for profit. No longer content with multi-volume "systems" and other "standard" works, progressive teachers and practitioners wanted the latest reports from hospitals and researchers, book notices, references to articles in other journals, news of the profession and of persons. Valedictory addresses to graduating medical students now often contained, in addition to admonitions against entering politics, reading "the light dissipating literature of the day," and countenancing homeopaths, earnest advice to subscribe to a few good journals. (It would be an additional blessing of marriage if the doctor's wife were intelligent enough to go through them first, marking those articles and reports a busy practitioner might read with profit.)[13]

With the increasing demand for current journals some of the old medical libraries experienced a revival. The College of Physicians of Philadelphia, for example, hired a librarian, ordered that its collection be open daily from 11 a.m. to 2 p.m., and catalogued the many periodicals it received in exchange for its *Transactions and Studies*, revived in 1846 after a long period of dormancy. Such evidences of increased activity had the expected effect: by gift and bequest fellows and their widows added to the collection.[14] In Baltimore, after more than a decade of sporadic activity the Medical and Chirurgical Faculty published a library catalogue in 1852, opened the library twelve hours daily, and laid thirteen current journals on the table. But a few years later the library's appropriation was cut, all the subscriptions were cancelled, and the society entered upon a long period of "feebleness," as John Shaw Billings told them.[15] On the other hand, more modest efforts to assemble a working collection of periodicals sometimes proved more successful. The Medical Association of the New York Dispensary, formed in 1834, had that objective: four "indigenous journals of the country"[16] were subscribed, and as each issue came in a member was assigned to report on its contents. The physicians of the German Dispensary in New York City did the same thing, taking in a number of German journals. And in 1864 the New York Medical Journal Association was formed.[17]

Meanwhile some private physicians, no less influenced by the new currents than the medical societies, responded to them. To assemble files of periodicals was the original aim of several large collectors, and several such collections became the foundations of modern medical libraries.[18]

Samuel Lewis was one of these private collectors. A native of Barbados, a medical graduate of Edinburgh in 1840, he practiced medicine in Philadelphia for half a century until his death in 1890.[19] He began to collect books while still a student and continued to do so after settling in book-rich Philadelphia. Rather early he seems to have decided that his collection should go to the College of Physicians, and thereafter he made his purchases with reference to the college's holdings. In 1864 Lewis presented 2,500 volumes to the college and another 2,000 the next year. During the next quarter century he constantly added to the collection, until his gifts numbered 10,000 volumes. "He longed to fill in the gaps of journals," Dr. S. Weir Mitchell remembered of him, "and disliked to see a man who needed a book unable to find it here." A colleague once mentioned in a letter to Lewis, who was then abroad, that he had been unable to find a certain volume in any Philadelphia library; in his next shipment of books from Europe Lewis included three different editions of the work. Inevitably Lewis acquired old books — his last gift to the college was a valuable edition of the works of Robert Fludd — but his interest in them was always that of a practicing physician and working scholar, not a mere collector, as his friend Dr. John Ashurst was at some pains to explain:

> Dr. Lewis valued books for their historical associations and for their real utility a great deal more than for mere beauty and rarity. He could appreciate a beautiful book, but did not value it on that account alone. . . . He was a lover of books, a bibliophile in the truest sense of the word, but in no sense was he a bibliomaniac. He did not care for a book because it had an additional third of a line in height, nor did he value it more because it had rough uncut edges, than if its edges were neatly trimmed and gilded. The greatest happiness of Dr. Lewis's life was in increasing the collection of books that he had placed in this College.

The stimulus that Lewis's gifts gave the college, the manifest increasing usefulness of the library to Philadelphia's practitioners and teachers, soon brought in other gifts. Journals from all over the country and from Europe received by local medical publishers and editors were regularly deposited in the college. In 1866 Dr. George B. Wood began to give $500 annually to pay a librarian so that the library might be kept open five or six hours a day, and in 1879 he bequeathed his library to the college. Other substantial gifts of books came from Drs. Alfred Stillé and Samuel D. Gross and from Mrs. J. F. Weightman. In 1880 S. Weir Mitchell created a journal fund with the first of two gifts of $1,000 each. The library was now seen as the principal activity of the college, and it was growing so rapidly that the college had to move, and move again, to larger quarters. "I do not know of any enterprise as popular in the Profession," one Philadelphia physician wrote a friend, "as the increase of the Library of this institution."

Samuel Smith Purple, like Lewis a physician and a collector, had a profound influence on New York and its Academy of Medicine.[20] Born in an upstate New York village, he attended a rural school and took over his father's tannery and shoe-making shop at the age of seventeen; but, encouraged by relatives to study medicine, he attended Geneva Medical College and opened a practice in New York City. He wrote several scientific papers and for ten years edited the *New York Journal of Medicine*. He took the opportunity his editorship afforded to collect and preserve files of journals received for review and in exchange. Encouraged by Dr. John B. Beck, a scholarly physician who had written on early American medical history and had a large library, Purple began to haunt the booksellers' shops and auctions. He corresponded with dealers, visited older doctors, and advertised his wants in the press. He liked to tell how in this way he turned up in a pile of old paper destined for pulping a copy of Samuel Bard's *Inquiry into the Nature, Cause, and Cure, of the Angina Suffocativa, or, Sore Throat Distemper* (New York, 1771).[21] His aim, he told Dr. Samuel D. Gross in 1875, had been to make "a depository of the writings of American physicians," that is, of the medical writings of the early American fathers, theses of American students here and abroad, "a complete file of the *regular* Medical Journals of America," the transactions of professional societies, and English, Scots, and Irish periodicals.[22]

To this end, for his own use, Purple compiled a number of lists and bibliographies. Among his manuscripts there are a "Bibliography of American Doctors and their Writings"; a "Bibliotheca Medica: A Bibliographical Account of the Medical Periodical Literature of the United States of America" (1860), with, in addition to bibliographical data, historical notes on the publications and biographical notes on the authors and editors; and a "Cronological [sic] List of Medical Periodicals in the Library..."(1858). This last contained 91 titles ranging from the *Medical Repository* of New York (1797–1824) and the *Philadelphia Medical and Physical Journal* (1804–1809) to journals published in Cincinnati; Lexington and Louisville, Kentucky; New Orleans; Buffalo, Utica, and Plattsburgh, New York; St. Louis; Chicago; Keokuk, Iowa; Richmond, Virginia; Nashville, Tennessee; Detroit; West Chester, Pennsylvania; and Burlington, New Jersey.[23]

Purple was also deeply interested in local history. He was a founder of the New York Genealogical and Biographical Society, whose president was another physician, Henry R. Stiles; edited the society's *Record* for a number of years; transcribed hundreds of pages of local records; and assembled a rich collection of historical and genealogical titles — 2,807 lots which it took eight sessions to disperse at public auction in Boston in 1909.[24]

Purple would assert afterwards that one of the original objectives of the New York Academy of Medicine at its founding in 1847 was to establish a medical library.[25] Whether or not this was the case, nothing was done until

1866, when a committee was named to report ways and means to secure funds for a permanent building. By way of stimulation Dr. Purple promised the academy his library, which he said he had been assembling "with some diligence." The campaign was not pressed, however, until 1875, when Purple, on assuming the presidency of the academy, revived the dormant effort. "It needs no argument here," he told the members, "to show the necessity or value of a great reference Medical Library, located in this city. . . ." Within months a house was purchased, the academy moved in, and Purple's books were installed.[26]

Joseph M. Toner, a practicing physician of Washington, was another indefatigable collector of medical books, especially journals, American imprints, and the classics of medicine and the profession.[27] Like Purple he scoured the bookstores and junkshops, bought old periodicals by the pound, and was often rewarded with some rare or unusual pamphlet among the bales of paper. By 1870 Toner's library was growing at the rate of 800–1,000 volumes a year, and he had a catalogue made. Soon Toner came to regard his private library as a national resource and its use as a public service. Upon the outbreak of cholera in 1865 he printed at his own expense a list of 68 titles from his personal library on the disease; offering the books to physicians for their use. Doctors stopped at his house for books they needed in their practice or study, and if he was not at home they scrawled a receipt on a prescription pad. Persons preparing scientific or historical papers asked him for information and references. "I know of no one else in the country to whom I could apply with any chance of being directed where I can obtain this information," William Pepper wrote him gratefully from Philadelphia in 1877. Even John Shaw Billings turned to Toner for materials and data not to be found in the Surgeon General's Library; and the *Index-Catalogue* was originally planned to begin in 1876 because Toner expected to publish his index of periodicals of earlier data.

Though he was a strong supporter of a national medical library, Toner offered his collection to any city that would erect a fireproof building to house it. Pittsburgh and Baltimore declined; Chicago failed to raise money for a site and building; Philadelphia seems to have been close to receiving the library when Ainsworth R. Spofford, librarian of Congress, recommended his institution — and to the Library of Congress it went: 25,000 volumes, as many pamphlets, and an estimated one million clippings.

In Boston the development of a modern medical library took a different course. As late as 1870 neither the Harvard medical library nor the library of the Massachusetts Medical Society was thought to be of much value to physicians. Noting that the Chicago Medical Society was attempting to form a public medical library, the *Boston Medical and Surgical Journal* in 1871 asked challengingly, "When will our local societies in New England do the same thing?" The gift by the Medical Society to the Boston Public Library of its collection of 1,687 volumes and 9,201 pamphlets in 1873 produced a strong reaction. Dr. Henry I. Bowditch and some others the next year formed the Boston Medical Library Association, elected Dr. Oliver W. Holmes as president, and obtained the services of an energetic young physician, James T. Chadwick, as director.[28] The success of the Library Association was instantaneous and phenomenal. Some 1,000 volumes of periodicals belonging to the Society of Medical Observation and another 500 from the Society of Medical Improvement were deposited with the new institution at once. The *Boston Medical and Surgical Journal* gave Chadwick its exchange files. The Boston Dispensary and Roxbury Athenaeum sent along their books, as eventually did the Boston Athenaeum, in which the old Boston Medical Library had placed its collection in 1826. The medical books of Harvard College were added, and also such titles as were not regularly required at the Harvard Medical School. Books flowed in from private persons as well—the libraries of E. H. Clarke, George C. Shattuck, Edward Jarvis, Calvin Ellis, Edward Wigglesworth. By the time the library opened in permanent quarters in December 1878 it numbered nearly 10,000 volumes, 5,000 pamphlets, and 125 journal subscriptions.[29]

Asked the secret of his success, Chadwick explained modestly, "The ways were numerous, but all natural. We started with about 1500 volumes loaned us by the two Societies [of Medical Observation and for Medical Improvement]...; with a list of these I personally visited every physician in town who was known to have a considerable library, and from these I solicited, and usually obtained, such as I wanted." It was the library's policy "to devote all our energy, and such small sums of money as could be spared from current expenses, to the department of periodicals as being the class of literature most in demand," especially since the inauguration of the *Index-Catalogue* and *Index Medicus*.[30] So strongly did some physicians feel on this point that when the library acquired some old texts, they protested what they saw as a diversion of resources and attention from the all-important periodicals. By 1900 the Boston Medical Library subscribed to 500 journals, and owned 20,000 volumes of periodicals and 15,000 bound books.

"It would seem," declared the *Medical Register* of Philadelphia editorially in 1882, "as if an era of medical libraries were now upon us."[31] It was indeed. Fully appreciating the value of a collection of current literature to physicians, and spurred by the examples of Philadelphia, New York, and Boston, physicians in smaller cities resolved to create similar libraries. Dr. Billings in the 1870s and 1880s tirelessly repeated the argument for libraries of journals— everything of value in medicine, he believed, could be found in publications of the previous 30 years;[32] and Dr. Chadwick frequently gave medical societies practical suggestions on how to begin.[33] The doctors of Pittsburgh, Grand Rapids, Michigan, and Wilkes-Barre, Pennsylvania, to take a few examples, made collections of journals, which became the bases of general medical libraries.[34] In Denver a collection assembled in this way was deposited in the public library, which supported it generously; and it was also in Denver that a local physician, Charles D. Spivak, made a union catalogue of the private libraries of doctors, which contained 6,000 volumes not otherwise accessible in the city. "Even in small cities," Spivak remarked on his experience, "there are enough books scattered among the practitioners to constitute a good reference library, if they were only supplemented with a good index."[35] In a list of the outstanding achievements of the century the president of the Rhode Island Medical Society named the discovery of anesthesia, the development of bacteriology, the revolution in hospital equipment and treatment, the advent of trained nurses, the growth of public health measures—and medical libraries.[36]

What encouraged the growth of medical libraries, indeed what made the establishment of new libraries to serve the current needs of the profession a reasonable enterprise, was that just at this time keys to collections of periodicals were provided by the *Index-Catalogue*, whose first volume appeared in 1879, and *Index Medicus*, which began publication soon afterward. These publications made libraries out of what might otherwise have been only flooding accumulations of journals. At the same time the existence of the *Index-Catalogue* and *Index Medicus* created a demand for public medical libraries. They assured an anxious practitioner or medical researcher that the answer to his question might be found in one journal or another. It was only good luck if the required article was in his own or a colleague's office; but, with a library within reach, there was no small probability it would be found. Hence the activity of the doctors of Pittsburgh, Grand Rapids, and Wilkes-Barre.

For the most part hospital and medical school libraries did not grow in the last quarter of the century as the societies' libraries did. Of the Pennsylvania Hospital Richard J. Dunglison wrote in 1867 that it had "never yet accomplished its full measure of usefulness; it is comparatively buried, its privileges actually enjoyed by but few, and its merits neither popularly known nor deservedly appreciated. . . [and] the rules prescribe that it shall be open only three times a week for an hour at a time."[37] In New York, Bellevue Hospital, with 200 beds, a permanent staff, and a school of nursing, had no library; and Mount Sinai was in operation twenty-eight years before one of its staff, collecting $500, made the first purchases toward a library.[38] Indeed, so small a part did libraries play in hospitals that, as Mrs. Koudelka has reported, Billings in his first plans for The Johns Hopkins Hospital made no provision for one.[39]

It was the same with medical schools. The president of the American Medical College Association, a professor in the Rush Medical College of Chicago, addressing medical educators in 1895 on "The Necessities of a Modern Medical College," spoke urgently of amphitheaters, laboratories, endowments, even gymnasiums, but made no mention of libraries.[40] Of fifty-nine "public medical libraries" reporting more than 10,000 volumes in 1891, none was in a medical school. Harvard, for example, with 399 medical students, reported only 1,500 volumes; yet the Law School, with 366 students, had 28,157 volumes, and the Divinity School provided its 86 students with a library of 23,360 volumes.[41] Utterly inadequate institutions, on which Abraham Flexner reported in 1910, owned but a handful of books, which were sometimes kept behind a counter in the business office or in a locked room to which the janitor kept the key. "The school grind," Flexner observed, "is merrily independent of medical literature."[42]

Medical professors did not always—or at least not often—regard such scanty library holdings as limitations. Where traditional methods of instruction by lectures and textbooks prevailed, students were neither encouraged nor required to read much. Even in better schools, emphasis on the laboratory and clinic thrust the library into second rank, making it seem hardly necessary. Thus The Johns Hopkins Medical School, Billings believed, would not need a large medical library because the Surgeon General's Library was only an hour away (which indeed it may have been when several score trains connected Baltimore and Washington daily, and a letter or package mailed in one city in the morning might be delivered in the other that afternoon).

Wide experience had convinced Billings that

> almost all attempts to establish medical libraries in connection with medical schools have been failures. Commenced with enthusiasm, they soon become antiquated, are rarely consulted, except by one or two species of beetles, are never properly catalogued or cared for, and dust and mould reign in them supreme. Students and teachers want the newest books and journals only. Libraries are used by the scholar and author [but not by the student and practitioner?], and for such are the true universities.[43]

The distinction Billings makes here explains the apparent inconsistency between his support and encouragement of collections of journal literature and his indifference to "libraries." It is a distinction others also made. "The medical classics, while retaining a certain historical importance or some living charm of literary form," declared Dr. George D. Hersey in 1900,

> are no longer safe guides to diagnosis or practice. The teachings of even twenty years ago are now backnumbery. The important topic of appendicitis, for example, can be studied for only a few years back. Treatises though high-priced and voluminous are shortlived, no matter how well edited, because they stop at a certain point in an advancing and rapidly developing science. The periodical is the only element of medical literature actually abreast of the times and alone supplies that up-to-date information that the up-to-date physician requires.[44]

Thus a collection of current journals, the core of any medical society library, was not simply a desideratum but a necessity for a modern medical school or hospital, required by student and teacher alike. A "library," on the other hand, if defined as a collection of books, mostly old and out-of-date—"backnumbery" in Hersey's phrase — and all of them growing older and more out-of-date every day, was, if not quite a luxury, hardly a necessity; something only "the author and scholar" consulted, possibly when writing the treatises that were already out-of-date the moment they fell from the press.

Needless to say, even among those who strongly and consistently urged the importance of current literature, the distinction was not sharp, nor was it long or generally insisted upon. Billings, for example, lectured on the history of medicine and said he would like to see on every doctor's shelves "a little group of books" such as the histories of Sprengel, Daremberg or Haeser, the letters of Guy Patin, Pettigrew's *Medical Portrait Gallery*, the writings of John Brown (author of *Rab and his Friends*) of Edinburgh, or a collection of works of local medical history.[45] And Dr. Hersey recommended that medical students should be required in their course "to look up thoroughly the history of some theory or medical event. This sifting and comparison of the labors of his predecessors, reaching his conclusions after painstaking study, is a most useful exercise and supplements class room and bedside work in a scholarly method too little appreciated."[46]

Among those who employed the historical approach in teaching, none was more effective, or more eloquent in his exposition, than William Osler.[47] Osler believed students should become acquainted with the library and be taught how to get at medical literature through bibliographical indexes and guides. Not every medical teacher, however, shared Osler's confidence that students would benefit from such instruction. Dr. Abraham Jacobi, who was by no means unfriendly to libraries, dissented strongly in remarks that show why, even early in the twentieth century, libraries were often little regarded in medical schools. Conceding that Hopkins students might be exceptional, Jacobi, on the basis of his own experience, warned that

> the drawing of the students' attention to medical literature [was] a very danger-ous practice in most cases. He thought that the students who read were the ones who neglected the clinics and left the college ill-equipped for the practical side of the professional life ahead of them. Moreover, he thought that when the stu-dent read the mass of unimportant literature and became cognizant with all the chaff that was published, the student himself was tempted to rush into print with something that was puerile and utterly valueless.[48]

At the opening of the century medical libraries had come to be recognized generally as one of the indispensable engines for the advancement and dissemination of knowledge. Despite reservations of clinical professors who prided themselves as "practical" men, libraries were seen to be as important as laboratories, to which they were in fact essential, "since no satisfactory investigation can be made that ignores the work of others or fails to profit by observations already recorded."[49] Dr. Jacobi, who did not encourage his students to use the library, nonetheless laid it down as axiomatic that "practice and learning do not exclude each other; on the contrary the former depends on the latter," and he argued that an erudite profession, which he regarded as desirable, required good libraries.[50] Nor did only medical science benefit. In professional societies, the library, as the principal activity, became a source of institutional strength, promoting good will. In the Medical and Chirurgical Faculty of Maryland, for example, as one member noticed, zeal and activity of the fellows rose and fell directly with their support or neglect of the library.[51] Even a normally uncommunicative colleague, Dr. Spivak discovered as he made his way among the doctors of Denver cataloguing their libraries, became "talkative and genial when the subject concerns his favorite books."[52] And Dr. Alfred L. Loomis, at ceremonies opening the building of the New York Academy of Medicine in 1890, expressed the belief that "there is an atmosphere about a large and well-selected library, which does not favor the growth of a mean, money-calculating spirit; it conduces to broadness, tolerance, and a love of the higher and nobler attributes of man."[53]

Another beneficent influence of medical libraries was mentioned in this place half a century ago. Regretting the fragmentation of medicine into a score of specialties. Harvey Cushing expressed the tempered conviction—perhaps it was but a hope—that the library would serve as a unifying force in the university and the profession. A library, he said in 1929, should be an active agency that "will serve as a common meeting ground, where the different streams of knowledge will coalesce," and in this service of reconciliation he gave primacy to the department of the history of medicine.[54]

Individual practitioners had contributed to the history of medicine by their writings—Thacher, Beck, Gross—and their collections—Toner, Purple, W. Kent Gilbert. Osler, Welch, and The Johns Hopkins Hospital Historical Club had encouraged physicians and students alike and set an example for other institutions. For several years before Cushing spoke, both a national medical historical association and a historical journal with national circulation had existed; now, in 1929, a chair of medical history was endowed. Those who appeared here half a century ago did not doubt the value of medical history, either to the medical profession or to the community at large. Although each viewed the Institute and its likely future from his own standpoint, they were united in this.

Abraham Flexner, after offering some reflections on American higher education—"our universities have...increased their genuine facilities and opportunities; they have simultaneously and needlessly cheapened and mechanized themselves"—declared firmly that since "an institute, devoted to the history of medicine, touches not only the medical faculty but equally the faculties of science, philosophy and history," it should be located not in the medical school but in the university.[55] However important the history of medicine is to physicians and medical scientists, it is no less so to other disciplines and the general public; and there seems to be no more reason to confine its study to the medical curriculum than to restrict the study of the history of art to painters and sculptors or the history of politics and economics to bureaucrats and politicians, labor leaders and businessmen. As public health and private medicine have become increasingly the concerns of individuals and the state, the history and sociology of medicine have increasingly engaged the attention of general historians; and so, while not losing their attachment to the medical school, they have found a place in graduate and undergraduate schools of arts and sciences.

Like Flexner, Welch believed that the history of medicine might best furnish the cultural background medical students and physicians should have. Such knowledge, he was confident, not only added interest to the work of physicians but also increased their influence and ability in practice.[56] And, perhaps too sensitive about his own lack of formal training in history, Welch entered a plea for those persons, amateurs in history but specialists in another field, who might profitably cultivate the history of medicine.

> While the professional historian...sometimes looks merely with tolerance, if not contempt, upon the productions of amateurs in the field of medical history, I would urge that historical studies by those who are specialists in other than historical lines and are fully abreast of the existing state of knowledge in their subject may have a significance surpassing that of contributions by the professional historian. Observations and facts, the meaning of which may not be apparent to the professional historian, may be found by the amateur in history, but a master in some other field, full of unsuspected significance. Every encouragement should be given to the pursuit of historical investigations by those whose principal interests may lie in other directions.[57]

One thinks at once of Dr. Ernest Caulfield's bringing the special knowledge of a pediatrician to the records of mortality preserved in New England graveyards.

What Welch told his audience in 1929 about amateurs in medical history is no less applicable to general history. Persons without formal historical training nonetheless do a great deal of research and writing, especially on local communities and institutions, with whose records they are usually intimately acquainted. Such amateurs, however, are no longer to be found in the American Historical Association, nor do they find other associations of professionals less uncongenial. That is a great loss all around. General history should not be written without knowledge of the local communities, whose particular experiences make up the national story. Nor should amateurs do their work without benefit of the professionals' enlarged views.

Perhaps Harvey Cushing had something like this in mind when, in the form of a question, he voiced the fear that medical history, like the specialties he hoped this library would bring together again, would itself become a specialty, separating itself from the practitioners:

> Will this foundation merely mean still another group of specialists having their own societies, organs of publication, separate places of meeting, separate con-

gresses, national and international, and who will also incline to hold aloof from the army of doctors made and in the making? Without lessening the opportunity and encouragement for historical and bibliographical research. . . . is there not something far more important for Medicine that can radiate from here?[58]

A good deal of importance for medicine and for our understanding of medicine has indeed radiated from "here" in the past half century, as well as from other departments and institutions established across the country in emulation of this. Many medical historians here present can recall a time when no gathering like this, none so large or so scholarly, could have been assembled in this country. The professionalization of medical history has occurred within our own lifetimes, much as the advent of scientific medicine had arrived mostly in the lifetimes of our predecessors of 1929. Yet amid the many reasons that this semi-centennial affords for satisfaction and confidence, we may ask again the questions that Flexner and Welch and Cushing put at the inauguration of the professional study of the history of medicine. They are worth remembering at the beginning of the second half-century, for they are an encouragement, a warning, and a guide.

NOTES

[1]The proceedings on the occasion of the dedication were published in *Bull. Johns Hopkins Hosp.* 46 (January 1930): 3–153, and reprinted in a small volume entitled *The William H. Welch Medical Library of the Johns Hopkins University* (Baltimore: Williams & Wilkins, 1930).

[2]Baltimore *Sun*, 16, 17, 18, 19 October 1929. Sudhoff was saluted editorially, 16 October, as "the notable representative of the German scholar class, which, within the last century, has labored so prodigiously to enrich the world." Of Welch the editorial writer asserted, 18 October, "It is impossible to estimate what the enlistment of such a man under the banner of medical science does for the growth of general respect for the scientific attitude."

[3]Thomas H. Morton and Frank Woodbury, *A History of the Pennsylvania Hospital: 1751–1895* (Philadelphia, 1895), pp. 345–56; Whitfield J. Bell, Jr., "The Old Library of the Pennsylvania Hospital," *Bull. Med. Lib. Assoc.* 60 (1972): 543–50.

[4]John Morgan, *Discourse upon the Institution of Medical Schools in America* (Philadelphia, 1765), p. 33; Whitfield J. Bell, Jr., *John Morgan: Continental Doctor* (Philadelphia: University of Pennsylvania Press, 1965), p. 162.

[5]W.S.W. Ruschenberger, *An Account of the Institution and Progress of the College of Physicians of Philadelphia* (Philadelphia, 1887), pp. 161–69.

[6]Walter L. Burrage, *A History of the Massachusetts Medical Society . . . : 1781–1922* (privately printed, 1923), pp. 388–415.

[7]D. Hayes Agnew, "The Medical History of the Philadelphia Almshouse," in *History of Blockley: A History of the Philadelphia General Hospital*, ed. John W. Croskey (Philadelphia: F. A. Davis, 1929), pp. 45–46.

[8]John P. Harrison, for the Committee on Medical Literature, "Report," *Trans. A.M.A.* 2 (1849): 417–18.

[9]Burrage, *History of the Massachusetts Medical Society*, p. 409.

[10]Richard J. Dunglison, *The Public Medical Libraries of Philadelphia* (Philadelphia, 1871), pp. 13–14.

[11]Eugene F. Cordell, *Medical Annals of Maryland: 1799–1899* (Baltimore: Medical and Chirurgical Faculty of Maryland, 1903), pp. 94, 108–9, *et passim*.

[12]Agnew, "Medical History of the Philadelphia Almshouse," pp. 45–46.

[13]Whitfield J. Bell, Jr., "The Medical Institution of Yale College," *Yale J. Biol. and Med.* 33 (1960): 176–77.

[14]Dunglison, *Public Medical Libraries*, pp. 21–31.

[15]Cordell, *Medical Annals*, pp. 124, 127, 132, 135, 137; John Shaw Billings, *Selected Papers*, ed. F. B. Rogers (Chicago: Medical Library Association, 1965), p. 159.

[16]Philip Van Ingen, *A Brief Account of the First One Hundred Years of the New York Medical and Surgical Society* (privately printed, 1946), p. 192.

[17]Herman G. Klotz, "A Brief History of the Library of the Physicians to the German Hospital and Dispensary of the City of New York," *Med. Lib. and Hist. J.* 2 (1904): 42–46.

[18]Samuel D. Gross, *History of American Medical Literature: From 1776 to the Present Time* (Philadelphia, 1875), pp. 74–76; Gross to Samuel S. Purple, 9 July 1875; Purple to Gross, 17 July 1875 (draft), New-York Historical Society (photocopies in New York Academy of Medicine). On this subject generally see Genevieve Miller, "In Praise of Amateurs: Medical History in America before Garrison," *Bull. Hist. Med.* 48 (1973): 586–615, and Whitfield J. Bell, Jr., "Practitioners of History: Philadelphia Medical Historians before 1925," ibid., 50 (1976): 73–92.

[19]"Remarks Commemorative of Samuel Lewis, M.D.," *Trans. and Studies College of Physicians of Philadelphia*, 3d ser., no. 12 (1890), pp. xci–ciii.

[20]Stephen Smith, "Memorial Address on the late Samuel Smith Purple, M.D.," *Med. Lib. and Hist. J.* 1 (1903): 102–16; "In Memoriam: Samuel Smith Purple, M.D.," *New York Genealogical and Biographical Record* (January 1902).

[21]Purple, *Medical Libraries: An Address Delivered before the New York Academy of Medicine, January 18, 1877* (New York, 1877).

[22]Purple to Gross, 17 July 1875.

[23]These manuscripts are in the New York Academy of Medicine.

[24]Purple, "Historical Sketch of the Society," *Twenty-Fifth Anniversary of the New York Genealogical and Biographical Society* (New York, 1895); *Catalogue of the Genealogical Library . . . to be Sold at Auction . . . Feb. 16th to 19th, 1909* (Boston: C. F. Libbie, 1909). A marked copy of the catalogue is in the New York Academy of Medicine.

[25]Purple, *Objects and Purposes: An Inaugural Address . . . January 21, 1875* (New York, 1875); "Address," in *The Celebration of the Semi-Centennial of the New York Academy of Medicine* (New York: printed for the Academy, 1903), pp. 12–15.

[26]Purple, *A Valedictory Address . . . January 16, 1879*; Philip Van Ingen, *The New York Academy of Medicine: Its First Hundred Years* (New York: Columbia University Press, 1944), pp. 155–72, *et passim*.

[27]Whitfield J. Bell, Jr., "Joseph M. Toner (1825–1896) as a Medical Historian," *Bull. Hist. Med.* 47 (1973): 1–24.

[28]John W. Farlow, *History of the Boston Medical Library* (privately printed, 1918), pp. 14–15, 32–34, 52–53, *et passim*; James R. Chadwick, "Address [at the dedication of the new building of the Boston Medical Library]," *Boston Med. and Surg. J.* 144 (1901): 56–58.

[29]Holmes's address on "Medical Libraries," on the opening of the library in 1878, is in his *Medical Essays: 1842–1882* (Boston, 1891), pp. 396–419.

[30]Chadwick, "The Boston Medical Library," *Med. Lib. and Hist. J.* 1 (1903): 127–35.

[31]"Medical Libraries," *Med. Register* 1 (1882): 27–28.

[32]Billings, *Selected Papers*, pp. 76–89, 159, 247; Chadwick, "Remarks," pp. 61–63; Fielding H. Garrison, *John Shaw Billings: A Memoir* (New York: G. P. Putnam's Sons, 1915), p. 236.

[33]Lewis H. Taylor, "Medical Libraries in Small Cities," *Med. Lib. and Hist. J.* 2 (1904): 187–92; Reuben Peterson, "The Need of More Medical Reference Libraries and the Way in Which They Can Be Established," *Bull. Amer. Acad. Med.* 2 (1895–97): 129–37; T. C. Christy, "A Plea for a Medical Library," *Pittsburgh Med. Rev.* 1 (1886–87): 87–88.

[34]Chadwick, "Medical Libraries," *Trans. Maine Med. Assoc.* 14 (1901–3): 266–80; "Medical Libraries: Their Development and Use," *Trans. Med. & Chirurgical Faculty of Maryland* (1892–96); pp.131–41.

[35]Charles D. Spivak, "How Every Town May Secure a Medical Library," *Med. News* 71 (1897): 443–44; "The Medical Libraries of the United States," *Phila. Med. J.* 2 (1898): 851–58; Francis D. Tardy, "The Colorado Medical Library Association: An Historical Sketch," *Colorado Med. J.* 4 (1898): 181–89; George M. Gould, "The Union of Medical and Public Libraries," *Phila. Med. J.* 2 (1898): 237–40; "Colorado Medical Library Association," *Trans. Colorado State Medical Society* 27 (1897): 386–87.

[36]George D. Hersey, "The Medical Library as a Factor in Medical Progress," *Trans. Rhode Island Medical Society* 6 (1899–1903): 162–70.

[37]Dunglison, *Public Medical Libraries*, p. 44.

[38]Robert W. Culp, "The Mount Sinai Hospital Library: 1883 to 1970," *Bull. Med. Lib. Assoc.* 60 (1972): 471–78.

[39]Janet B. Koudelka, "A History of the Johns Hopkins Medical Libraries: 1899–1935," (Master's thesis, Catholic University of America, 1963).

[40]E. Fletcher Ingals, "The Necessities of a Modern Medical College," *Bull. Amer. Acad. Med.* 2 (1895): 235–46.

[41]Bayard Holmes, "The Medical Library for the Medical School of Small Community," ibid., pp. 247–56.

[42]Abraham Flexner, *Medical Education in the United States and Canada: A Report to the Carnegie Foundation*, Carnegie Foundation for the Advancement of Teaching Bulletin, no. 4 (New York, 1910), p. 82.

[43]Billings, "Literature and Institutions," in *A Century of American Medicine: 1776–1876*, ed. Edward H. Clarke (Philadelphia, 1876), p. 351.

[44]Hersey, "The Medical Library as a Factor in Medical Progress," pp. 162–63.

[45]Billings, "Literature and Institutions," p. 350; *Selected Papers*, p. 168.

[46]Hersey, "The Medical Library as a Factor in Medical Progress," p. 169.

[47]Much was being thought and written about medical history at this time. In 1902 Dr. Eugene Cordell, author of *Medical Annals of Maryland*, proposed the establishment of "an American Medical Historical Society." *Med. Lib. and Hist. J.* 1 (1903): 49. See his eloquent plea for "The Importance of the Study of the History of Medicine," ibid. 2 (1904): 268–82. An editorial on "The Teaching of Medical History," ibid, pp. 52–58, sets forth all the arguments.

[48]Ibid, p. 185.

[49]Hersey, "The Medical Library as a Factor in Medical Progress," p. 170.

[50]Abraham Jacobi,"The Influence and Work of the Academy," *Trans. New York Academy of Medicine*, ser. 2, 6 (1890): 118–21.

[51]Cordell, *Medical Annals*, p. 91.

[52]Spivak, "How Every Town May Secure a Medical Library," pp. 443–44.

[53]*Trans. New York Academy of Medicine*, ser. 2., 7 (1891): 390, 413.

[54]*William H. Welch Medical Library*, pp. 30–31.

[55]Flexner in ibid., p. 96. See the Baltimore *Sun's* editorial "Eternal Quandary" on Flexner's remarks, 20 October 1929.

[56]Welch in *William H. Welch Medical Library*, pp. 92–93.

[57]Ibid., p. 94.

[58]Ibid., p. 38.

MEDICINE AS SOCIAL HISTORY: CHANGING IDEAS ON DOCTORS AND PATIENTS IN THE AGE OF SHAKESPEARE

Charles Webster

Links between Johns Hopkins and Oxford in the history of medicine extend back as long as this subject has existed as an identifiable specialism in either institution. Presiding over the prehistory of our discipline in the two institutions stands Sir William Osler, a figure whose ineradicable mark is etched into the fabric of the two medical schools on either side of the Atlantic. Especially in his later years Osler argued that medical history should be adopted as a unifying principle in the study and practice of medicine. Osler took practical steps towards the recognition of the history of medicine as a separate area of study at Oxford. By 1912 he was looking for a specialist medical historian to work in Oxford, with a view to rivaling German scholarship in this field. Two years later he persuaded Charles Singer to leave his clinical post in London in order to take up a research post in Magdalen College, nominally intended for pathology, but in practice permitting work in any field of medicine. With Osler's encouragement, Singer plunged himself into research and teaching in the history of biology and medicine.[1]

Singer's work was complemented by that of R. T. Gunther, also a senior member of Magdalen College, who was to build up the magnificent Museum of the History of Science, and whose writings embraced every aspect of science and medicine in Oxford. Gunther's biography testifies to the importance of Osler's support at the planning stage of the museum, and the exhibition of early scientific instruments arranged by Gunther in connection with Osler's presidential address to the Classical Association in 1919 was the first public demonstration of these collections.[2] Again with Osler's support, Singer persuaded curators of the Bodleian Library to set aside a small section of the Radcliffe Camera as a study area for the history of science and medicine.[3] Singer's own direct part in this work was interrupted by service in the First World War, but the activity continued, Osler himself in 1917 contributing the preface to the first volume of the group's research. This was shortly followed by a second volume, edited by Singer.[4] Singer became Oxford's first lecturer in the History of Biology, then the first lecturer in the History of Medicine at University College, London.

For many years Singer's name dominated all facets of the history of science and medicine and ultimately even the history of technology in Britain.[5]

He was also active on the international scene. In 1924 he coedited with Henry Sigerist the collection of essays presented to Karl Sudhoff on the occasion of his seventieth birthday, thus establishing a cordial relationship with the future director of The Johns Hopkins Institute. In 1929, at the request of William H. Welch, Singer was invited to deliver the first series of Hideyo Noguchi lectures at Johns Hopkins on "The Transition of Medieval to Modern Science." There was some chance that Singer might succeed Welch as director of the Institute of the History of Medicine.[6] At this time Baltimore was also visited by Sir D'Arcy Power, the leading British historian of medicine of the older generation, whom Welch also invited to deliver at the Institute a series of lectures on medical history.[7]

The lectures delivered by Singer and Power in Baltimore took place at a watershed in the history of science and medicine in the United States and Britain. A sharp reminder of change within these subjects came with the publication in 1931 of *Science at the Cross Roads*, the collection of papers given by the Soviet delegation at a session chaired by Singer at the Second International Congress of the History of Science and Technology held in London.[8]

Power and Singer emerge as representative figures of their respective generations, showing obvious points of contact and common interest, but also revealing fundamental differences of emphasis, with Singer pointing firmly to medicine as a major ingredient in the modern scientific enlightenment, whereas Power and his contemporaries had been much more appreciative of the independent character of medicine as an art pursued by an unbroken lineage of erudite craftsmen. This shift in perspective was accompanied by few explicit historiographical pronouncements. Nevertheless the difference of outlook evident from any comparison of the works of Power and Singer is indicative of a broader pattern of change in the center of gravity of the subject, not strikingly clear over the short term, but evident over a longer period in the course of the present century. I would argue that the history of medicine, perhaps especially in Britain, underwent a fundamental change in character in the hands of Singer's generation, and that more recently it has become subject to a further significant reorientation. This change in character could be illustrated with reference to any facet of modern medicine, but it is particularly well exemplified by writings on the sixteenth and seventeenth centuries, always one of the areas of major interest among historians of medicine. The age of Shakespeare is recognized as one of unparalleled intellectual creativity in the fields of science and medicine. The representative geniuses of the period, Gilbert, Bacon, Harvey, Burton, and Browne, were collectively apostrophized by Osler as "the transmuters" who "have given to man his world dominion."[9]

It would be a mistake to adopt a dismissive attitude towards the work of the pioneers of our subject at the turn of the century. Reference to Creighton's masterly survey of historical epidemiology, a work consulted more now than ever before, induces a sense of respect for the scale and versatility of

Victorian scholarship. Despite the now fashionable interest in major crises of health, no individual researcher or research group has succeeded in superseding Creighton over any part of his field of coverage, notwithstanding distortions of perspective in Creighton's work deriving from his eccentric epidemiological viewpoint.[10]

Creighton's work is not an isolated example. Young's account of the Barber Surgeons' Company, Barrett on the Society of Apothecaries, Munk's collective biography of the College of Physicians, Moore's history of St. Bartholomew's Hospital, Ferguson's bibliography of works on alchemy, are notable examples of scholarship in our field which have remained of permanent value.[11] Remarkably little has been added to this pioneer work, despite strongly expressed reservations concerning its defects and idiosyncrasies. These early writers were predominantly concerned with the history of institutions and medical specialisms with which they were intimately involved. Their work conveys a sense of authenticity, difficult for modern outsiders to recapture. They wrote with sympathy and commitment, recognizing a strong sense of organic continuity with previous generations involved with the same specialism or institution.

Histories produced at this stage contained many permanently useful ingredients. They provided particularly full insight into the structure of the medical profession and the evolution of medical institutions in London from the late Middle Ages onwards. Any aspect of the professional and corporate life of nascent medical organizations was likely to be handled in detail, albeit without the systemization we would now expect. The leading pioneer medical historians were contributing to the wider investigations of London civic life. As much as William Morris and George Unwin, they subscribed to the view that the ancient guilds lay at the heart of the best traditions within English culture.

By the turn of the century important steps had been taken towards the compilation of individual and collective medical biographies. Osler was the master of the biographical essay, believing that the exercise of total involvement with the author of a medical classic constituted a fundamental character-building experience for the medical student.[12] A more documentary approach towards collective biography had been taken by Munk in compiling his biographies of the fellows and licentiates of the Royal College of Physicians. A similar roll of the freemen and apprentices of the Barber Surgeons' Company or Society of Apothecaries would have been a vast undertaking. The nearest approach were the 2,800 biographies of fellows of the Royal College of Surgeons compiled under the editorship of D'Arcy Power, who regretted that the existence of ten to fifteen thousand members of his college at any one time precluded this group being included in the enterprise.[13] Moore and Power made a substantial contribution to collective medical biography in entries commissioned for the *Dictionary of National Biography*, arguably the most remarkable monument to the scholarship of that generation.

Biography was closely linked with biobibliography in the work of the pioneers. Few pursued this joint study with the vigor or systematic detail of John Ferguson, who, in his areas of interest, approached the erudition of Karl Sudhoff. Other medical historians came to appreciate the value of exhaustive biobibliographical surveys. This bibliographical thoroughness earned numerous minor medical authors of the age of Shakespeare a place in the *Dictionary of National Biography*. Osler was deeply impressed by the combination of detailed bibliographical description and condensed biography advocated by Ferguson, whose model was adopted in the long-term work on the bibliography of Osler's own library.[14]

This early work generated minor bibliographical discoveries, many of which have been overlooked, or only latterly acknowledged. Power was the first author to investigate the complex history of early works concerning midwifery: *Aristotle's Masterpiece*, other spurious writings attributed to Aristotle, and the *Birth of Mankind*. Power fully appreciated the place occupied by such works in popular culture. In a piece of intelligent detective work Power concluded that the celebrated black letter printing of *The Order of the Hospitalls of King Henry the VIIIth*, dated 1557 on its title page, was actually issued in 1691.[15] There is no reason to believe that there was any earlier printing of this document. Ferguson gave a more adequate account of the first English translations of Paracelsus than any later writer, among other things making the important observation that the first work of Paracelsus to be translated into English was a millennial tract. Ferguson drew attention to the interest of such minor authors as John Hester, the Paracelsian, distiller and medical translator.[16]

The success of this early work in medical bibliography owed much to the medical man's appreciation of work in this field undertaken by students of early English literature. The London Bibliographical Society and a constellation of exclusive bibliographical clubs provided a forum for a variety of special bibliographers.[17] The way was thus paved for the definitive bibliographies, such as those compiled by Fulton and Keynes, and for S. V. Larkey's summary bibliography of early modern medical literature contributed to the *Cambridge Bibliography of English Literature*.[18]

Bibliographers and literary scholars, either in association with medical historians or independently, have developed the work undertaken at the turn of the century in various directions. One outstanding contribution is F. P. Wilson's *The Plague in Shakespeare's London* (1927). More accessible than Creighton's account, it is an early example of urban demography and a model description of the cultural impact of plague on the seething population of the capital. The Herford and Simpson edition of Jonson, another major piece of literary scholarship, provides not only a model for scholarly standards, but also a yet unexploited source concerning disease and popular medicine.

Despite the totally informal structure of research undertaken before 1930 on medicine in early modern England, such work assumed consistency, char-

acter, and stature. While little of the historical analysis was to prove of enduring value, except as a reflection of the mentality of Edwardian and Victorian
medical elites, the biobibliographical data compiled has provided a permanent reference point. By this stage the bibliographical foundations were laid
for the study of popular medicine, and the medical practitioners of London
were more comprehensively investigated than their counterparts in any other
major city. Yet at every point this program was incomplete, as admitted in
1931 when Power appealed for the new Institute at Johns Hopkins to "place
the history of medicine on a sound scientific basis." There was need for a
more rigorous and exhaustive approach with respect to many of the topics
investigated by the pioneers, and for a synthesis and reappraisal of their
findings, in the light of the newly emerging fields of economic and social
history. The concern that medicine should not fall outside the purview of
modern historical studies and the social sciences was central to the conception of the history of medicine being articulated by Henry Sigerist and his
coworkers. In a celebrated and characteristically audacious aphorism Sigerist
argued that the history of medicine should not "limit itself to the history of
science, institutions, and characters of medicine, but must include the history of the patient in society, and that of the physician and the history of the
relations between physician and patient. History thus becomes social history."[19]

Working intuitively, medical men and laymen writing on English medicine of the period under consideration had addressed themselves conscien-
tiously to the dimension of this program relating to the medical practitioner.
Little had been said concerning the patient, although printed sources relating to popular medicine were exploited to a limited extent by bibliographers
and editors. Paradoxically, little was done after 1930 to bring the earlier
work to a natural conclusion, or to amplify it along the lines proposed by
Sigerist. Indeed, quite contrary to the spirit of Sigerist's remarks, research in
the history of medicine moved firmly in the direction of the history of science. This transition is evident in the writings of Singer. Before 1920 he had
written on a variety of subjects, including Anglo-Saxon medicine and her-
bals; he was also interested in the relations of magic and medicine. Thereafter, he became predominantly concerned with the emancipation of medicine
from magic and the emergence of modern medical science. From the date of
his influential *Short History of Medicine* (1928), his major writings were to
concern themselves with the rise of modern science. Singer came to view the
history of science primarily as a contribution to modern scientific thinking.
The subject was used as a didactic device for demonstrating the mental attitudes and methodological procedures most conducive to the advancement of
science. Singer wanted to instill among specialists a clear idea of the unity of
scientific knowledge and to preserve a platform for the defense of biological
ideas and metaphysical beliefs which were in danger of becoming outmoded.
He was insistent that scientific credentials should be uppermost in the selec-

tion of the international leadership of the history of science. The 1931 congress was dominated by the debate between vitalists and mechanists among the biologists. Singer declared: "We must prevent the History of Medicine from becoming a high and dry speciality. It is as material for the emergence of modern scientific problems that the History of Science can be most fruitfully presented today. This I have sought to bring out alike in the title, introduction, and text of my *Short History of Biology*. . . . If the History of Science does not help the scientific worker. . . it does nothing."[20] Early in his career Singer aimed to institute a *Journal of the History and Method of Science*. His aim was largely fulfilled with the establishment in 1936 of *Annals of Science* — a journal closely associated with University College, London, and devoted to the "origins and growth of Modern Science." In 1946, Singer became the first president of the British Society for the History of Science, which eventually established its own journal. There was at this stage no suggestion that the history of medicine should have its own parallel national society or independent journal. Perhaps more than Singer intended, the history of medicine became subordinate to the history of science. The History of Medicine Section of the Royal Society of Medicine founded by Power, Singer, and others in 1912 flourished temporarily, but along with other similar medical clubs, failed to make an impression outside a closed circle.

The above trend was perhaps the inevitable consequence of a phase of dominance and assertiveness of the pure sciences. A byproduct of this process was the professionalization of the history of science within universities, usually in association with science departments, and the new subject was taken up predominantly by those trained as scientists. This development involved a change in the sociological pattern of practitioners of the history of medicine, away from clinicians and towards scientists. Medical schools found this trend to be compatible with the increasing tendency of pure science to dominate medical education and medical research. A final element in this situation was the reaction in scientific circles against the Marxist idea of science and its history implicit in *Science at the Cross Roads*, this movement being spearheaded in Britain by the Society for Freedom in Science. In the shorter term very little comment on historical themes emanated from the Marxist side in academic circles. In Britain, by contrast with other countries, there was no call for the separate development of the history of medicine within medical schools. Whatever academic and professional development has occurred in the history of medicine has taken place predominantly in the shadow of the history of science. The pursuit of the history of medicine on an organized basis, without respect to the history of science, is still scarcely possible in Britain.

Increasing dominance of the history of science has had profound consequences for the study of medicine of the period under consideration. Because of the accelerating rate of progress of science, the earlier the period concerned, the greater likelihood of its being seen as devoid of interest. Somewhat awkwardly, medical men were out of step much of the time with major conceptual advances in the physical sciences which are traditionally taken as the yardstick of values in the history and philosophy of science.

The search for a meaningful field of contact with mainstream science has thus generated a relatively narrow area of focus in the history of medicine. Students of English medicine of the period between 1500 and 1700 have been predominantly concerned with William Harvey and the circulation of blood, and to a lesser extent with the broader field of experimental physiology. When just embarking upon research, I was persuaded to study Henry Power as an experimental philosopher rather than Henry Power as a Yorkshire medical practitioner. Many others in the field were similarly directed. One characteristic result of this bias has been the great disproportion in the research effort devoted to William Harvey compared with Thomas Sydenham.[21] Acceptance of the circulation of blood tends to be regarded as the measure of intellectual enlightenment in the seventeeth century. This factor has elevated many minor figures to a place in the history of science, whereas by this standard Sydenham appears inexplicably and embarrassingly reactionary.[22] Failure to exploit experimental physiology has been a license for neglect of the English Hippocrates in recent history of medicine. Apart from William Harvey, Francis Glisson was arguably the most important English physiologist of the seventeenth century. He was also a voluminous writer; his published works are matched by a complete and readily accessible body of manuscript notebooks. In his case almost total neglect of all but his ideas on irritability can be attributed to his opposition to "modern" forms of physiochemical reductionism, to his philosophical eclecticism, and to his tendency to adopt more explicitly biological and teleological forms of explanation. Thus Glisson, despite his intellectual kinship with William Harvey, is left out of account because he fails to fit into the supposed main line of Harveian science, which is somewhat arbitrarily identified as the application of the varieties of mechanical philosophy to physiology.[23] We find it uncomfortable to be obliged to recognize that the most sophisticated and sensitive scientific effort within medicine often occurred in directions not relevant to what we regard as main lines of scientific development.

Even attempts to explore new ground have been unduly conditioned by reference to scientific innovation. For instance, much of the creditable effort to draw attention to the influence of Paracelsus has been conducted on the basis of isolating a limited set of "modern" elements in the Paracelsian system. By this means, Paracelsus and his followers are depicted as contributors to the simplification and clarification of ideas on the theory of matter, proponents of ideas concerning respiration which place them in the lineage of John Mayow, and advocates of pragmatic and experimental methods reminiscent of Baconianism. Hence Paracelsus, Van Helmont, and other major representatives of Hermeticism are successfully emancipated into the modern world by maximizing their affinities with mainstream science.[24]

The history of science has not exercised a totally destructive influence. Even in its narrower forms it has repaired the previous neglect of the history of physiology. Michael Foster's *Lectures on the History of Physiology* (1901) had drawn attention to the profitability of this subject, but it was a long time before the case studies by Foster were superseded, and before the works of such original and able experimentalists as Lower and Mayow received detailed consideration.

Particularly during the last two decades the horizons of the history of science have expanded — not entirely an autonomous trend, but one accelerated by the growing influence of professional historians who have become increasingly concerned with the interrelationship between intellectual and social change. At the same time there has been a further sociological change within the history of science, as the subject becomes less dominated by lapsed career scientists. Finally the values of science are no longer taken as the single unquestioned standard of reference among historians of the subject.

It is no longer tenable to discuss scientific change in descriptive terms, or to regard innovation as the product of the inspired labors of fortuitously gifted individuals. The cycle of events previously consigned to a hurriedly compiled and compressed introductory biography, is now recognized as offering invaluable insights into intellectual development. Scientific innovation emerges as a process to a large degree capable of explanation. It is no longer an isolated phenomenon assigned to a class of inexplicable idiosyncrasies.

In the course of this work, factors such as social class, education, vocational association, religious affiliation, and philosophical outlook become germane to the understanding of intellectual biography. Scientists are recognized as operating in groups rather than as isolated individuals, scientific knowledge and innovative urges being as much the property of the group as of the individual. The processes of social, political, and economic change are seen to be potent forces in the affairs of the scientific community. Eventually, continued investigation exposes general patterns of change within the sciences; it brings to light connections between science, medicine, and events that are occurring at the institutional, educational, or economic level. Only at this stage could there have emerged within the history of science a serious appreciation and amplification of the dissertation on the sociology of seventeenth-century English science published by R. K. Merton in 1938, along with renewed interest in the sociology of religion of Max Weber and Ernst Troeltsch.[25] The above factors are increasingly taken into account as a matter of course in studies of the medical sciences in the seventeenth century.[26]

A more rigorously sociological approach to scientific change is no guarantee of arriving instantaneously at definitive and sweeping explanations. We are at the stage when major technical difficulties stand in the way of any intelligently conceived research program. Virtually any inquiry concerned with the early modern period is handicapped by major gaps in the evidence.

We have paid too little attention to the conceptual difficulties involved in the assessment of early scientific work. Even the utilization of the terms "science," "physics," "chemistry," or "physiology" may involve the questionable assumption that the seventeenth-century intellectual was a specialist who would perceive these subjects, if not their content, in the manner in which they are currently conceived. We are only just coming to realize the difficulties in translating into modern expressions the conceptual categories and terminology concerning natural philosophy and medicine used by generations of intellectuals still operating within a context of ancient philosophy and patristic theology. With respect to popular knowledge we pay lip service to anthropology, and to the notion that society in early modern Europe bears comparison in its belief systems with present-day non-Western traditional societies, but in practice the history of science makes too little concession to this point of view. It has also too readily been assumed in the absence of direct evidence that institutions function very much as do their modern counterparts. It comes as a surprise to find that professors of medicine at Oxford and Cambridge universities were unlikely to deliver their statutory lectures or perform statutory dissections and that teachers and their students are likely to be absentees.[27] Fellows of the Royal Society were unlikely to attend its meetings, contribute to its *Philosophical Transactions*, or pay the stipulated fees. Overall both universities and learned societies functioned very little like their modern counterparts.[28] Such basic considerations need to be taken into account before embarking on facile sociological or numerical exercises concerning such institutions.

The value of framing scientific innovation in its full intellectual context is aptly demonstrated by the reconstruction of William Harvey's biological philosophy undertaken by Walter Pagel.[29] Pagel's work highlights the impoverishment involved in ritually repeating the story of the discovery of the circulation of blood. Harvey emerges as a challenging biological thinker over the whole range of his writings, and one whose ideas were not unchangeable or invariably moving in the direction of modern science. Jerome Bylebyl of Johns Hopkins has demonstrated that *De motu cordis* must be viewed as a composite document, its parts embodying major shifts of emphasis, the chronology of which is still uncertain.[30] Similarly, Harvey's "precursors" emerge as more than cardboard figures having had the good fortune to stumble across a few useful pieces of data that they were unable to appreciate, and which awaited synthesis by the master. Not only anatomists, but chemists, philosophers, and even humble mechanics can be shown as contributing to the dialectic in which Harvey was engaged.[31] It is thus possible to build up a unified picture of a figure of the stature of William Harvey, demonstrating that his achievements as an innovator are in no way diminished by the acknowledgement that he was genuinely a figure of the culture of the Baroque.[32]

The cultural historical approach to the history of medicine when executed as above, or when carried further, as in cases where scientific knowledge is related more explicitly to its socioeconomic context, or even subsumed under a deterministic economic framework, is by no means uncontroversial. Moves in these directions are seen as undermining traditionally held beliefs concerning the independence or sanctity of scientific inquiry. While it is now universally accepted that a biographical approach to knowledge, carried out very much in the spirit of Osler, is necessary for a satisfying contextual appreciation of scientific creativity, there is resistance to regarding significant innovations or major currents of scientific change as predictable outcomes of a particular stage of economic development, or facets of the process of class conflict. Yet much of the research currently undertaken is undermining any conception of the autonomous nature of scientific knowledge. A dualistic mode of interpretation has been introduced in some circumstances to preserve the notion of an "internal" element in science irreducible to "external" factors, but it is doubtful whether this internalist/externalist distinction will prove of any lasting value. Especially with respect to the early modern period there are major problems of defining boundaries between external and internal factors, and it can be argued that this distinction is anachronistic, being arbitrarily and artificially imposed on a unified set of phenomena. Ultimately every case ought to be decided on its merits.

It will perhaps be accepted that the formation of Linacre's College of Physicians in London was not simply a reflection of progress in medical humanism, but was connected with the crisis in public health facing the capital city at the date of the college's foundation.[33] Similarly the famous *Pharmacopoeia Londinensis* was not primarily an exercise in promulgating Paracelsian innovations in pharmacy, but was a necessary response to social conflict in an urban setting, involving the struggle for power between organizations of physicians, apothecaries, and grocers.[34] In a wider context it has been argued that the appeal of Paracelsianism and Baconian natural history in mid century becomes more meaningful when considered in the light of the ethos of the reforming party during the English Revolution.[35]

There is much less agreement when, for instance, it is proposed that William Harvey's change of mind with respect to the primacy of the heart was a manifestation of the influence of emergent republicanism, or that the remarkable revival of scientific and medical studies at the English universities was an expression of recovery from the decadence of the Laudian regime, or that the Royal Society was indebted to the Office of Address Project of the Republicans.[36] The precise connection between the religious and scientific movements of the seventeenth century is likely to be contested well into the future, raising as it does in this crucial area the precise nature of the relationship between the scientific revolution and other factors in the process of modernization. Whatever the outcome with respect to specific issues under debate, the general exercise is productive as a contribution to the demythologization of the history of science. It must now be positively proved, rather than assumed, that the scientific process is entirely independent of the mode of production and social processes connected with any stage of economic development.

Current work is increasingly examining innovations in the medical sciences in a balanced historical context. It will now be more difficult to wrench elements out of this context for the convenience of producing simple linear accounts of scientific change of the kind recently in fashion. We are thus in process of attaining a more genuinely historical view of the medical sciences. But it must be borne in mind that this perspective relates to a highly selected intellectual elite within medicine, while the topics with which we are most familiar tend to have only a remote connection with the practice of medicine. For example, the program for a practical application of the new anatomy and physiology in the field of medical practice never came near to realization in the seventeenth century.

Despite genuine steps towards liberalization, preoccupation with the history of science has continued to deflect attention away from medicine as it was practiced by the great majority of practitioners. Consistent with this omission, the patient has been almost entirely disregarded, despite the fact that the patient's presence constitutes a necessary precondition for the very existence of medicine. The "patient," perceived as more than a passive vehicle of disease, establishes a fundamental point of distinction between science and medicine. In accordance with the view of Sigerist, the history of medicine possesses validity as an independent specialism rather than as a subsidiary aspect of the history of science when it is addressed as much to the province of the patient as to the ideas and vocational activities of medical practitioners.[37] The twin pillars of history of medicine, with respect to any defined cultural situation, should be the investigation of the human subject in all states of health and disease, and the study of medical practice in all of its forms. Medical history, then, would become more concerned with abiding features of medical systems and much less with linear development in the medical sciences. This objective may seem like a truism, but it has proved remarkably difficult to attain.

Apart from such isolated examples as Creighton's studies of major infectious diseases, our insight into patients and their ailments was negligible until the recent rise of historical demography. Even evidence deriving from demography will prove to have serious limitations from a historical point of view unless it is viewed in the broader context of historical epidemiology and social history. Knowledge of demographic change in early modern England still rests to a great extent on an exemplary study of one parish in Devon.[38] Effort in the demographic field revolves around questions of longterm drifts in fertility, mortality, and population, especially with respect to the industrial revolution — the so-called modern rise of population associated with economic modernization. There is relatively less concern with more static demographic situations such as that existing before 1700. Here the scene tends to be described as one of "demographic stagnation." The rise of the population in the later sixteenth century was not consolidated into an accelerated increase in the seventeenth. By comparison with France, England before 1700 seems unremarkable with respect to crises of subsistence and disease. Infant mortality was generally not as great as experienced elsewhere. Even major epidemics are now recognized as little more than minor perturbations in the demographic process.[39] But for the social historian, populations are not consigned to the demographic scrapheap because of the absence of major secular trends. Stagnation is largely an artifact of types of aggregative analysis, which serve to reduce the statistical impact of a whole host of minor fluctuations that may have exercised a profound effect at the local level. The villages and towns of Shakespeare's England represent a mosaic of ecological niches, each displaying its characteristic pattern of demographic fluctuation, each involving a succession of crises that seemed very real to the inhabitants, but may not necessarily have been in phase with crises elsewhere. Thus Flinn has documented severe famine in various parts of Scotland between 1621 and 1636 amounting to a "natural catastrophe" in 1623; Appleby has distinguished reasons why famine struck Cumbria particularly severely, while Skipp detects a Malthusian situation in three Warwickshire villages, at a time when there is no evidence of national food shortages.[40]

Epidemics struck with similar diversity. On closer investigation the great London Plague of 1665 emerges as less damaging demographically than the plagues of 1603 and 1625, while none of the seventeenth-century outbreaks was as serious as that of 1563.[41] Bristol, Exeter, and Norwich—three of the largest cities in England—experienced regular outbreaks of plague, but with strikingly different patterns of virulence. Even within towns, parishes were often differently affected according to their geographical and social characteristics.[42] For local inhabitants, pestilences assumed the character of a Great Plague according to their immediate impact and feared consequences. To the social historian the anxieties aroused by threats of epidemic visitation are as relevant as the mortality induced by visitations themselves.

From the medical historian's point of view crude mortality rates give very little insight into the state of health of the various social strata and age groups comprising any community. The importance of paying attention to age-specific mortality rates is demonstrated in a recent study that indicates not only the distinction between trends in adult and child mortality patterns, but also the clear difference between infant and child mortality rates.[43] Such research provides promising insights into the epidemiology of the different age groups. Current work shows that in Shakespeare's England, infant and child mortalities fluctuated greatly, but were often alarmingly high, and in general they constituted the dominant element in the bills of mortality.[44] The distinction between endogenous and exogenous mortality rates, made possible by family reconstitution methods, has been exploited in the study of the relevance of weaning practices to infant mortality and birth spacing, so providing a useful demographical parallel between early modern Western society and present-day non-Western societies.[45]

Utilization of such distinctions serves to break down the exclusive concern with crude rates of mortality and to draw attention to specific causes of death and related morbidity factors. Crude birth and death rates and estimates of average life expectancy are among the most accessible demographic indices, but they can be uninformative concerning the underlying pattern of morbidity and general quality of life. Indeed, it would be easy to produce a model that would generate an increase in average life expectancy explained on the basis of a decrease from high levels of infant mortality (associated for instance with the decline of smallpox, improvements in midwifery, or changes in infant-rearing practices), but which would involve a declining state of health of the population owing to increasing incidence of such factors as typhus, tuberculosis, sexually transmitted diseases, malnutrition, cumulative poisoning, long-standing dermatological conditions, and occupational diseases. Variants of this model must frequently have occurred, especially in expanding urban communities. The possibility of a "demographic upturn" combined with a mounting crisis of health has not been sufficiently taken into account in current theorizing concerning the association between modern population growth and presumed improvements in standards of living.

Recent work by Forbes indicates the usefulness of paying attention to the causes of death, as recorded in the Parish Registers of St. Botolph without Aldgate from 1583 to 1599.[46] Such detailed records are exceedingly rare, but they could be supplemented by evidence from a variety of other sources, the most important of which are the London Bills of Mortality. These records cannot in all cases be taken as an authoritative statement of the cause of death, but they possess validity as an indication of the major conditions concomitant with the direct cause of death. This evidence accordingly provides a valuable insight into prevailing problems of ill-health. The causes of death recorded in the bills of mortality have hitherto been little exploited, largely owing to the supposed unreliability of the searchers—those "ancient matrons, sworn to their office," censured by Graunt for understating the numbers of deaths occasioned by syphilis.[47] But it should be recalled that this was the only major reservation expressed by Graunt, while the reputation of the searchers was defended by the well-informed witness, John Bell, in 1665.[48] Both Graunt and Heberden made constructive use of the tabulations of the causes of death in the bills of mortality.[49] We are still some long way from a precise understanding of the epidemiology of Shakespeare's England, but with more effective exploitation of available evidence it will be possible to establish a good impression of the factors that made towns such as London effective incubators of disease. The experience of ill-health was an important factor in the social situation, as is evident from innumerable personal records, reinforced by the evidence of drama and literature. Smallpox and syphilis were taking on ever more importance as disfiguring diseases, while the inhabitants were infested by a rich flora and fauna of external and internal parasites. Bodies were wracked by pain deriving from stone, hernia, gout, and syphilis. The drastic remedial action to which the patients were driven often exacerbated the problems, as in the case of mercury, which provided effective treatment for syphilis, but at the cost of generating a whole range of physical and mental side effects. As appreciated by Graunt, the full epidemiological picture is only incompletely reflected in the records of mortality.[50]

Personal ill-health and experience of disease and death within the family and social circle must have been a potent cause of anxiety. Mental disorder was contributed to by a variety of factors, some of universal experience, others characteristic of the seventeenth century. The study of the intractable area of mental disorder constitutes an important challenge, and it provides crucial evidence relating to the mentality of the period, relating as it does to a whole range of questions of interpersonal relations. Psychiatry in the early modern period has hitherto been the subject of little more than disconnected comment, the major element of coherence coming from the direction of English literature.[51] An opportunity to exploit the notebooks of Simon Forman as a means of illuminating this subject has fallen prey to trivialization.[52] The first constructive insight into the epidemiology of anxiety and mental disorder in preindustrial England is contained in the important study of Macdonald based on the intensive analysis of more than two thousand cases of mental disorder extracted from the diaries of Richard Napier, the most expert practitioner in this field in the early seventeenth century.[53] Macdonald's study, like other current work with a medical bearing relating to such issues as sexuality, menstruation, childbirth, lactation, infanticide, and infant care, provides the stabilizing elements urgently needed to balance certain impressionistic insights and numerous wild speculations concerning the presumed emotional impoverishment of family relations in the premodern period.[54]

Very little has been done to extend the encouraging pioneer work on medical practice in Shakespeare's period undertaken at the turn of the century. Work in this area has noticeably lagged behind demography in the exploitation of quantitative and systematic methods. Goodall's seventeenth-century account of the London College of Physicians has been filled out by Sir George Clark, but the perspective of the two studies is remarkably similar, each striking a strongly apologetic note with respect to the college, while being censorious of inferior medical organizations, and sarcastically dismissive of practitioners lacking formal medical credentials. Clark, like Goodall, falls back on stigmatizing competitors of the college as "ignorant, mercenary and fraudulent," "criminal impostors," or "crows and magpies."[55] A radically different perspective emerges from the analysis of the interminable legal disputes between the college and its rivals undertaken by R. S. Roberts.[56] With further examination the college appears less prestigious, powerful, and influential in London medicine than would be anticipated from its statutory position. Beyond a small number displaying genuine distinction, the educational and intellectual record of the fellows of the college was not imposing, at least until the generation of the dominance of William Harvey's disciples. Linacre's dream of his college as a supreme and coherent medical elite, united by subscription to a humanistic Galenism, was to be largely unfulfilled.[57] A more accurate assessment of the college awaits a more comprehensive study in collective biography than has so far been undertaken.[58] In the meantime it would be a mistake to attribute to the fellows of the college too many of the professional and intellectual characteristics of their modern counterparts, on the basis of a thin line of institutional continuity. There is also little point in using terms such as "empiric" or "mountebank" as freely as they were applied by the college to designate virtually all practitioners lying outside its membership, as if the fellows were the only persons competent to engage in the responsible practice of medicine. This construction might be defensible in some narrow legalistic sense, but it is unrewarding from the historical point of view insofar as it prevents appreciation of the numerical strength and quality of medical practice outside the College of Physicians. The citizens of Shakespeare's London accorded the fellows of the college no monopoly of medical practice, and they recognized that responsible and irresponsible practice were diffused throughout the ranks of medical practitioners.

We are slowly coming to appreciate the great numerical strength of medical practice outside the College of Physicians. Clark greatly understated the number of practitioners prosecuted by the college. Between 1550 and 1640, the first extensive period for which reasonably reliable records survive, the college enrolled 130 fellows (19 of them after prosecution), and in addition 56 individuals registered as licentiates (10 of them after prosecution). There were never more than 50 practitioners associated with the college in practice at any one time. For the same period incomplete records describe prosecutions against some 650 practitioners who never became fellows or licentiates. This figure probably represents no more than a significant proportion of the men and women involved in medical practice in London. Data relating to surgeons and apothecaries suggest that each group comprised some 120 freemen by 1600. Between 1540 and 1640 the records of the Barber Surgeons' Company witness to the activities of more than 900 individuals, most of them freemen and apprentices.[59] Our estimates suggest that there was likely in Shakespearian times to be at least one identifiable medical practitioner for every 400 individuals in London.[60] This calculation excludes midwives, nurses, and the like, many of whom probably engaged in medical practice. Such evidence indicates an unexpectedly high incidence of medical practitioners in the capital. Perhaps even more surprisingly, sample studies in Norwich and East Anglia suggest similar levels for small towns and rural communities.[61] The directory compiled by Raach is found to represent only a small fraction of medical practitioners in rural England.[62]

Even the above preliminary estimates indicate an unexpectedly high level of demand for specialized medical assistance among urban and rural populations in Shakespeare's England. Our findings justify the anxiety of such experienced surgeons as William Clowes that medical practice was becoming invaded by tradesmen from virtually every known trade, from rat catchers to sow gelders, whom he collectively castigated as "rotten and stinking weeds."[63]

The numerous and diverse tribes of medical professionals admit no simple categorization according to the educational or vocational criteria traditionally applied in the sociology of medicine. Although regularly accused of being "illiterate empirics," practitioners prosecuted by the college turn out to have had a higher educational standing than would be supposed from the evidence presented by Clark. Indeed, on certain occasions, such "illiterates" metamorphosed into reputable fellows of the college![64] Of the 650 prosecuted practitioners, 126 are known to have received a university education; over half of this group were in possession of a medical degree. It may also be reasonably supposed that the bulk of the 249 surgeons and apothecaries prosecuted were well educated, since they often came from good families, and were vocationally successful, articulate, prosperous, and active in civic affairs. It was surgeons and apothecaries and unlicensed practitioners in Shakespeare's England rather than collegiate physicians who contributed most actively to the medical literature. Within this group, such well-known figures as Bullein, John Dee, Elyot, and Hester avoided prosecution, while other well-known authors such as Baker, Bannister, Bright, Arthur Dee, Mouffet, Parkinson, Penny, and Surphlet were censured for unlicensed practice.[65]

Illiterates may have been common among the 103 women prosecuted by the college, but it would need to be proved that illiteracy was necessarily a handicap for the type of medical practice in which women engaged. Preliminary findings suggest that women from all classes were playing a significant part in the practice of medicine throughout this period, despite their virtual absence from the emerging professional organizations.[66] Indeed, it is likely that males and females identified as "practitioners in physick and surgery" — that is; general practitioners — most of them unlicensed and unattached to any professional organization, dominated medical practice throughout the sixteenth and seventeenth centuries. On the other hand, the strict division of labor between physicians, surgeons, and apothecaries favored by the humanistic physicians was, despite the prominence accorded to this tripartite arrangement in histories of medicine, never more than imperfectly realized, even in London.

The above instances illustrate the importance of subjecting evidence concerning medical practice to numerical analysis. By this means it becomes evident that medical practice was not effectively confined to a small body of physicians in London attached to a single institution, or to licensed graduates in the provinces. Other practitioners should not be dismissed as a handful of illiterate quacks in an exploitative relationship with the public. The strength of traditional medicine lay in its heterogeneity. Any physician subscribing to Galenic medicine found himself in competition with humanistically educated Paracelsians such as Thomas Mouffet, or with humble practitioners exploiting a handful of simple cures, often administered in a magical context. William Bullein, himself a lay medical practitioner, could not help noting that an old empiric like John Preston, although entirely ignorant of Galen or Hippocrates, was "greatly sought unto," and by virtue of his cheap cures "custom hath commenced him amongst the common people to be their doctor."[67]

Concern to eliminate the magical element in midwifery and medicine had been basic to the medical legislation from its outset in 1511. It was a constant complaint against empirics as well as learned alchemists that they resorted to conjuring. Although the modern medical historian finds greater appeal in the intellectual rigor of humanistic Galenism and its anatomical and physiological progeny, by all sections of the sixteenth-century public magical systems were accorded high intellectual and practical value. It would be quite unrealistic to claim that magical beliefs persisted simply because of the apparent practical value of chemical therapy. In the context of the pattern of diseases afflicting the community, Galenic medicine drew upon fewer resources than its rivals. In situations where no physician possessed adequate therapeutic tools, the system having the deeper, richer, and more varied psychological dimension would be at an advantage. Even if there were doubts at the level of authority about the efficacy of many of the practices of Paracelsians and natural magicians, there was too little confidence in the Galenic option for prudence not to demand the preservation of alternative forms of practice. If these factors are borne in mind it can be better appreciated why on the one hand the College of Physicians was established and given the unambiguous backing of law, while on the other, it received so little support in realizing its plan for the professionalization of medicine in London; at the same time the college was legitimated, the protection of authority was extended to a body of seemingly eccentric empirics. By giving formal sanction to the organization of humanistic physicians, authority was dutifully acknowledging the highest expression of rationalistic medicine; by protecting alternative traditions, society was insuring against the premature suppression of magical beliefs, and thereby contributing to the stability of a new type of urban culture.

The precise role played by medical practitioners in providing health care to the various social groups in Shakespeare's England is still largely conjectural. The sceptical attitude towards physicians expressed by Margaret Paston in 1464 must have been reiterated on countless occasions among those classes capable of affording the services of the medical elite.[68] The lower classes were perhaps no less vigilant concerning the cures peddled by simple empirics. Much of the medical care needed by families and communities must have been derived from intrinsic cultural resources. Gifted neighbors, or the wives of ministers and gentlemen, regularly dispensed medical assistance to those in need. Much of this wisdom was transmitted orally. The outlook of this domestic medicine was essentially magical. Full reconstruction of the system of medical beliefs and popular practices prevailing at this period must be based on the collation of fragmentary evidence deriving from a variety of sources: the voluminous published literature of popular medicine, and also a variety of manuscript sources, such as medical notebooks, recipe books, diaries, civil and ecclesiastical records, and local history materials. Apart from this direct evidence, some light is cast on traditional medical practices by information derived from later records of folk belief, present-day oral testimony, and structural insights derived from studies of non-Western societies.

Until recently the materials and methods applied in this field have been outside the frame of reference of medical historians, the initiative for the exploration of this important area having derived from anthropologically sensitive social historians investigating popular religion and witchcraft.[69] Magic, astrology, and alchemy provide important connecting links between medicine and religion, and between popular culture and scientific speculation. It is only recently that magical belief systems in Western Europe have come, among historians of science and medicine, to be regarded as anything more than a legacy of superstition awaiting elimination in the course of the scientific enlightenment. The danger now is that magic is becoming the object of an undiscriminating curiosity as subversive to any critical historical evaluation as the simplistic linear histories of science. While in general the seventeenth century is regarded as a watershed for the rise of science and decline of magic, it has proved by no means easy to drive a wedge between magic and legitimate science. Nonmechanistic philosophies of nature were tenaciously defended in the later decades of the century. Rather than being abandoned, magic became more sophisticated. Alchemical literature was exerting an undiminished hold on the attention of Newton and his contemporaries. Belief in witchcraft was reluctantly abandoned by leading intellectuals. All classes persisted in following traditional magical practices in medicine. The elimination of magic at the village level in Western Europe is a phenomenon of the recent past, if it can be said to have occurred at all.

This review of the historiography of medicine with respect to the age of Shakespeare ends on no note of complacency. During the last fifty years the major energies applied to the subject have done little to advance the conception of the social history of medicine developed in embryo by pioneers before 1930, and by Henry Sigerist at The Johns Hopkins Institute. We have remained too preoccupied with problems dictated by the history of science. Extension of our horizons beyond questions relating to innovation, precursors, and priorities has been made with timidity rather than determination. Mounting concern with "relevance" is serving to devalue the full historical record of medicine in favor of new priorities dictated by new masters. Major grant-giving bodies have on occasion acted as a drag on initiative. The most active steps towards the realization of a social history of medicine have been taken by social historians and social scientists, rather than medical historians. It remains to be seen whether medical historians will at this stage take the final imaginative leap to exploit the social history of medicine to its fullest extent. It would be disappointing if the subject that they pioneered ultimately achieved its full fruition in entirely different hands. To advance the social history of medicine along the lines indicated above would be to make a major contribution to medical thinking and to the social sciences. Failure to contribute to this study would be to the impoverishment of our discipline, and would perhaps incur risk of institutional redundancy. On the issue of contributing to the enduring goals of scholarship, Osler cited Sir Thomas Browne. He might also have cited Francis Bacon's interpretation of the Fable of Atalanta, who sacrificed the race for the sake of the golden apples. Bacon warned of the penalties of "continually stopping short, forsaking the track, and turning aside to profit and convenience, exactly like Atalanta. Whence it is no wonder that art gets not victory over nature, nor, brings her under subjection."[70]

NOTES

[1]Osler to R. T. Gunther, 5 June 1912, Old Ashmolean Letter-Book 1912–1933, History of Science Museum, Oxford; E. A. Underwood, ed., *Science Medicine and History: Essays on the Evolution of Scientific Thought and Medical Practice Written in Honour of Charles Singer*, 2 vols. (London: Oxford University Press, 1953), 1: introduction; Harvey Cushing, *The Life of Sir William Osler*, 2 vols. (Oxford: Clarendon Press, 1925), 2:445, 558, 560, 595, 637.

[2]A. E. Gunther, *Early Science in Oxford*, vol. 15 *Robert T. Gunther: A Pioneer in the History of Science, 1869–1940* (London: Dawson's, 1967), pp. 154–195; Cushing, *Life of Osler*, 2:640, 648–49.

[3]C. Singer, *Studies in the History and Method of Science* (Oxford: Clarendon Press, 1917), preface; *Life of Osler*, 2:444–45. Singer worked closely with his wife Dorothea Waley Singer, herself a major historian of early science. E. A. Underwood, "Obituary of Dorothea Waley Singer (1882–1964)," *Br. J. Hist. Sci.* 2 (1965): 260–62.

[4]C. Singer, *Studies in the History and Method of Science*, 2 vols. (Oxford: Clarendon Press, 1917–1921).

[5]Underwood, *Science, Medicine and History*, 1: introduction; idem, "Obituary of Charles Joseph Singer (1876–1960)," *Med. Hist.*, 8 (1960): 353–58.

[6]C. Singer and H. E. Sigerist, eds., *Essays on the History of Medicine Presented to Karl Sudhoff on the Occasion of his Seventieth Birthday* (London: Oxford University Press; Zurich: Verlag Sedwyla, 1924). Singer's Noguchi lectures were delayed until 1932, and were delivered in part by Mrs. Singer owing to Singer's illness. They were not published; Singer to Welch declining the Johns Hopkins appointment in the History of Medicine, 27 March 1931, Welch Papers, folder 27, Alan Mason Chesney Medical Archives of The Johns Hopkins Medical Institutions.

[7]Sir D'Arcy Power, *The Foundations of Medical History* (Baltimore: Williams & Wilkins, 1931).

[8]*Science at the Cross Roads* (London: Kniga, 1931); 2d ed. with a foreword by Joseph Needham and an introduction by G. Wersky (London: Cass, 1971). The best known Russian delegates were N. I. Bukharin, N. I. Vavilov, and B. Hessen. J. D. Bernal regarded Hessen's contribution as "the starting point for a new evaluation of the history of science," *The Social Function of Science* (London: Gollancz, 1939), p. 406. For a similar view, see J. G. Crowther, *Soviet Science* (London: Kegan Paul, 1936), pp. 325–26. Welch wrote of the Russian "appearance as most sensational, and possibly at most of historical significance," Diary, vol. 38, pp. 120–21, Welch Papers. For the immediate impact of *Science at the Cross Roads*, see G. Wersky, *The Visible College* (London: Allen Lane, 1978), pp. 139–49.

[9]*Selected Writings of Sir William Osler* (London: Oxford University Press, 1951), p. 5.

[10]C. Creighton, *A History of Epidemics in Britain*, 2 vols. (Cambridge: At the University Press, 1891); reprint ed. with additional material (London: Cass, 1965). For a fierce review of Creighton and his modern editors, see R. S. Roberts, "Epidemics and Social History," *Med. Hist.*, 12 (1968): 305–16.

[11]S. Young, *Annals of the Barber Surgeons of London* (London: Blades, East & Blades, 1890); C.R.B. Barrett, *The History of the Society of Apothecaries of London* (London: Elliot Stock, 1905); W. Munk, *The Roll of the Royal College of Physicians*, 2d ed., 3 vols. (London: Royal College of Physicians, 1878); N. Moore, *The History of St. Bartholomew's Hospital*, 2 vols. (London: C. A. Pearson, 1918); J. Ferguson, *Bibliotheca Chemica*, 2 vols. (Glasgow: J. Maclehose, 1906).

[12]Osler, *Selected Writings*, p. 61.

[13]Sir D'Arcy Power, ed., *Plarr's Lives of the Fellows of the Royal College of Surgeons of England*, 2 vols. (Bristol: J. Wright, 1930); see Sir Z. Cope, *The Royal College of Surgeons of England* (London: A. Blond, 1959), pp. 268–69, for a brief account of this collaborative venture.

[14]Cushing, *Life of Osler*, 2:417–18; *Bibliotheca Osleriana* (Montreal and London: McGill—Queen's University Press, 1969), p. x. The first edition of this bibliography, edited by W. W. Francis, appeared in 1929.

[15]Power, "Notes on the Bibliography of Three Sixteenth-Century English books connected with London Hospitals," *The Library*, 4th ser., 2 (1921): 73–94; idem, "The Birth of Mankind or the Woman's Book: A Bibliographical Study," *The Library*, 4th ser., 8 (1927): 1–36; idem, *Foundations of Medical History*, pp. 134–38, 147–78; Power is cited by Janet Blackman, "Popular Theories of Generation: The Evolution of Aristotle's Works. The Study of an Anachronism," in J. Woodward and D. Richards, eds., *Health Care and Popular Medicine in Nineteenth Century England* (London: Croom Helm, 1977), pp. 64, 86.

[16]J. Ferguson, *Bibliographia Paracelsica*, 5 parts (Glasgow: privately printed, 1877–93). Ferguson's work is noticed in Sudhoff's *Bibliographia Paracelsica* (1894), but not by P. H. Kocher, "Paracelsian Medicine in England (c. 1570–1600)," *J. Hist. Med.* 2 (1947): 451–80, or A. G. Debus, *The English Paracelsians* (London: Oldbourne, 1965).

[17]See Cushing, *Life of Osler*, 2:414–18, for various bibliographical societies with which Osler was involved. Among his many projects, Osler encouraged Medical Librarians' Associations in Britain and America; *Life of Osler*, 2:184, 237.

[18]J. F. Fulton, *A Bibliography of the Honorable Robert Boyle* (Oxford: Oxford Bibliographical Society, 1932). Bibliographies compiled by G. Keynes extend from *A Bibliography of William Harvey* (Cambridge: University Press, 1928) to *A Bibliography of Sir Thomas Browne* (Oxford: Clarendon Press, 1968); S. V. Larkey, "A Critical Bibliography of English Medicine and Biology: 1477–1603," *Archeion* 14 (1932):

533–43; idem, "Science and Pseudo-Science," in *Cambridge Bibliography of English Literature*, ed. F. W. Bateson (Cambridge: At the University Press, 1941), 1:879–94.

[19]H. E. Sigerist, "The Social History of Medicine," *West. J. Surg., Obst. and Gyn.*, 48 (1940): 715–16.

[20]Singer to Welch, 27 March 1931, Welch Papers, folder 27.

[21]For a review of recent work on Harvey, see W. Pagel, *New Light on William Harvey* (Basel: Karger, 1976). The only important modern study of Sydenham is D. G. Bates, "Sydenham and the Medical Meaning of 'Method'," *Bull. Hist. Med.* 51 (1977): 324–38.

[22]See. L. J. Rather, "Pathology in Mid-Century: A Reassessment of Thomas Willis and Thomas Sydenham," in *Medicine in Seventeenth Century England*, ed. A. G. Debus (Berkeley and Los Angeles: University of California Press, 1974), pp. 71–112, especially pp. 75–76.

[23]O. Temkin, "The Classical Roots of Glisson's Doctrine of Irritation." *Bull. Hist. Med.* 38 (1964): 297–328; the only recent major paper on Glisson's biological ideas. See also Temkin's entry on Glisson in *Dictionary of Scientific Biography*, ed. C. C. Gillispie (New York: C. Scribner's Sons, 1972), 5:425–27. As Professor Mani's contribution in the present volume, and other current work by Boss, Brown, and Cunningham indicate, neglect of Glisson is at an end.

[24]See particularly the writings of A. G. Debus, gathered into *The Chemical Philosophy: Paracelsian Science and Medicine in the Sixteenth and Seventeenth Centuries* (New York: N. Watson, 1977).

[25]R. K. Merton, "Science, Technology and Science in Seventeenth Century England," *Osiris* 4 (1938): 360–632; 2d edition with a new introduction (New York: H. Fertig, 1970). Merton throughout this work gracefully acknowledges a debt to Hessen's contribution to *Science at the Cross Roads*.

[26]R. G. Frank, Jr., *Harvey and the Oxford Physiologists: A Study of Scientific Ideas* (Berkeley: University of California Press, 1980). See also T. M. Brown, "The Mechanical Philosophy and the Animal Oeconomy," (Ph.D. diss., Princeton University, 1968); idem, "Physiology and the Mechanical Philosophy in Mid-Seventeenth Century England," *Bull. Hist. Med.* 51 (1977): 25–54.

[27]C. Webster, "The Medical Faculty and the Physick Garden," in *History of the University of Oxford: 1688–1800*, ed. L. Sutherland (Oxford: Oxford University Press, forthcoming).

[28]M. 'Espinasse, "The Decline and Fall of Restoration Science," *Past and Present* 14 (1958): 71–94; M. Hunter, "The Social Basis and Changing Fortunes of an Early Scientific Institution...the Royal Society, 1660–1685," *Notes and Records of the Royal Society* 31 (1976): 9–114.

[29]W. Pagel, *William Harvey's Biological ideas* (Basel, New York: Karger, 1967); idem, *New Light on William Harvey*.

[30]J. J. Bylebyl, "The Growth of Harvey's *De Motu Cordis*," *Bull. Hist. Med.* 47 (1973): 427–70.

[31]W. Pagel, "Giordano Bruno. The Philosophy of Circles and the Circular Movement of the Blood," *J. Hist. Med.* 6 (1951): 116–24; C. Webster, "William Harvey and the Crisis of Medicine in Jacobean England," in *William Harvey and His Age: The Professional and Social Context of the Discovery of the Circulation*, ed. J. J. Bylebyl (Baltimore: The Johns Hopkins University Press, 1979), pp. 1–27.

[32]H. E. Sigerist, "William Harvey's Stellung in der Europaischen Geistesgeschichte," *Arch. f. Kulturgeschichte* 19 (1928): 158–68; Pagel, *William Harvey's Biological Ideas*, pp. 24–28.

[33]A. S. MacNalty, "Sir Thomas More as a Student of Medicine and Public Health Reformer" (Chadwick Lecture, 1945), in Underwood, *Science, Medicine, and History*, 1:418–36; C. Webster, "Thomas Linacre and the Foundation of the College of

Physicians," in *Linacre Studies: Essays on the Life and Work of Thomas Linacre c. 1460–1524*, ed. F. Maddison, M. Pelling, and C. Webster (Oxford: Clarendon Press, 1977), pp. 198–222.

[34]C. Webster, "Physicians and Magicians in London: 1550–1640" (lectures delivered at Adelaide University, June 1979).

[35]C. Webster, *The Great Instauration: Science, Medicine and Reform, 1626–1660* (London: Duckworth, 1975); P. M. Rattansi, "Paracelsus and the Puritan Revolution," *Ambix* 11 (1963): 23–32.

[36]C. Hill, "William Harvey and the Idea of Monarchy," *Past and Present* no. 27 (1964); the article is included with debate between Hill and G. Whitteridge in *The Intellectual Revolution of the Seventeenth Century*, ed. C. Webster (London: Routledge & Kegan Paul, 1974), pp. 160–96; M. Curtis, *Oxford and Cambridge in Transition* (Oxford: Clarendon Press, 1964), pp. 227–60; C. Hill, *Intellectual Origins of the English Revolution* (Oxford: Clarendon Press, 1965), pp. 301–14; B. J. Shapiro, *John Wilkins 1614–1672: An Intellectual Biography* (Berkeley and Los Angeles: University of California Press, 1969), pp. 81–147; Webster, *The Great Instauration*, pp. 51–99; M. Hunter, *Science and Society in Restoration England* (Cambridge, At the University Press, 1981).

[37]H. E. Sigerist, "The History of Medicine and the History of Science: An Open Letter to George Sarton, Editor of *Isis*," *Bull. Inst. Hist. Med.* 4 (1936): 1–13 (a reply to Sarton's second preface to *Isis* 23 (1935): 313–20, entitled "The History of Science Versus the History of Medicine"); More recent statements concentrating on the nineteenth century, roughly consistent with the views of Sigerist, include J. Woodward and D. Richards, "Towards a Social History of Medicine," in Woodward and Richards, *Health Care and Popular Medicine* pp.15–55; G. Grob, "The Social History of Medicine and Disease in America," *J. Soc. Hist.* 10 (1977): 391–409.

[38]E. A. Wrigley, "Family Limitation in Pre-Industrial England," *Ec. Hist. Rev.*, 2nd ser., 19 (1966): 82–109; idem, "Mortality in Pre-Industrial England: The example of Colyton, Devon over Three Centuries," *Daedalus* 97 (1968): 246–80.

[39]Particularly influential are a series of contributions by T. McKeown, starting from McKeown and R. G. Brown, "Medical Evidence Related to English Population Changes in the Eighteenth Century," *Population Studies* 9 (1955–56): 285–307, to the most recent *The Modern Rise of Population* (London: Arnold, 1976). For the most detailed survey of the demographic impact of famine and epidemic disease, see J. D. Post, "Famine Mortality and Epidemic Disease in the Process of Modernisation," *Economic History Review* 29 (1976): 14–37. The most adequate general survey of the preindustrial period is J. D. Chambers, *Population, Economy, and Society in Pre-Industrial England* (London: Oxford University Press, 1972). The most detailed regional study is M. Flinn, ed., *Scottish Population from the Seventeenth Century to the 1930s* (Cambridge: At the University Press, 1977), pp. 107–200.

[40]A. B. Appleby, "Disease or Famine? Mortality in Cumberland and Westmorland: 1580–1640," *Economic History Review* 26 (1973): 403–32; V. Skipp, *Crisis and Development: An Ecological Case Study of the Forest of Arden: 1570–1674* (Cambridge: At the University Press, 1978), pp. 37–38; M. Flinn, ed., *Scottish Population History*, pp. 116–32.

[41]C. Morris, "Plague in Britain," in *The Plague Reconsidered: A New Look at the Origins and Effects in 16th and 17th Century England*, Local Population Studies Supplement (Matlock, Derbyshire, 1977), pp. 37–48; I. Sutherland, "When Was the Great Plague?: Mortality in London, 1565–1665," in *Population and Social Change*, ed. D. V. Glass and R. Revelle (London: Edward Arnold, 1972), pp. 287–320.

[42]P. Slack, "The Local Incidence of Epidemic Disease: The Case of Bristol 1540–1650," in *The Plague Reconsidered*, p. 59; idem, "Mortality Crises and Epidemic Disease in England: 1485–1610" in *Health, Medicine and Mortality in the Sixteenth Century*, ed. C. Webster (Cambridge: At the University Press, 1979), p. 19.

[43]R. Schofield and E. A. Wrigley, "Infant and Child Mortality in the Late Tudor and Early Stuart Period," in Webster, *Health, Medicine and Mortality*, p. 61–95.

[44]F. West, "Infant Mortality in the East Fen Parishes of Leake and Wrangle," *Local Population Studies* 13 (1974): 41–44; C. Cunningham, "Christ's Hospital: Infant and Child Mortality in the Sixteenth Century," *Local Population Studies* 12 (1977): 37–40. R.A.P. Finlay, "The Accuracy of the London Parish Registers: 1580–1653," *Population Studies* 32 (1978): 95–112; R. E. Jones, "Infant Mortality in Rural North Staffordshire: 1561–1810," *Population Studies* 30 (1976): 305–17.

[45]D. McLaren, "Fertility, Infant Mortality, and Breast Feeding in the Seventeenth Century," *Med. Hist.* 22 (1978): 378–96.

[46]T. R. Forbes, *Chronicle from Aldgate: Life and Death in Shakespeare's London* (New Haven: Yale University Press, 1971), pp. 86–118; idem, "By What Disease or Casualty: The Changing Face of Death in London," in Webster, *Health, Medicine and Mortality*, pp. 117–39.

[47]John Graunt, *Natural and Political Observations upon the Bills of Mortality* (London, 1662), chap. 3.

[48]John Bell, *Londons Remembrancer* (London, 1665).

[49]Graunt, *Natural Observations*; William Heberden, Jr., *Observations on the Increase and Decrease of Different Diseases, and Particularly of the Plague* (London, 1801).

[50]Graunt, *Natural Observations*, chap. 3.

[51]L. Babb, *The Elizabethan Malady: A Study of Melancholy in English Literature from 1580 to 1642* (East Lansing: Michigan State University Press, 1951); B. G. Lyons, *Voices of Melancholy* (London: Routledge & Kegan Paul, 1971); R. L. Colie, *Shakespeare's Living Art* (Princeton: Princeton University Press, 1974).

[52]A. L. Rowse, *The Case Books of Simon Forman* (London: Weidenfeld and Nicolson, 1974).

[53]M. Macdonald, *Mystical Bedlam: Madness, Anxiety and Healing in Seventeenth Century England* (New York: Cambridge University Press, 1981).

[54]The barbarism of family relations in the early modern period contrasted with affective individualism in recent times is articulated in strikingly different ways by P. Ariès, *L'Enfant et la vie familiale dans l'ancien regime* (Paris: Plon, 1960); E. Shorter, *The Making of the Modern Family* (New York: Basic Books, 1975); L. Stone, *The Family, Sex, and Marriage in England: 1500–1800* (London: Weidenfeld and Nicolson, 1977). For a rival, if controversial view, see A. Macfarlane, *Origins of English Individualism* (Oxford: Blackwell, 1978).

[55]Sir George Clark, *History of the Royal College of Physicians* (Oxford: Clarendon Press for the Royal College of Physicians, 1964), 1:111–21, 143–47, 261–64.

[56]R. S. Roberts, "The London Apothecaries and Medical Practice in Tudor and Stuart England" (Ph.D. diss., London University, 1964).

[57]Webster, "Physicians and Magicians in London."

[58]A useful trial exercise is W. J. Birken, "The Fellows of the Royal College of Physicians of London, 1603–1623: A Social Study" (Ph.D. diss., University of North Carolina, 1977), primarily useful for its exploration of the Puritan religious associations of the families of many Fellows.

[59]Above estimates derived from: C. Webster, M. Pelling et al., "Biographical Index of The Annals of the College of Physicians 1550–1640 and "Biographical Index of Records of the Barber Surgeons' Company 1540–1640," Wellcome Unit for the History of Medicine, Oxford.

[60]M. Pelling and C. Webster, "Medical Practitioners," in Webster, *Health, Medicine and Mortality*, pp. 166–89.

[61]Pelling and Webster, "Medical Practitioners," pp. 205–33.

[62]J. H. Raach, *A Directory of English Country Physicians: 1603–1643* (London: Dawson, 1962).

[63]William Clowes, *A Brief Treatise of Morbus Gallicus* (London, 1585), fol. 8. r.

[64]The most notorious case is perhaps that of Leonard Poe, who was vigorously prosecuted by the College between 1589 and 1606. He built up an aristocratic practice and was appointed physician to the royal household in 1609. Thereafter he was admitted fellow of the college in 1609, and was granted a doctorate of medicine at Cambridge in 1615. See Royal College of Physicians of London, MS Annals, cited by kind permission of the President and Fellows.

[65]Royal College of Physicians, MS Annals.

[66]Webster, "Physicians and Magicians in London."

[67]William Bullein, *Bulwarke of Defence againste All Sickness* (London, 1564), pp. 56 v–57 r.

[68]Margaret Paston to John Paston, 8 June 1464: "God's sake beware what medicines you take of physicians in London," who had killed both his father and her uncle, N. Davis, ed., *Paston Letters and Papers of the Fifteenth Century: Part I* (Oxford: Clarendon Press, 1971), p. 291. For a similar warning concerning the dangers of medicine see Sir John Salusbury's poem, "Certaine Neccessary Observations For Health" (1603), in *Poems by Sir John Salusbury and Robert Chester*, ed. C. Brown (London: Early English Text Society, 1914), p. 28.

[69]K. V. Thomas, *Religion and the Decline of Magic* (London: Weidenfeld and Nicolson, 1972); A. Macfarlane, *Witchcraft in Tudor and Stuart England* (London: Routledge & Kegan Paul, 1970).

[70]Francis Bacon, *De sapientia veterum* (London, 1609), Fable 25, "Atalanta sive lucrum."

Commentary

Don G. Bates

Professor Webster began by speaking of Sir William Osler. He was, Webster said, "a figure whose ineradicable mark is etched into the fabric of [Hopkins and Oxford] on either side of the Atlantic." Now this is at least one statement on which I can easily comment. The institution from which Osler received his primary medical education, to which he gave the first ten years of his professorial career, and upon which he bestowed his magnificent library of the history of medicine would not forgive me if I did not add the name of McGill University to the list of those places upon which Osler has left his "ineradicable mark."

Making this amendment to Professor Webster's opening remarks was easy. After that, however, I find myself in difficulty. There is much in his essay with which I agree and much else by which I am impressed and persuaded. In particular, I enjoyed his review of the literature on sixteenth- and seventeenth-century medicine and the rich documentation of this story that he has furnished in his notes. If he had done nothing more, this would have been an eminently useful exercise.

As I see it, there are three phases to Webster's history of British historiography of medicine in Shakespeare's England: before 1930, when members of the medical profession cultivated biobibliography and the history of particular institutions and specialties; after 1930, when professionalization of the field occurred largely under the umbrella of the history of science; and the very recent past, when the cultivation of a social historiography of medicine has gradually increased in sophistication.

Webster feels that the earliest period left compilations of permanent value but a historical analysis that has not endured except as a "reflection of the mentality of the Edwardian and Victorian medical elites." The trend to the history of science after 1930 receives Webster's severest criticism, it having focused too narrowly on one aspect of medicine and, for a long time, having wrenched even that part out of its social context. More recently, along with the history of science in general, this context is being restored, but it remains a fact that, as reflected in British academic institutions, the history of medicine continues to be seen as the history of medical sciences, a perspective that relates "to a highly selected intellectual elite within medicine." Meanwhile this has "continued to deflect attention away from medicine as it was [typically] practised" while "the patient has been almost entirely

127

disregarded." This neglect has gone on despite the fact that Henry Sigerist called for this approach as early as 1936.

Webster then deals with the third phase by reviewing recent efforts to make good this deficiency, but observes that the most active "steps towards the realization of a social history of medicine have been taken by social historians and social scientists, rather than medical historians." The latter, he maintains, still languish in the grip of the history of science, however broadly conceived.

I have no fundamental disagreement with this thesis but would like to add a greater emphasis to some points that Webster has only touched upon.

With respect to institutional developments, it is instructive to compare the British experience with that of North America. As Webster has noted, medical institutions in Britain did not provide an academic base for medical history. Had they done so, would the story have come out differently?

On the face of it, the experience of North America, from about 1930 to 1960 (roughly Webster's middle phase), would seem to argue that it would have. Hopkins harbored Sigerist, and then Shryock. Wisconsin had its Ackerknecht.[1] Still, despite these and other notable exceptions, it seems fair to say that the social history of medicine was not pursued in medical centers in North America during this time with either the sophistication or the breadth that Professor Webster has called for, nor in a volume that greatly exceeds that of Great Britain.

What about the obverse proposition? Was North American historiography less influenced by the institutionalization of the history of science than that of Great Britain during this time? It is impossible to answer with any assurance. Certainly the history of science increased its academic base enormously and there was a feeling in some quarters in the 1960s that the history of medicine might be swallowed up by departments of the history of science.[2]

More important, to my mind, is the fact that a science orientation, similar to that which Webster described for Great Britain, is very much in evidence within the subject matter of medical history in North America.[3] In other words, had British medical historiography not had to contend with the strong institutional embrace of the history of science, nor the simultaneous absence of its own professional development in medical schools, it still seems likely that things would have turned out much the same as they did.

On both sides of the Atlantic, the rapid professionalization of the history of science had a strong influence on the history of medicine for other reasons besides institutional arrangements. Webster mentions, in passing, "a changing balance of values within medical schools as the pure sciences came to dominate medicical education and medical research." Surely this trend deserves greater emphasis. It led not only to the leaving out of the patient and society, it also meant the ignoring altogether of vast realms of clinical medicine, at least by many professional historians of medicine. Medical history was not just science oriented, it was basic science oriented.

Then too, in its fondness for the history of ideas during this period the history of science offered an attractive approach to medical historiography. This more or less rigorously internalist viewpoint had the advantage of being able to use present-day scientific knowledge as a seemingly firm reference point for posing questions, measuring progress, and giving a special *raison d'être* to those historians with a knowledge of current scientific and technical medicine. Perhaps unconsciously, this type of history also seemed more polished and valid when set over against the amateur form from which an increasingly professionalized medical history was trying to distance itself.

In short, I would be inclined to give a little more emphasis to the values then internationally current in medicine and among medical historians than to the unique institutional developments in Britain: in view of the fact that even the institutional voices of a Sigerist, a Shryock, or an Ackerknecht were not often heard, or at least heeded, before the 1960s.

There is another factor that is muted in Webster's account, and that is the influence of professional orthodoxy on medical historiography; that is, the selective fostering of that set of values which redound to the legitimation and reinforcement of the profession's image of itself and the neglect of, or opposition to, those that do not. One of the medical profession's strongly held values during the thirties, forties, and fifties has already been mentioned — the belief that what is scientific in medicine is good. The value placed on science, however, was by no means peculiar to the medical profession. It was ubiquitous in the larger society. Indeed, partly because of this widespread reverence for science, the medical profession stood to benefit from any connection that resided in the public mind between the healing art and medical science.

There is, however, a subtle but important difference in valuing science for its instrumental utility, and valuing it for the symbolic worth it bestows upon its possessors and producers. For example, interest in William Harvey reflects, it is true, the influences of the history of science. But it also reflects the profession's desire to celebrate a great medical luminary. This interest existed before 1930 and after 1960, within the history of science, within academic medical history, and also among avocational historians.[4] I doubt that the history of science has been any more responsible for Harvey's great popularity than the fact that he is a gem in the crown of a medical profession proud of its contribution to a publicly valued science.

My point, then, is that it is not always possible to distinguish between the impact of the history of science and the influence of medical orthodoxy, since there has been, during the time in question, a social reason, as well as an instrumental one, for making the profession eager to associate medicine with science.

This same orthodoxy is possibly even more important in accounting for the lack of growth of social history. No student of that era can seriously argue that medical orthodoxy was oriented to, or even very friendly with, the social dimensions of medicine in the way in which Webster perceives them. Even public health and preventive medicine eventually had to change their names before they could join "the club."[5]

One can also see the workings of orthodoxy in Sir George Clark's *History of the Royal College of Physicians*. Webster criticizes, quite rightly in my opinion, the overly narrow definition of what constituted a competent, as distinct from a legitimate, healer in this work. In explaining Clark's bias, Webster would have been justified in pointing out that Clark was invited by the Royal College to write this history, and that people quite closely associated with the college's leadership were involved in its preparation. In Clark's *History*, then, I see the influence of orthodoxy even when science is not directly involved.[6]

There is another way in which professional values have influenced medical historiography. Webster has traced the largely profession-supported tradition of biography, biobibliography, and histories of particular specialties and institutions up to about 1930. But any full account of the medical historiography of Shakespeare's England must take some notice of the continuation of that earlier tradition through the next three decades. Some mention would have to·be made, for example, of people like Keynes, Cope, Guthrie, Franklin, and Bishop.[7] The list would have to include Copeman's *Doctors and Disease in Tudor Times*, and Keevil's twin volumes, *Hamey the Stranger* and *The Stranger's Son*. Most particularly, it could not leave out that same author's *Medicine and the Navy: 1200–1900*.[8]

The reason why Webster left these out, I presume, is that he felt that they do not represent any advance on the generation of Power and Osler to whom they looked for inspiration. The implication is that, like their predecessors, they gained their enduring value largely as a reflection of the mentality of a medical elite. If this is Webster's view, I find the judgment that this was their *chief* value a little harsh. But I would agree that such writings continue to manifest, as did those of their renowned forebears, the values of a medical profession, or what I have called professional orthodoxy.

What are the values that these works reflect? I would argue that they include those of individualism and humanism and that these lie even closer to the core of the profession's self-image than does the value of science, particularly for that part of the profession which is associated with clinical practice.

Reference to these values is, I think, important. For example, while such values are tolerant of science, on the whole they relate (though unconsciously perhaps) more to its symbolic than to its utilitarian role. More importantly, the chronic tension between basic scientists and clinicians, between research clinicians and practitioners, between science-oriented gown and practice-oriented town, suggests that science has its limits in the eyes of the practicing profession. Within medical history, this same limit of toleration has been shown towards the professionalization of that subject, which has been received with some ambivalence, even when it manifests itself in the otherwise attractive garb of the history of medical science.

Indeed, the argument might be pushed further. In Britain, where science and technology have not, perhaps, weighed as heavily against these entrenched values of individualism and humanism within medicine, it could be argued that the very vigor of these latter has played as important a role in resisting the professionalization of medical history in medical schools as it has in sustaining the remarkably strong avocational interest in that subject that clinicians and their organizations have shown up to the present day.[9]

In summary, I believe that the three decades after 1930, while marked by some notable exceptions of course, were, on both sides of the Atlantic, not only science oriented but "professionocentric."[10]

The decades of the sixties and seventies are more complex as far as comparison of Britain and North America is concerned. There does seem to have been, temporarily at least, a fostering of the social history of medicine in the U.S., on a scale not found in Britain before the 1970s. (Whether many of its practitioners qualify in Webster's mind as *bona fide* medical historians and not social historians or social scientists, I am not clear. And, of course, their contributions are not particularly oriented to Shakespeare's England.)

Probably this U.S. interest in the social history of medicine had something to do with the influx of substantial support for training and research from the National Institutes of Health, a large federal granting agency that was quite flexible in defining the nature of the field. But it is also possible that the rapid growth of social and behavioral sciences within medical schools played a part, a phenomenon that does not appear to have had as great a counterpart in Britain.

Whatever the case may be, by Webster's own testimony, a full range of studies is now appearing that reflects the social history of medicine in its manifold expression — the social history of scientific thought, of lay views on health and disease, of the practices of the unorthodox but more typical practitioner, of medical professionalism, and the history of the patient himself.

This being so, I am left finally with a problem about the thrust of Webster's remarks concerning the future. When he says that "the most active steps towards the realization of a social history of medicine have been taken by social historians and social scientists, rather than medical historians," I wonder what he means exactly by "medical historians."[11] Throughout this commentary, I have taken him to mean a professional historian focusing on aspects of medicine and health and based either in a quasi-autonomous medical history academic unit or in a medical school, as distinct from a historian based in a history or social sciences academic unit. But I find this unsatisfactory, not only because I am not sure that this is what Webster means but also because I do not see its significance. Unfortunately, Webster does not make clear the connection between such institutional affiliations and the making of "a major contribution to medical thinking and to the social sciences," or between the lack of such connections and "the impoverishment of our discipline and . . . risk of institutional redundancy."

As for the 1970s, this is the only part of Webster's account with which I frankly disagree. There are, I believe, encouraging signs that the social history of medicine is coming of age in Britain. The process may be slow—there may still be discouraging impediments for those most closely involved—but there are clear indications of change. The Society for the Social History of Medicine and the work of Thomas McKeown, to pick out only two examples best known on this side of the water, suggest a promising future. More particularly, the work of the Wellcome Unit at Oxford, under Webster's direction, is a sign that this future is already here. Indeed, the publications of Webster himself make him an outstanding exception to his own argument.

NOTES

[1]George Rosen's career is not straightforward enough to serve as a clearcut example.

[2]Cf. D. G. Bates, "The History of Medicine as Part of the University Complex," in ed. John B. Blake, *Education in the History of Medicine: Report of a Macy Conference*, (New York: Stechert-Hafner, 1968), pp. 85–92.

[3]Webster himself noted that Singer was invited to the post at Hopkins before Sigerist and cites work by Rather, Debus, (note 24), Frank, Brown, and Bylebyl as research that is still oriented to science, however sophisticated it may be as to social context. Commenting on the failure of Hopkins to appoint a successor to him, Sigerist told George Rosen that he thought it opportune to double the scope of the Institute by introducing both the sociology of medicine and possibly the history of science "for which there is so much interest in America at the moment." Arthur J. Viseltear, "The George Rosen—Henry E. Sigerist Correspondence," *J. Hist. Med.* 33 (1978): 281–313; letter of 13 February 1948, p. 295.

[4]Harvey's name was used in the interests of the beleaguered Royal College of Medicine as early as the 1670s. Robert G. Frank, Jr., "The Image of Harvey in Commonwealth and Restoration England," in *William Harvey and His Age: The Professional and Social Context of the Discovery of the Circulation*, ed. Jerome J. Bylebyl (Baltimore: The Johns Hopkins University Press, 1979), pp. 103–43; see especially the section "Harvey and the Harveians for the Defense of Physicians," pp. 124–29, and p. 135. At that time, however, the value of science for medicine (in the form of anatomical studies) had to be argued for against opponents who apparently had much public support for the view that such knowledge did not cure sick people.

[5]I refer to terms like "community medicine," or "community health sciences." To this day, in North America, the term "social medicine" is assiduously avoided in professional circles.

[6]In vol. 1, 1964, Clark says that the "invitation to write this book. . . was conveyed by its former President, Lord Moran," (p. [v]) who, he continues, gave much advice and stimulation throughout its progress. He also received hospitality from Lady Moran and research assistance from Lady Frank. The officers of the college, he reports, expedited his work but never exercised any censorship nor saw anything he had written. Given the shared values and world view of Clark and his college assistants, such restraints would hardly have been necessary. Indeed, as a relative newcomer to the medical profession when this book first came out, I too was not sensitive to its professionocentric perspective. It is only the insights of the social sciences to which I have been subsequently exposed that have made me wonder how I could have missed this orientation at the time.

[7]The very extensive biobibliographical work of Keynes is taken notice of by Webster (note 18). That of W. R. Le Fanu would have to be included if other periods of history were being considered. Institutional histories include not only Zachary Cope's *The Royal College of Surgeons of England, A History* (London: Anthony Blond, 1959), but also lesser known works such as Maurice Davidson, *Medicine in Oxford: A Historical Romance*, The Fitzpatrick Lectures of 1952–53 (Oxford: Basil Blackwell, 1953); and Walter Langdon-Brown, *Some Chapters in Cambridge Medical History* (Cambridge: At the University Press, 1946). A general work is Douglas Guthrie, *A History of Medicine* (London: Thomas Nelson & Sons, 1945). Guthrie also collaborated with R. Scott Stevenson to produce the history of a specialty, *A History of Oto-Laryngology* (Edinburgh: E. & S. Livingstone, 1949). Other British examples of the genre are Harvey Graham, *Surgeons All* (London: Rich & Cowan, 1939; 2d ed. 1956); Kenneth J. Franklin, *A Short History of Physiology* (New York: Staples Press, 2d ed., 1949, having first appeared in 1933). W. J. Bishop not only contributed to specialty histories (*The Early History of Surgery* [London: Robert Hale, 1960]), he also compiled, with Hamilton Bailey, the biographies for *Notable Names in Medicine and Surgery* (London: H. K. Lewis, 3d ed. 1959), which was preceded by editions of 1944 and 1946.

[8]Copeman's book was published in London by Dawson's of Pall Mall, 1960, Keevil's three books, also in London, by George Blas (1952), George Blas (1953), and E. & S. Livingstone, vol. 1, 1957, vol. 2, 1958, respectively. Other works specifically related to the period include Arthur S. MacNalty, *The Renaissance and its Influence on English Medicine, Surgery, and Public Health*, The Thomas Vicary Lecture for 1945 (London: Christopher Johnson, 1946); idem, *Henry VIII, A Difficult Patient* (London: Christopher Johnson, 1952); K. D. Keele, *Leonardo da Vinci on the Movement of the Heart and Blood* (London, 1952); *Selected Writings of William Clowes: 1544–1604*, ed., with intro. and notes by F.N.L. Poynter (London: Harvey & Blythe Ltd., 1948); Kenneth J. Franklin, *William Harvey, Englishman: 1578–1657* (London: MacGibbon & Kee, 1961); and *Movement of the Heart and Blood in Animals, An Anatomical Essay by William Harvey*, trans. Kenneth J. Franklin (Oxford: Blackwell, 1957). In both this footnote and the previous one no attempt has been made to give a complete list of works produced by British authors but only a sampling of the monographic literature which illustrates that both the types of literature under discussion and Shakespeare's England were well represented between 1930 and 1960. It will be appreciated that, although some valuable and important contributions are included, my list is uncritical. However, the quality of the work is not the point. What is being argued is that this is largely the work of those who, like Osler and Power before them, were either physicians or, if not, then gainfully employed in medical institutions at occupations other than that of historian of medicine. They demonstrate that the old tradition, the Oslerian tradition as it is often called, of avocational medical history has continued to thrive in the British medical community.

[9]These views and attitudes are clearly discernable in Douglas Guthrie, "Whither Medical History?" *Med. Hist.* 1 (1957): 307–17. As he suggests, the history of medicine is to be cultivated as an antidote to the evils of specialization. Another common motive for avocational historians is to emphasize the art, the humanistic dimension of the medical enterprise.

At the risk of confusing the argument, I might mention that Osler expended a great deal of time, energy, and words to increase and improve the use of science in medical practice and medical education, but he is now universally celebrated as a great humanist physician and his interest in history is now imitated partly as an antidote to the over-emphasis on science in medicine.

[10]If such a horrible word may be allowed to live! The more commonly used "iatrocentric" is less clumsy but also not quite as suggestive of the meaning given to it. See

J. Woodward and D. Richards, cited by Webster (note 15). These British authors, although dealing with the historiography of nineteenth-century medicine, complain of an "iatrocentric" rather than a history of science focus (see Webster, note 37). The other survey to which Webster appeals, that of Grob, also has little to do with the impact of the history of science. It is really a complaint that social historians have not interested themselves in medical and health issues and activities.

[11]A difficulty that I also find with the article by Grob.

ON THE SOURCE AND DEVELOPMENT OF METAPHORICAL LANGUAGE IN THE HISTORY OF WESTERN MEDICINE*

L. J. Rather

The phrase "Western medicine" in my title refers to a system of theory and practice that took form among the physicians and philosophers of ancient Greece. It then spread to encompass the entire Mediterranean world and eventually reached Western Europe, where it became ensconced in the medieval universities as one of the traditional four faculties: theology, philosophy, law, and medicine. In this tradition—and it is, of course, not the sole Western medical tradition—"practice" is more or less confined to the cure of ailments of the *body*, by means of hygienic measures, drugs, and surgery. Correspondingly, "theory" deals with the material constitution of the body, of its mode of functioning, and of its interaction with the physical environment. Our university medical schools continue to maintain this tradition. It is, for example, easy to show that the present-day "basic medical sciences" cover the same ground as the several elements of "theory" in the medical writings of Galen; that is, the field of studies has remained unchanged in scope, despite the enormous development of the sciences (anatomy, physiology, biochemistry, and pathology) in question.[1] Due to a slightly deviant course taken in England and North America, the tie between medicine and the universities there was not secured until, historically speaking, a short time ago. I should add that I use the word "ensconced" in the above account deliberately, for at the present time Western academic medicine, while still triumphantly asserting its superiority, finds itself forced to take serious account of medical claims asserted by adherents of nonacademic or non-Western systems. Indeed, for someone miraculously transported from a university medical school of fifty years ago to one of today this might prove to be the most surprising development of all.

The above remarks are made in order to define the limits, geographical and temporal, within which my interest in the use of metaphor, analogy, simile, and the like in the language of medicine has been contained. A small body of literature on this topic already exists.[2] For the sake of brevity I shall use the term "metaphor" here in an all-inclusive sense, and I begin with a striking instance of what is in fact a full-fledged analogy. In the mid seventeenth century Thomas Willis, the great physician of Oxford University, wrote:

135

We are not only born and nourished by means of Ferments; but we also Dye; Every Disease acts its Tragedies by the strength of some Ferment...Yea we also endeavour the Cure of Diseases by the help of Fermentation; For to the preserving or recovering the Health of man, the business of a physician and a Vintner is almost the same: the blood and humours even as Wine, ought to be kept in an equal temper and motion of Fermentation; wherefore when the blood grows too hot, even as Wine, it is usual to empty out some of the Vessels, and to allay its Fervor with temperate things....I could easily unfold the Curatory intentions, as also the effects and operations of every Medicine, according to the Doctrine of Fermentation....[3]

In calling attention to this passage in 1971 at a symposium held in honor of the late Charles D. O'Malley, I remarked that in it the locus of the medical model for physiological and pathological processes had been shifted from the kitchen to the winery, and that Willis was presenting us here with the prospect of a complete oinophysiological, oinopathological, and oinotherapeutic system of medical thought and practice. "Fermentation" is, for Willis, a process of change induced by ferments in the chemical "principles," namely "salt, sulfur, spirit, earth, and water," constitutive of all material bodies.[4] We recognize here biochemistry at an early stage of its development, but freed nevertheless from its still earlier humoral trappings. For Willis, the language is still to some degree metaphorical, but for a modern biochemist nothing of metaphor remains: enzyme chemistry is one and the same thing, whether it deals with blood or wine. Surviving from Willis's time into the present day, however, are metaphors such as that of the blood "boiling" or "effervescing" in the veins. These are sometimes called "dead" metaphors, but they might better be called "undead," since they do in fact live on, deprived of real substance, like shadows without Peter Schlemihls. The really dead metaphor simply vanishes, as such. Another instance: Theodor Schwann, in 1838, spoke of the "analogy" between the cellular structure and growth of plants and animals, while for us today cells are cells, whether in plants or animals, and there is no "analogy" about it.[5]

Not long ago I conceived the idea of carrying out a historical survey of the use of metaphor in the language of Western medicine. I drew up a tentative table of contents in which I grouped metaphors in accordance with the sources from which they appeared to have been drawn. The list came to occupy five or six closely typewritten pages, and it threatened to go on expanding indefinitely. When I began with this project I seemed to myself to be working at a high level of abstraction. As time went on my view gradually underwent inversion. I now saw myself engaged in a search for the *roots* of abstract thought in the earthy, material conditions of human life on this planet, a life in which human beings are required, to an extent completely unknown among other animals, to produce their food, clothing, shelter, and other immediate necessities of life, as well as their complicated networks of family, social, economic, and political relations. Five things became evident to me as I continued to marshal, group, and study my metaphors. First, that a thorough knowledge of the history of technical procedures—the history of technology, so-called—was necessary in order to recognize and fully appreciate them as metaphors. Although some were derived simply from nature observed, a larger part came from human activities in the home, the hearth, the kitchen, from homecrafts such as cooking, baking, weaving, from the arts of the agriculturalist's field and the hunter's forest, from the workshops of tool-makers, machine-builders, chemists, and metallurgists, from mining, brewing, wine making, and a host of other technical procedures. Second, that an understanding of political, social, and economic history was called for as well, since the metaphors were at times drawn from the social roles played by individuals in society, from the structure of society itself, and from the great human preoccupation with war making, with defense, invasion, rebellion, civil strife, and so on. Third, that when new techniques became available and new natural forces exploitable, or when social relations changed, older metaphors were often displaced by new ones. Fourth, that metaphors employed in the languages or special vocabularies of medicine, science, politics, economics, and the study of human social life in general tended to shift back and fourth and roundabout, with the result that their precise place of origin was frequently uncertain. Finally, that while some metaphors were "mere" metaphors—this is, mere means of description—others anticipated the fusion of fields of thought hitherto considered separate, while still others were operative in solution of specific problems, or in the interpretation of the findings obtained.

Apropos of the revolution in the weaving industry in England brought about in 1745 by John Wyatt's spinning machine, Karl Marx commented in 1867:

> A critical history of technology would show how little any of the inventions of the 18th century are the work of a single individual. Hitherto there is no such book. Darwin has interested us in the history of Nature's Technology, *i.e.* in the formation of the organs of plants and animals (*Pflanzen- und Tierorgane*), which organs serve as instruments of production for sustaining life. Does not the history of the productive organs of man, of organs that are the material basis of all social organisation, deserve equal attention?... Technology discloses man's mode of dealing with Nature, the process of production by which he sustains his life, and thereby also lays bare the mode of formation of his social relations, and of the mental conceptions that flow from them.

I add that the translation "formative history of the productive organs of the social human being" is closer to the original "Bildungsgeschichte der produktiven Organe des Gesellschaftsmenschen" than the one given above.[6]

In this passage Marx identifies natural productive "organs" or "instruments" with artefactual "organs" or "instruments" of production constructed by human beings. Among other things, we have here a version of the old microcosm-macrocosm analogy, the "social human being" as the individual human being writ large. There is nothing new in this metaphorical assimilation of anatomical organs to instruments or tools produced by human hands. Marx was undoubtedly aware that the word "organ" is simply the Greek word *organon*, which means an organ, instrument, tool, or, alternatively, a part of a living body. *Organon* is cognate with the English word "work," by way of the Greek *ergō*, meaning "I work." As I have suggested elsewhere, the application by the early Greek anatomists of the term *organon* to the internal as well as the external parts—the latter are, quite obviously, working instruments—suggests that from the beginning the Greeks regarded the internal parts as functioning structures, or structures with functions; that is, as instruments intended for specific purposes.[7] What these purposes were was of course not always evident. The stomach and gut, perhaps, never presented a problem. But the heart, that most "noble " of organs, was seen variously as a center of heat, life, or emotional force, or as a kind of pressure-cooker where blood was mixed with inspired air, and "fuliginous vapors" of combustion were discharged to the exterior. Not until the seventeenth century did William Harvey lower its kingly status to more or less that of a lowly pump. It is somewhat disquieting to recall that Harvey's royal patron, Charles I, who is exalted as "the sun of the world" and "the heart of the republic" in the opening words of Harvey's disquisition on the motion of the heart and blood in animals, was shortened by a head only twenty-one years after the publication, in 1628, of *De motu cordis*.

Let us consider the word "tissue." Before the eighteenth century it was rarely used with reference to anything other than an actual fabric or cloth woven with threads spun by human hand. The word was used less frequently, even in this sense, at the beginning of the seventeenth century than might be supposed. Shakespeare employs it on one occasion only: he refers to a pavilion or tent on Cleopatra's barge as of "cloth of gold, of tissue." The translators of the King James Version of the Bible do not appear to have employed it at all. Nor does Shakespeare use the words "texture" or "fiber" in this or any other connection.[8] But in 1665 Robert Hooke called animal substance a "text of filaments," comparing it to "the infinite company of small filaments every way contexted and woven together, so as to make a kind of cloth" constituting the substance of mushrooms. He suggested that the "texture" of both plant and animal substance was fibrous throughout. And in 1671 Nehemiah Grew stated that plants "consist of fibers...wrapped and stitched (though in divers manners) together."[9] Bichat is said to have revived the Old French word *tissu* at the beginning of the nineteenth century and used it with reference to the metaphorical "tissues" or "membranes" of the body.[10] (In fact, the phrase *tissu cellulaire* was already well-enough known for Voltaire to have used it in his poem *La Pucelle*.) Bichat's contemporaries were aware that he had revived, expanded, and modified Albrecht von Haller's eighteenth-century doctrine of the tissues, in particular that of the *tela cellulosa* or "cellular tissue." Haller too was aware of the historical antecedents of his doctrine, namely the medieval and early modern anatomical doctrine of the "similar" and "dissimilar" parts of the body. These two terms—roughly corresponding to present-day "tissues" and "organs"—come, by way of the Arab translators and students of ancient Greek medicine, from the Aristotelian terms *homoiomere* and *anomoiomere*. A thorough and easily available exposition of the doctrine of the similar and dissimilar parts may be found in Robert Burton's *Anatomy of Melancholy*, a work first published in 1621, five years after Shakespeare's death and seven years before the appearance of Harvey's *De motu cordis*. The fountainhead of the doctrine of similar and dissimilar parts is of course Aristotle's treatise on anatomy, best known by its Latin title, *De partibus animalium*. In 1819, at the University of Bonn, A.F.J.K. Mayer coined the term "histology" (*Histologie*)—from the Greek *histos*, meaning "web"—for the study of the tissues of animal bodies, the Greeks having no word for it. Mayer's histology, like Bichat's study of the tissues, made no use of the microscope.[11]

How far back into the past can we trace the metaphorical assimilation of the natural fabric of human beings, animals, and plants to artefacts woven, plaited, or strung from plant and animal fibers by human hands? Can we be certain that natural fabrics were assimilated to man-made fabrics, rather than the other way around? The possibility that examination of the natural structure of plants and animals inspired some early human being to fashion a roughly similar artifact cannot be ruled out, but it seems highly unlikely. (The same holds true for the assimilation of man-made tools or instruments to the "organs" of the body, although in this case it would not be far fetched to imagine a clever primitive fashioning a pair of pincers after having closely observed a crab.) Weaving, spinning, plaiting, and their allied pursuits are among the oldest and most ubiquitous of the domestic arts.[12] Sooner or later the notion of comparing these man-made artifacts to the "tissues" of plants and animals from which their actual substance was derived would have to assert itself, but we must leave it to medical anthropologists to tell us whether and how often this occurred in cultures other than our own. We are told by William Laughlin, who has studied the anatomical vocabulary of various Eskimo tribes, that the organization of the mammalian body "provides a basis for intellectual organization," and that "anatomical analogies and reasoning are found in all cultures."[13] The problem, of course, is to get at the process in the beginning. Once intellectual structures have been built a ready interchange of metaphor may occur. The starting point of the metaphor may then be difficult or impossible to ascertain.

I should add that I use the term "man-made" here in a generic sense only. In the case of most domestic arts, the "makers" were not men but women. Direct evidence for this claim is easy to find, and an interesting bit of indirect evidence is the fact that the metaphorical spinners of human destiny— the Moirai and Parcae of the Greeks and Romans (Clotho, Lachesis, and Atropos) and the three Norns (Urd, Verdandi, and Skuld) of the Northern

Europeans—are always female, and are often depicted with spindle, distaff, and thread in hand. The same may be said of the arts of brewing and wine making. According to R. J. Forbes, the art of brewing in Old Babylonia stood under the tutelage of two goddesses. The rise to preeminence of all-powerful male deities, and the shift of certain activities from the home to the outside world, led to the displacement of women from this and other fields. "With the semitization of the country [Old Babylonia], and with the advent of mass-production of beer," says Forbes, "the female brewer made place for her male counterpart, as she did in practically all other countries."[14]

We turn now to the word "cell." In 1858 Friedrich Engels, who kept himself very well-informed on developments in the natural sciences, wrote to Karl Marx that during the past two decades the whole of physiology had been revolutionized by Schleiden and Schwann's "discovery" of the cell, and by the enormous progress of organic chemistry.[15] Marx duly took note of his friend's letter. In 1867, in the preface to Volume I of the first edition of *Das Kapital*, we find him using Schwann's cell—by then more important than ever—to highlight the importance of his own discovery of the ultimate economic unit of capitalist organization, namely the "money-form" assumed by all human products and relations in a capitalist economy. Marx writes that "neither microscopes nor chemical reagents" are of use in the analysis of the minutiae of economic forms; only by means of the "force of abstraction" has he discovered that the money-form of a commodity is in fact the "economic cell-form" of the capitalist organism.[16] The passage as it stands is little more than one of the innumerable witty plays of fancy to be found scattered throughout Marx's writings. I shall develop Marx's metaphor a bit further, in order to foreshadow the third part of my essay.

For Schwann, the cell is the primary constitutive unit of plant and animal organisms. In its earliest manifestation the cell exists as a relatively simple, rounded, or polyhedral microscopic body. The key to the understanding of structure and function in living organisms is, he says, the fact that these simple objects multiply and undergo metamorphosis in the course of growth and development to yield the multiform units constitutive of tissues and organs. For Marx, on the other side, the multiform products of human minds and hands are the units of any economic organism, and the characteristic feature of the capitalist organism is that in it the "product" undergoes metamorphosis into a "money-form"; this is the key to the understanding of the way the capitalist system works. Metamorphosis takes place in reverse, so to speak, from the complicated to the simple: the "product" becomes a "commodity," the commodity casts off its "use-value" to become "exchange-value," and exchange-value finally reveals itself as that universal commodity and master of human relations, money. For Marx, we must remember, a commodity is a disguised form of human relationship; and, according to Marx, as the capitalist organism matures, *all* relations between human beings caught up in it tend to become transformed into money relations. This is, of course, the omnipresent "cash nexus" made famous, or rather infamous, by Thomas Carlyle, a generation before Marx subjected it to closer scrutiny.

Usually—and this is a qualification to which we shall return later—the cells of living organisms work harmoniously together for the benefit of the "unified commonwealth" (as Rudolf Virchow called it in 1859), of which they are integral parts.[17] According to Marx, the situation is quite otherwise in the case of the economic cell-form of the capitalist organism. In Marx's terms a "contradiction"—which means a *real*, not merely a *logical*, conflict— arises because of the necessity of positing all products doubly, as both "commodity" and "money-form." As commodities, products retain their naturally inherent qualities as useful objects; in the money-form, however, all such qualities have disappeared (except insofar as money itself is a useful commodity). The contradiction of which Marx speaks manifests itself when the economic laws regulating the movement of useful commodities come into conflict with those regulating the movement of money; for example, when grain or coffee is burnt or dumped in order to keep up the price, or when pigs are plowed under, as we used to say in the 1930s. For this and other reasons, Marx, as is well known, thought that capitalism was an inherently unstable, ultimately self-destructive system, despite its truly remarkable productive accomplishments over the past few hundred years.[18]

Every feature of nature perceived, every human product, procedure, or mode of relationship—from the simplest tool to the most complicated mechanisms of interrelationship of whole societies—acquires in the course of time a metaphorical value. A king's scepter is only a sublimated form of the club still wielded by the hand of the policeman. The metaphorical use of words was called "catachresis," or misuse, by older grammarians who, as Darmesteter has pointed out, failed to see that so-called catachresis was an act of emancipation for words, one of the vital forces directing the growth of language.[19] The object, product, procedure, or form of interaction, whether economic, social, political, or military, is used as a model to aid in the explanation and manipulation of some thing other than itself. A case in point is inflammation. Both the pathophysiological nature of the inflammatory process and its meaning for the economy of the whole organism have been perennial subjects of interest since the earliest years of Western medicine. A large number of interesting changes in the interpretation of the overall significance of inflammation have occurred. During the past fifty years yet another significant change has taken place, to which I shall devote some attention in this section of my paper.

The Latin word *inflammatio*, which has come directly into English as "inflammation," was rarely used in its technical medical sense until the late sixteenth or early seventeenth century: this, despite the use of it by Celsus in the first century of our era as the equivalent of the Greek *phlegmonē*. The great Latin dictionaries of the sixteenth century do not list the medical meaning of the word.[20] In classical Latin *inflammation* means a "conflagration," the result of something having been set on fire: hence the use of it as a trope by Cicero and others — "inflamed by desire," "inflammatory words," and so on. As for the equivalent word in Greek, it is interesting to find that Plato used it in both the general sense and the technical medical sense. He discusses inflammatory diseases in the *Timaeus*, for example, while in the *Republic* (II, 372, E) he contrasts an "inflamed" (*phlegmainousan*) city with a "healthy" (*hygiēs*) city. (Modern translators seem to prefer "fevered" or "feverish" to "inflamed.")

What I wish to discuss here is not the metaphor involved in naming "inflammation" as such, but the metaphors involved in the *interpretation* of inflammation. Is inflammation a helpful or harmful process, a disease or a reaction against disease, a defensive reaction? Today we have become almost as familiar with metaphorical wars as with real wars — wars against poverty, high prices, oil shortages, as well as wars against specific disease, such as cancer, heart disease, muscular dystrophy, or whatever — partly, I suppose, because the word "war" seems to unleash a money-be-damned kind of behavior in many people. The notion of a metaphorical war against disease waged by the forces of the human body seems hardly metaphorical when it is expressed in the form of the "defense reactions" of the body. This notion is, however, relatively new. It has little part in the Hippocratic-Galenic tradition, although Max Neuburger was able to trace the therapeutic use of induced fever back to the first century, in Rufus of Ephesus. Early in the sixteenth century Pierre Brissot spoke of the expulsion of "foreign substances" from the body, of "the neighboring parts uniting and sending, as it were, auxiliary troops to beat down the common enemy."[21] The idea that disease is, or is caused by, something that can be "cast out" is, of course, an ancient and ubiquitous one, but I am speaking here of official, academic medicine in the West.

Even to our own way of thinking, fever and inflammation are closely related processes; in the minds of the older medical writers they are almost indissoluble. The first full use of military metaphor in medical thought known to me occurs in connection with fever and inflammation. It is to be found in the medical writings of the philosopher Thomas Campanella, author of that famous depiction of a utopian state, *The City of the Sun*. The collection of essays in which the military metaphor is used seems to have been written between 1610 and 1613, although not published until 1635. Campanella develops the idea inherent in the phrase *bellum contra morbum*, "the war against disease," at some length. It seems clear that he was opposed by regular physicians because of his belief that "fever is not a disease, but a war against disease" — but we must always remember the tendency of an outsider to exaggerate the strength of the opposition from within the establishment. Campanella's pathophysiology, which is largely Galenical in spirit, does not concern us here. I call attention rather to the way in which he assesses the inconveniences to the body often occasioned by the inflammatory process. Campanella argues that such disturbances of bodily function as do occur are mere accidental concomitants of the beneficial process. They occur, he says, *"per accidens,* for while spirit is fighting against disease it is hardly able to attend to other functions." In order to make himself fully understood, Campanella adds that "when a state is fighting against an enemy, public works, agriculture, schools and festivals are held up." By means of this somewhat jesuitical maneuver, Campanella, and those who follow him, can write off all undesirable concomitants of the "defense" effort as not being parts of the effort per se.[22]

At the beginning of the eighteenth century, Georg Ernst Stahl of Halle again proposed that the inflammatory process was essentially therapeutic in intent. Stahl's pathophysiology, unlike that of Campanella, is post-Harveian; the inciting cause of inflammation is a circulatory block in the small vessels, and this is to be overcome by pumping blood into the inflamed region in greater amount and intensity. Both patient and physician should know, admonishes Stahl, that the discomforts of inflammation are little in comparison to the evil results of its absence. From a poem appended to a dissertation carried out in 1705 under Stahl's direction, we may infer that the view of inflammation as a disease rather than a cure was still dominant. Two of its lines are: *Quae tanta invidia est, ut quod Natura saluti/Consulit, hoc medicus damnet et aeger idem* — it is a pity that both physician and patient condemn nature's means of restoring health. Another poem, appended to the same dissertation, warns, however, that the physician must take care to moderate the inflammatory process if it seems to be getting out of hand. Stahl's views, adopted by his successor at Halle, Michael Alberti, who called inflammation an *actus salutarius,* or salutary act, made themselves felt in England later in the eighteenth century. They are evident to some extent in John Hunter's frequently quoted claim that inflammation is not a disease, but a "salutary operation consequent to some violence or disease." Hunter's "salutary operation" is not the overcoming of a vascular block, as it is for Stahl and Alberti; it is, instead, a tissue-reparative process involving the so-called "coagulable lymph" of the blood. It is evident that neither Stahl nor Hunter employ the military metaphor here: inflammation, for them, is not a defensive but a therapeutic measure.[23]

Riches of metaphor and analogy abound in the medical literature of Germany throughout the Romantic period and far into the first half of the nineteenth century.[24] A single instance, one that is peculiarly pertinent to our topic, must suffice here. In 1845, long before the bacteriological era, Carl Heinrich Schultz (1795–1871), a many-sided naturalist and physician, continued — in what was by that time an outmoded fashion frowned on by scientific physicians such as Jacob Henle and Rudolf Virchow — to formulate much of his pathophysiology in terms of the metaphorical "battle against disease" (*Krankheitskampf*) and "defensive processes" (*Wehrprozesse*) of the body. The two key terms in Schultz's metaphorical construct are *Heerde* and *Keim*, respectively the "focus" of the body and the "germ" of the disease. The "germ" is a hostile *force* of undetermined nature; it is not, of course, a bacterial organism. The "focus" is the part of the body affected. The metaphorical construct here is not that of the familiar seed, sower, and soil — which might perhaps have been expected from Schultz, since he began his scientific career in the field of botany. *Heerde* is the German word for "hearth," the seat of warmth and life of the home, the sun of its little microcosm, a *force* in its own right. What Schultz has in mind is a battle between opposing forces, a battle of life against death — an idea later resurrected by the psychoanalytic school. The "germ" interferes with the life-functions of a part or the whole of the organism attacked. The affected part reacts in a threefold manner, first by expulsive actions (coughing, vomiting, diarrhea, etc.), second by assimilative actions, the purpose of which is to render the "germ" harmless, and third by what Schultz calls the defensive processes proper, namely certain general reactions on part of the circulatory and nervous systems, perhaps the most important of which are inflammation and fever.

Schultz's "defensive reactions proper" are of special interest to us here not the least because of his presentation of their two-edged character. Primarily, he says, they are protective in character. But under certain circumstances they lose their protective character and become destructive. Or, as Schultz puts it, the reactions change from "healing-forces" into "death-forces" (*die Reaktionen anstatt zur Heilkraft zur Todeskraft werden*), a change in character that Schultz believes has so far gone unrecognized. For this reason it is difficult at times, he says, to draw a line between the manifestations of disease due to the attacking agency and those due to the defensive agency. In some instances, according to Schultz, the defense activities may have from the very beginning a "biolytic," that is, life-destructive character. Further, even where the "germ" of the disease has been successfully repelled, the so-called biolytic response may persist in the form of local or general "hyper-arousal" (*Hochregung*) or "exhaustion" (*Erschöpfung*).[25]

To physicians of the postromantic school of strict science such language was almost anathema, and its use was vigorously opposed by Henle, Virchow, Gabriel Andral, Rudolph Lotze, and many others.[26] It persisted, nonetheless, and there is some historical irony in the fact that Henle's essay of 1840 on miasmatic and contagious diseases can be seen as the theoretical framework on which a later generation of investigators, most notably Henle's former pupil Robert Koch, rested their studies of bacterial agents of disease. Bacteria, of course, became the enemy agents par excellence. So strong was the defense metaphor that in 1869, before a convincing case had been made for the germ theory of disease, and only two years after Julius Cohnheim's account of the source of white blood cells in inflamed tissues, a Philadelphia pathologist by the name of Joseph Richardson proposed that the white cells had, in this instance, the office of collecting "germs of bacteria" and subsequently eliminating them from the body.[27] And twenty years earlier, in 1847, Richardson's interpretation had already been written off in advance as anachronistic by Virchow, with the words: "We no longer regard the pus corpuscles as gendarmes ordered by the police state to escort over the border some foreigner or other who is not provided with a passport."[28] Three years later, oddly enough, Virchow was himself the subject of a police expulsion from Berlin, when he returned there in 1850 on the occasion of his wedding.[29]

Despite his early skepticism as to the protective role of white blood cells, Virchow encouraged Ilya Metchnikov's studies on phagocytosis, and in 1885 he wrote an early and favorable assessment of Metchnikov's theory of inflammation entitled, appropriately, "The Battle of Cells and Bacteria."[30] Metchnikov summed up his theory of inflammation in 1892 in his *Lectures on the Comparative Pathology of Inflammation*, and again in 1901, in his *Immunity in Infectious Diseases*. His theory of immunity is coextensive with his theory of inflammation. As Metchnikov sees it, the inflammatory-immune apparatus has arisen through natural selection in the course of evolutionary development to become a survival system of the highest importance, a system of "organs of attack and defense" directed at invading parasites; these are dealt with by digestion and expulsion. In this defense system, the production of humoral antibodies is secondary in importance. Although some of the antibodies produced do indeed have bactericidal properties, for the most part they serve only to further the activities of the real defenders of the body, the white cell phagocytes of the blood and tissues. Moreover, the antibodies themselves are the result of the intracellular digestion by the phagocytes of invading organisms.[31]

Metchnikov, who compared phagocytes vis-à-vis microorganisms to an "army hurling itself against the enemy," thus gave the military metaphor a new lease on life by precisely defining the aggressors and the defenders at the dawn of the bacteriological era. His overall interpretation of the inflammatory-immune process as protective in intent was not as simplistic as is sometimes supposed. From the beginning, he recognized the need for checking it in certain uncommon instances.[32] Nevertheless, his claims were regarded, with some justice, as highly one-sided by most pathologists and bacteriologists of the time. An enormous, now almost forgotten, debate on the subject of inflammation at once arose among German pathologists, who were then, of course, the pacesetters for the world. It continued for nearly forty years, subsiding only after the general catastrophe of the Great War. We cannot pause here to examine in detail the conflict of evidence and points of view.[33] Summing up, it is fair to say that the proponents of the military metaphor carried the day, and by the 1920s most textbooks of pathology in the United States had accepted the dogma that the inflammatory process was *essentially* defensive in intent. Where tissue damage did occur, it was written off — to borrow Campanella's words — as damage *per accidens* rather than *per se*. When it was found that repeated exposure to initially harmless agencies could elicit harmful responses, including destructive inflammation, on part of the body, new words were coined. Thus Portier and Richet wrote in 1902: "We term *anaphylactic* (the contrary of phylaxis) the property of a toxin to diminish instead of reinforcing immunity, when it is injected in non-fatal doses." Anaphylaxis is thus "negative protection." Maurice Arthus, in 1903, showed that repeated injections of horse serum into rabbits, although harmless at first, eventually elicited destructive local inflammation. In 1906 Clemens von Pirquet took note of this paradox and suggested that the term "allergy" should be used for all instances of this kind, in which the so-called "immune" response was in fact harmful to the body.[34]

W. C. MacCallum, a graduate of The Johns Hopkins University School of Medicine who returned to it in 1917 as professor of pathology and bacteriology, was the author of a textbook of pathology that went through seven editions between 1916 and 1940. In the sixth edition (1936) MacCallum defined inflammation as a "complicated vascular and cellular response [to injury]...adapted...to prevent the extension of the injury, hold in check the injurious agent, or even destroy it." Immunity, likewise, he defined as a "response adapted to annul and prevent the inroads of a [particular] injurious agent." MacCallum qualifies the apparent simplism of his approach on the following page, however, noting that inflammation is a "complex phenomenon, elaborated to *a certain degree of perfection*," the aim of which *"seems* to be the prevention of further injury," but which may, on occasion, "produce unsatisfactory or even *harmful results*" (my emphasis).[35] Curiously enough, a similar and even more simplistic definition — I emphasize here that I speak only of the *definition* of inflammation, and not of the whole treatment of the subject — is to be found in an authoritative textbook of pathology published in 1977. It is as follows: "Inflammation is the characteristic response of mammalian tissue to injury. Wherever tissue is injured by laceration, burning, chemicals, bacteria, or allergy, there follows at the site of injury a series of events that tend to destroy or limit the spread of the injurious agent."[36] An unwary reader might conclude that nothing had occurred to shake the dogma during the sixty years since the first edition of MacCallum's textbook; if anything, it appeared to have become more firmly established than ever.

In fact, a great deal had occurred, of which only the merest sketch can be given here. Dissatisfaction with the dogma that inflammation was always in essence a defense reaction to foreign injurious agents had never disappeared from among the ranks of German pathologists. One of the most radical critics of the dogma in the 1940s and 1950s was Siegfried Gräff, a pathologist in Hamburg. Gräff was, as it happens, the son-in-law of Ludwig Aschoff, the well-known professor of pathology at Freiburg who had done so much to justify the now standard view of inflammation. Gräff argued that the weakness of the ruling concept was most evident in connection with so-called chronic inflammatory processes, such as "chronic hepatitis," "chronic nephritis," "chronic thyroiditis," and "chronic arthritis," where no good evidence had ever been brought forward to show that the long-standing inflammatory response characteristic of these tissue lesions was in any way a helpful "response" or "reaction" to a foreign injurious agent. The diagnosis of inflammation, and all that term implied, was made in a mechanical fashion on the basis of histopathological appearances, and, in an equally mechanical fashion, a search for foreign agents was carried out, solely on the basis of the ruling dogma that inflammation was a reaction to injury.[37]

Gräff's critique was linguistic and conceptual in character, and he himself did not offer any more fruitful procedure for solving the problem posed by this group of diseases. Furthermore, he was very much an outsider among German pathologists; he was regarded, in fact, as somewhat of an eccentric. In my opinion he has nonetheless been to some extent vindicated by the subsequent course of events. During the past twenty years or so, enough evidence has accumulated to convince most of us that precisely the group of chronic inflammatory diseases to which he made reference—chronic arthritis, chronic nephritis, chronic thyroiditis, and so on—fall into the ever-growing class of diseases now called "diseases of immunity," the chief feature of which is the development of "immunity" against one's own tissues and cells. Expressed in terms of the military metaphor, what happens then is that the ostensibly protective forces of the organism launch a full-scale attack not against some foreign agent of disease but against some vulnerable part of the organism itself. An articulate antibody, or the white cell that had responded to its call, might perhaps be inclined to defend this patently self-destructive procedure on the ground that in order to save the part it had to destroy it.

An René J. Dubos pointed out in 1955, the original critics of Metchnikov's views objected to the teleological interpretation of life processes inherent in regarding the "phagocytes as a police force," and the inflammatory response as "a sort of mobilization," but the objection was readily countered by Metchnikov's appeal to the Darwinian principle of natural selection. The critics also called attention to diseases, such as leprosy, in which the phagocytes appeared to harbor and spread the invading microorganisms rather than destroy them. Dubos himself thought that more attention should be given to the possible role of the inflammatory "micro-environment" in checking or even preventing the multiplication of microbial agents. Where the protective effect, however mediated, of the inflammatory response was achieved at the cost of tissue destruction, Dubos spoke of a "scorched earth" policy.[38] Given the total irrationality of human warfare, such a policy is not without an element of rationality. But what if we ourselves are the enemy? In this case, clearly, inflammation begins to manifest itself—to borrow Karl Kraus's famous *mot* on psychoanalysis—as the disease for which it is supposed to be the cure. In Hans Selye's pioneering concept of "diseases of adaptation," inflammation sometimes appears as an inverted protective mechanism. In Pierre Dustin's textbook of pathology, published in 1966, a subsection of the chapter on inflammation and the phenomena of defense deals with "diseases of defense" (*maladies de défense*). And in 1970, at a symposium on the adaptive aspects of inflammation, Lewis Thomas compared the results of the "self-destructive mechanisms" operative in chronic inflammatory diseases such as rheumatoid arthritis to "those sometimes observed in human affairs when war-making institutions pretend to be engaged in defense."[39]

In mid-nineteenth-century Germany, when the bourgeoisie was attempting to throw off the remnants of aristocratic centralism, Virchow argued that the human body itself was a "democratic cell state," a "federation of cells," and a "free state of equal individuals." Commenting on this in 1953, Erwin Ackerknecht remarked that Virchow's political and biological opinions had a way of giving each other mutual reinforcement. He then asked: "Is it a mere accident that we have moved away simultaneously from the ideas of the independence of the cell in the body and of the individual in society?"[40] Likewise, we may now ask whether it is a mere accident that the role of apparently self-destructive mechanisms in human social arrangements, in the body politic as it were, and apparently self-destructive mechanisms in the body proper, as well as in the human mind, have at the same time gradually moved to the center of interest in Western thought today. Without pretending to offer an answer to the question of whether we are in fact the victims of blind programs that, given an appropriate change of circumstances, accomplish our destruction rather than assure our salvation, I would reply that it *is* no accident.[41]

How, then, does the simultaneity of expression come about? In the body of my paper, I have already suggested what little I have to offer with respect to a general explanatory proposition. The first formulation of it, that of Karl Marx, is familiar enough. The material basis of human life—that is, the productive forces available at a given time, together with the corresponding property relations then obtaining—constitute the foundation on which social, political, legal, religious, artistic, philosophical, and, in general, ideological superstructures are raised, and when changes in the substructure take place they are sure to be followed by corresponding changes in the superstructures.[42] To this statement, Engels added in 1890 the qualification that in the materialist conception of history the "production and reproduction of real life" should be understood to be no more than the "*ultimately* determining factor," the *primum agens*, and that "ideological spheres" could influence it in turn.[43]

The second formulation of the general explanatory proposition is the one that I offer here. It is, I suppose, "idealist" rather than "materialist" in char-

acter. It can best be stated in the form of two postulates: (1) human language determines as well as reflects our thoughts and actions, to an extent
varying with the individual case; it is itself, of course, a kind of expressive action or behavior; (2) early in the course of human history metaphors arise at
the base of the pyramid of human needs and activities. Subsequently they
spread upward and outward to all levels of human thought and activity; at
a more advanced stage of human development, metaphors are drawn from
all levels and spread in all directions, but the lower level metaphors continue, in general, to carry the most force. It is not surprising, then, that parallel movements occur at different levels, more or less simultaneously. But it
must always be remembered that every particular claim made in the pursuit
of the natural or humane sciences must be judged in the light of the evidence on which it purports to rest, and not on the basis of its ideological fit-
ness.[44] To do otherwise, whether in the name of religion, country, or political
party, is, for the scholar, a betrayal of trust.

NOTES

*Supported in part by National Institutes of Health Grant LM 02058.

[1] L. J. Rather, "Systematic Medical Treatises from the Ninth to the Nineteenth
Century: The Unchanging Scope and Structure of Academic Medicine in the West."
Clio Med. 11 (1976): 289–305. See Arthur M. Kleinman, "Medicine's Symbolic Reality: On a Central Problem in the Philosophy of Medicine," *Inquiry* 16 (1973):
206–13, for a cross-cultural perspective on the symbolic, language-centered character
of the emphasis on biophysical "reality" characteristic of academic Western medicine.
For the origins and development of the bias of Western medicine toward treatment
of the *body* — even where the role of emotional factors in disease causation was recognized — see Pedro Lain-Entralgo, *The Therapy of the Word in Classical Antiquity*,
ed. and trans. L. J. Rather and John M. Sharp (New Haven: Yale University Press,
1970); also, L. J. Rather, *Mind and Body in Eighteenth Century Medicine: A Study
Based on Jerome Gaub's De regimine mentis* (Berkeley and Los Angeles: University
of California Press, 1965).

[2] See, for example, "Analogy in the History of Science," by Agnes Arber, in
Studies and Essays in the History of Science and Learning, ed. M. F. Ashley-Montagu
(New York: Schuman, 1947); Owsei Temkin, "Metaphors of Human Biology," in
Science and Civilization, ed. Robert C. Stauffer (Madison: University of Wisconsin
Press, 1949); Peter Niebyl, "The Helmontian Thorn," *Bull. Hist. Med.* 45 (1971):
570–95; L. J. Rather, "Towards a Philosophical Study of the Idea of Disease," in *The
Historical Development of Physiological Thought*, ed. C. McC. Brooks and P. F.
Cranefield (New York: Hafner, 1959); idem (and J. B. Frerichs), "On the Use of
Military Metaphor in Western Medical Literature: The *Bellum Contra Morbum* of
Thomas Campanella (1568–1639)," *Clio Med.* 7 (1972): 201–8; idem, "Some Aspects
of the Theory and Therapy of Inflammation: From William Harvey to Clemens von
Pirquet," *Proc. 22nd Int. Cong. Hist. Med.* (London: Wellcome Institute, 1974);
idem, "Alchemistry, the Kabbala, and Analogy of the 'Creative Word' and the
Origins of Molecular Biology," *Episteme* 6 (1972): 83–103.

[3] Thomas Willis, *Dr. Willis's Practice of Physick. Being the Whole Works of that*

Renowned and Famous Physician: Containing these Several Treatises, viz. I. Of Fermentation. II. Of Feavers. III. Of Urines. IV. *Of the Accension of the Blood. V. Of Musculary Motion. VI. Of the Anatomy of the Brain. VII. Of the Description and Use of the Nerves. VIII. Of Convulsive Diseases. IX. Pharmaceutice rationalis, the First and Second Part. X. Of the Scurvy. XI. Two Discourses Concerning the Soul of Brutes* (London, 1684); Thomas Sydenham, *The Works of Thomas Sydenham, M.D., Translated from the Latin Edition of Dr. Greenhill, With a Life of the Author by R. G. Latham, M.D.*, 2 vols. (London, 1848, 1850).

⁴L. J. Rather, "Pathology at Mid-Century: A Reassessment of Thomas Willis and Thomas Sydenham," *Medicine in Seventeenth-Century England: A Symposium Held at UCLA in Honor of C. D. O'Malley*, ed. Allen C. Debus (Berkeley and Los Angeles: University of California Press, 1974), pp. 71–112.

⁵Theodor Schwann, "Ueber die Analogie in der Structur und dem Wachstum der Thiere und Pflanzen," *Neue Notizen aus dem Gebiete der Natur- und Heilkunde* 93 (January 1838): 33–37.

⁶Karl Marx, *Capital: A Critique of Political Economy*, 3 vols. (New York: International Publishers, 1967), 1:372; idem, *Das Kapital: Kritik der politischen Ökonomie*, 3 vols. (Berlin: Dietz Verlag, 1957), 1:389. Expanding the macrocosm-microcosm analogy used here by Marx, John McMurtry argues that a society is above all concerned with the "preservation of the stage of development of its productive forces," hence will "select out" whatever is incompatible with this concern: "Just as, to follow Marx's own course of analogue, the individual is governed before all else by the natural law to preserve his 'organs' of person, so society is governed before all else to preserve its 'organs' of technology" (*The Structure of Marx's World-View* [Princeton: Princeton University Press, 1978], p. 218). In a brilliant essay, which unfortunately did not come to my attention until after the present paper had been completed, Benjamin Farrington has argued convincingly that some of the pre-Socratic philosophers and Hippocratic physicians adopted as a methodological postulate the interpretation of physical and physiological processes in the light of technical procedures employed by human beings, for example, the techniques of the smith, the weaver, the fuller, the cobbler, the basket-maker, the gold-refiner, etc. Their central idea was, writes Farrington, that technical processes themselves are really "copies or imitations of natural processes" (*Head and Hand in Ancient Greece: Four Studies in the Social Relations of Thought* [London: Watts & Co., 1947], p. 14).

⁷L. J. Rather, *The Genesis of Cancer: A Study in the History of Ideas* (Baltimore: The Johns Hopkins University Press, 1978), p. 47.

⁸Marvin Spevack, *The Harvard Concordance to Shakespeare* (Cambridge: Harvard University Press, 1973), s.v. "Tissue"; James Strong, *The Exhaustive Concordance of the Bible* (Nashville: Abington, 1976).

⁹Robert Hooke, *Micrographia* (London, 1665), Obs. XXII: Nehemiah Grew, *The Anatomy of Plants* (New York: Johnson Reprint Co., 1965), pp. 120–21.

¹⁰Charles Singer and E. Ashworth Underwood, *A Short History of Medicine*, 2d ed. (New York: Oxford University Press, 1962), p. 320.

¹¹See Rather, *The Genesis of Cancer*, chap. 2, for the literature and a recent discussion of these topics.

¹²Grace M. Crowfoot, "Textiles, Basketry, and Mats," *A History of Technology*, ed. Charles Singer, E. J. Holmyard, and A. R. Hall, 5 vols. (London: Oxford University Press, 1954), 1:413–55.

¹³William Laughlin, "Acquisition of Anatomical Knowledge by Ancient Man," in *Social Life of Early Man*, ed. Sherwood L. Washburn (New York: Viking Fund, 1961). Of course an Aleut of today, or even of three hundred years ago, is far from being an "ancient man."

[14]R. J. Forbes, "Chemical, Culinary, and Cosmetic Arts," in Singer et al., *A History of Technology*, 1:238–98.

[15]Friedrich Engels, in *Marx Engels Selected Correspondence*, trans. I. Lasker and ed. S. W. Ryazanskaya (Moscow: Progress Publishers, 1975), letter dated 14 July 1858.

[16]Marx, *Capital*, vol. 1, chap. 8.

[17]Rudolf Virchow, "Atoms and Individuals," trans. in *Disease, Life, and Man: Selected Essays by Rudolf Virchow* (Stanford: Stanford University Press, 1959), pp. 120–41.

[18]The classic account of the way in which capitalism "self-destructs" is of course that given in Marx and Engels's *Manifesto of the Communist Party* (1848). My examples are instances of a conflict or "contradiction" between "price" and "use-value," and, since Marx carefully distinguishes "price" from "exchange-value," perhaps not quite to the point. For a detailed account of the contradictions that arise when financial operations become increasingly independent of actual trade in commodities, see Roman Rosdolsky, *The Making of Marx's Capital*, trans. Pete Burgess (London: Pluto Press, 1977), pp. 97–166.

[19]Arsène Darmesteter, *A Historical French Grammar*, trans. Alphonse Hartog (London: MacMillan and Company, 1934), p. 533.

[20]For literature see notes 60 to 63 in L. J. Rather, "Disturbance of Function (*Functio Laesa*): The Legendary Fifth Cardinal Sign of Inflammation, Added by Galen to the Four Cardinal Signs of Celsus," *Bull. N.Y. Acad. Med.* 47 (1971): 303–22.

[21]For literature see L. J. Rather, *Addison and the White Corpuscles: An Aspect of Nineteenth-Century Biology* (Berkeley and Los Angeles: University of California Press, 1972), pp. 187–89, nn. 3, 4.

[22]Rather and Frerichs, "On the Use of Military Metaphor in Western Medical Literature," pp. 201–8.

[23]For literature see Rather, *Addison and the White Corpuscles*, p. 17, nn. 11, 12; p. 148, n. 26; idem, "Some Aspects of the Theory and Therapy of Inflammation: From William Harvey to Clemens von Pirquet," *Proc. 23rd Cong. Hist. of Med.*, 2 vols. (London: Wellcome Institute, 1974), 1:8–12.

[24]See Werner Leibbrand, *Romantische Medizin* (Hamburg: Govaerts Verlag, 1937), esp. chap. 4, "Das 'Gut und Böse' der Krankheit,"

[25]Carl Heinrich Schultz-Schultzenstein, *Lehrbuch der allgemeinen Krankheitslehre*, 2 vols. (Berlin, 1844–1845), 1:215–25, 248–52.

[26]Henle refers disparagingly to the "old and poetic idea" that the organism engages in battle with disease. He even rejects the term "reaction"; all is "cause and effect." For a study of his *Pathologische Untersuchungen* (Berlin, 1840), in which these topics are considered, see Max Neuburger, *Die Lehre von der Heilkraft der Natur im Wandel der Zeiten* (Stuttgart: Enke Verlag, 1926), pp. 182–89. Virchow accepts the existence of organismic regulatory mechanisms, but points out that in some instances, in particular inflammation, the regulatory process itself produces further damage. For a complete account of Virchow's concept of inflammation see my "Virchow und die Entwicklung der Entzündungsfrage in neunzehnten Jahrhundert," *Verhandlungen des XX. Internationalen Kongresses für Geschichte der Medizin, Berlin, 22.–27. August 1966* (Hildesheim: Georg Olms Verlag, 1968), pp. 161–78. Rudolf Hermann Lotze's *Allgemeine Pathologie und Therapie als mechanische Naturwissenschaften* (Leipzig, 1842) might be described as an attempt to "demythologize" (in keeping with the spirit of the time) pathology. Gabriel Andral, in 1829, suggests that metaphorical terms such as *cancer* and *inflammation* be eliminated from the language of science. "Created in the infancy of science," he writes, "this quite metaphorical term...inflammation...is like a worn-out effaced coin

which ought to be withdrawn from circulation" (*Précis d'anatomie pathologique*, 3 vols. [Paris, 1829], 1:9).

[27]See "The White Cells as Phagocytes: Metchnikov's Biological Theory of Inflammation," in Rather, *Addison and the White Corpuscles*, pp. 179–93, for the work of Richardson and others on the role of white cells vis-à-vis bacteria in the period before Metchnikov.

[28]Rudolf Virchow, "Ueber die Reform der pathologischen und therapeutischen Anschauungen durch die mikroskopischen Untersuchungen," *Arch. F. path. Anat., Physiologie, u.f. klin. Med.* 1 (1847): 207–55.

[29]Erwin H. Ackerknecht, *Rudolf Virchow, Doctor, Statesman, Anthropologist* (Madison: University of Wisconsin Press, 1953), p. 22.

[30]Rudolf Virchow, "Der Kampf der Zellen und der Bakterien," *Arch. f. path. Anat., Physiologie, u. f. klin. Med.* 101 (1885): 1–13. For Virchow's relations with Metchnikov, see Rather, "Virchow und die Entwicklung der Entzündungsfrage im neunzehnten Jahrhundert."

[31]The *Lectures on the Comparative Pathology of Inflammation*, trans. F. A. and E. H. Starling, with a new introduction by Arthur M. Silverstein, has been reprinted by Dover Publications (New York, 1968); *Immunity in Infectious Diseases,* trans. F. G. Binnie, with a new introduction by Gert H. Brieger, has been reprinted by the Johnson Reprint Co. (New York and London, 1968). See my review of both volumes in *Med. Hist.* 14 (1970): 409–12, for remarks on the medical-historical background of Metchnikov's work.

[32]In 1884, for example, Metchnikov stated that the use of drugs to inhibit white cell migration should be "limited to cases where the phagocytes were devouring elements important for the integrity of the whole, as, for example, in atrophic diseases of the central nervous system" (see Rather, *Addison and the White Corpuscles*, p. 193, for literature).

[33]Julius Cohnheim, whose paper on leucocytic emigration was published in 1867, reversed his views on the subject in 1873, claiming then that the presence of white cells in zones of inflammation was due to a "molecular lesion" of capillary vascular walls. At this time he did not regard inflammation as in any way a protective reaction, and accorded no importance to bacteria. For the literature, s.v. "Cohnheim," in Rather, *Addison and the White Corpuscles*. The debate over the nature and significance of the inflammatory process took a new turn in the 1880s with the work of Metchnikov. All the leading pathologists of Germany tried to come to terms with the problem, some of them over periods of twenty-five years or more. Ernst Neumann's publications on the subject extend from 1889 to 1918, those of Otto Lubarsch from 1896 to 1922, and those of Felix Marchand from 1900 to 1922. Richard Thoma's publications extend from 1886 to 1922, and from the beginning he called for the elimination of the concept of inflammation (independently, he says, of Andral). Ludwig Aschoff, who was somewhat younger than any of these men, came to the debate toward its close as the proponent of a "biological" concept of inflammation, which was broader than, but not in conflict with, that of Metchnikov. On the other side, Lubarsch asserted that Aschoff's concept of inflammation was, *horribile dictu*, "evaluative" rather than "biological." See Lubarsch, "Ueber Entzündungsbegriffe und Entzündungstheorien. (Kurze Bemerkungen zu Aschoffs Aufsatz in Nr. 18 d. Wschr.)," *Münch. med. Woch* 69–74 (1922): 893. In 1921, Felix Marchand, then in his seventy-sixth year, argued in favor of the view that inflammation, although a process causally determined throughout, was nevertheless "to a certain degree" useful for the preservation of the organism. See Marchand, "Der gegenwärtige Stand der Entzündungsfrage," *Deutsche med. Woch.* 69 (1921): 893–94.

[34]See Rather, "Some Aspects of the Theory and Therapy of Inflammation," for the literature.

[35]W. G. MacCallum, *A Textbook of Pathology*, 6th ed. (Philadelphia: W. B. Saunders, 1936), p. 140. (The passages cited also appear in the first edition of 1916). MacCallum's *Textbook* is unique in that the "defense" metaphor enters into its structure: five successive chapters are entitled "Defenses of the Body against Injury." See also his *Inflammation* (Detroit: Wayne County Medical Society, 1922), a Beaumont Foundation Lecture. MacCallum studied under Felix Marchand at Leipzig in 1900. His predecessor in the chair of pathology at The Johns Hopkins University, William H. Welch, held more or less similar views on inflammation. "A burning question," Welch writes, "and one of perennial interest...is: How far are we justified in regarding acute inflammation as an adaptive or protective process?" He concludes that in some instances it is the best response possible. See Welch, "Adaptation in Pathological Processes," *Am. J. Med. Sci.* 113 (1897): 631–55.

[36]D. L. Wilhelm, "Inflammation and Healing," *Pathology*, ed. W.A.D. Anderson and John M. Kissane, 7th ed., 2 vols. (St. Louis: C. V. Mosby, 1977), 1:25.

[37]Siegfried Gräff, *Medizinische und pathologisch-anatomische Forschung und Lehre* (Hamburg: Stromverlag, 1950). See L. J. Rather, "Krankheit und Läsion," *Med. Heute* 4, no. 7 (July 1955), pp. 359–61, for a brief review of Gräff's ideas.

[38]René J. Dubos, "The Micro-Environment of Inflammation, or, Metchnikoff Revisited," *Lancet* 2 (2 July 1955): 1–5. A few years later, Dubos stated that the aggressive warfare waged by physicians against microbes "during the gory phase of Darwinism" had left no place for the view that an ecological equilibrium might somehow be reached (*The Mirage of Health* [New York: Harper, 1959], p. 61). Commenting on this statement in 1972, I suggested that physicians might thereby be led to search for "symbiotics," rather than, or in addition to, antibiotics (Rather and Frerichs, "On the Use of Military Metaphor in Western Medical Literature," p. 206).

[39]For Thomas's comments, and for Leslie Foulds's suggestion, made in 1969, that "military terminology and value judgments...should be excluded from discussions of invasion and other tumour-host relationships," see Rather and Frerichs, "On the Use of Military Metaphor in Western Medical Literature," p. 206. See also Lewis Thomas, "Inflammation as a Disease Mechanism," in *The Inflammatory Process*, ed. B. W. Zweifach, L. Grant, and R. T. McCluskey, 2d ed., 3 vols. (New York: Academic Press, 1974), 1:515–18.

[40]Ackerknecht, *Rudolf Virchow, Doctor, Statesman, Anthropologist*, p. 45.

[41]The phrase "it is no accident that—" epitomizes a characteristic feature of German thought in the nineteenth century. The classical formulation is that of Friedrich Schiller in *Wallensteins Tod* (2. *Aufzug*, 3. *Auftritt*):
> Es gibt keinen Zufall
> Und was uns blindes Ohnegefähr nur dünkt,
> Gerade das steigt aus den tiefsten Quellen.

[42]Cf. Karl Marx's statement of the thesis in 1859, in the passage beginning: "My inquiries led me to the conclusion that neither legal relations nor political forms could be comprehended whether by themselves or on the basis of a so-called general development of the human mind, but that on the contrary they originate in the material conditions of life..." (*A Contribution to the Critique of Political Economy* [New York: International Publishers, 1970], see preface, pp. 19–20).

[43]Friedrich Engels to Conrad Schmidt, 5 August 1890, and to Joseph Bloch, 21 September 1890, in *Marx Engels Selected Correspondence*.

[44]Cf. Appendix C, "Subsequent Fate of the Blastema Theory in England, France, Germany and the U.S.S.R.," in Rather, *Addison and the White Corpuscles*, pp. 217–27, for an account of a conflict in connection with the origin of plant and animal cells, and in between the demands of political ideology and those of strict science.

Commentary

Peter H. Niebyl

What is a metaphor? Within the realms of grazing cows, literary endeavors, and popularized medical science it has a well-defined place, but is it an inherent and necessary part of science and medicine? In her recent essay *Illness as Metaphor* Susan Sontag tried to rid disease of its popular connotations as if scientific knowledge was, or at least should be, without metaphor.[1] Whatever be the role of metaphor in science, it differs from that in the humanities in at least some respects. Whereas real literature abounds with fresh metaphors, a certain amount of historical research is required to find them in scientific literature. Once discovered these metaphors tend to be repeated almost *ad nauseum* over centuries. Whether it be the lamp, the thorn, the clock, or the boiling pot that is involved, the influence of these metaphors, as I have indicated elsewhere, rests on their role in a scientific model that has met with a certain amount of acceptance from the scientific community.[2] This is why, as Rather seems to acknowledge, scientific metaphors are often "dead" metaphors, or close to it, if they have been successful. The scientific physician, far from being poetic, tends to be pedantic and even plagiaristic in his use of metaphor.

To a large extent the established knowledge of medical science can be expressed in positivistic terms where morphologic patterns and reproducible relationships have been freed of the ambiguous metaphor—an ideal with benefits for both physician and patient. At the time of Willis, Sennert decried the use of metaphor in medicine as misleading and dangerous; and many physicians since have followed suit. In "real" literature, metaphor is of course the ideal—especially new metaphor. However, if this device can be seen as bridging the "two cultures," the water under the bridge is still there. Metaphor in science is most important and least dead during the process of discovery; that is, in dealing with the hypothetical. Here of course there is a high risk that a metaphor will turn out to be inappropriate.

An old military metaphor ultimately proved to be fruitful and appropriate. The length of time required indicates that there is more to science than metaphor. Rather finds its source in Brissot. The therapeutic use of fever per se hardly qualifies as a statement of this metaphor and is quite compatible with totally different lines of thought. Brissot was influenced by the controversies between Arabic and Humanist interpretations of Galenic medicine. The origin of the military metaphor can be found in the Aristotelian formu-

154

lation of Galenic medicine by Arabic physicians such as Averroes, especially in their discussions of variola and fever. This can be seen in Peter of Abano's influential *Conciliator controversiarum, Differentia CVII*, where a war between the body and the morbific material is compared to dueling boxers. Nature is identified with the Aristotelian innate heat as opposed to the extrinsic heat. The distinction is made in Aristotle's *De generatione*, V, vi, and *Meterologica*, IV, i, but without the belligerent connotations. Although Max Neuburger identified Campanella's military metaphor with the classical *vis medicatrix naturae*, classical nature was not an inherent part of the body that fought off external invaders. Conversely, in the macrocosm-microcosm metaphor, dominant from Antiquity to the Renaissance, the body was a relatively passive recipient of external factors that became internalized. The model of nature as a rugged individualist claims more the Protestant ethic or entrepreneurial spirit as its social origin than technological metaphors derived from some specific industry. The idea that the microcosm could stand on its own in a hostile macrocosm did represent a major shift in biomedical thought. It represented a kind of vitalism more neo-Aristotelian than Aristotelian. We probably have not seen the ultimate effects of the military metaphor in medicine, but it would appear to have reached new heights in a recently published medical text.[3] Here the skin, which, it should be kept in mind, separates the microcosm from the macrocosm, is called "a primary organ of defense" whose morphology, physiology, and biochemistry are all organized to defend against chemical agents, fluid loss, thermal stress, solar radiation, physical trauma, as well as microbial agents. Even personal hygiene, clothing, and working conditions are "cultural defenses" against environmental assaults. Occupational disease is then defined as a breakdown in these defenses. Ironically, instead of the occupation determining the metaphor as suggested by Rather, the metaphor determines how one looks at the occupation.

The idea that the defensive reactions of the body could be harmful — even self-destructive, as it were — was so well developed in Van Helmont's writings, with their depiction of the rage and indignation of the Archeus, that this tended to be the rule rather than the exception. C. H. Schultz also used the Helmontian term Archeus. Although, as Rather points out, Henle was critical of Schultz, in his famous essay of 1840 (which so accurately foreshadowed the bacteriologic era), Henle himself used the Helmontian metaphor of a thorn to exemplify the hostile invader.

If metaphor is more important for scientific discovery than it is for scientific knowledge, it is because metaphor provides a way of visualizing the as yet undiscovered phenomena. Rather mentions Marx's "discovery" of the money-form. Here it may be questioned whether the bourgeois class needed to be told by Marx that everything was money including time. Money was already the phenotypic appearance. If there was any discovery by Marx, it must have had to do with the labor theory of value, and the supposed human exploitation of that labor as the genotypic "reality" underlying the apparent money relationships. Schwann's cell, of course, played no role as a creative metaphor in Marxian discoveries; however, their mutual use of living beings, rather than inanimate elements, as the underlying basis for appearances seems more parallel than the cell-money comparison of Rather. Since the cell-metaphor was not an essential part of Marx's theory and since medicine, not economics, is the issue at hand, the point is made only to stress the importance of extending theoretically significant metaphors to the point where they reveal what the author is really trying to say. Casual metaphors may be very misleading. A case could be made for asserting that all language is ultimately metaphorical in origin, but trivializing metaphors to mere words can confuse the differences between research and established knowledge. Metaphor is perhaps best thought of as a tension between the imagined and the real worlds. Both worlds are a necessary part of creative thought. We can no longer praise one world by discrediting the other as metaphorical, and this is the important message of Rather's paper.

NOTES

[1] Susan Sontag, *Illness as Metaphor* (New York: Farrar, Straus and Giroux, 1978).

[2] Peter H. Niebyl, "Old Age, Fever, and the Lamp Metaphor," *J. Hist. Med.* 26 (1971): 352–68; idem, "The Helmontian Thorn," *Bull. Hist. Med.* 45 (1971): 570–95; idem, "Science and Metaphor in the Medicine of Restoration England," *Bull. Hist. Med.* 47 (1973): 356–74.

[3] Thomas B. Fitzpatrick et al., eds., *Dermatology in General Medicine*, 2d ed. (New York: McGraw-Hill, 1980), p. 1009.

THE MEDICALIZATION OF FRENCH SOCIETY AT THE END OF THE ANCIEN RÉGIME

Jean-Pierre Goubert

> *The distinguished French journal,* Annales: Economies,
> Sociétés, Civilisations, *celebrated its fiftieth birthday in 1979.
> In the very wide range of its interests it has not neglected
> biology and medicine. In The John Hopkins University Press
> series of volumes of translated selections from the* Annales *two
> belong in this category—the first of the set,* Biology of Man in
> History *(1975), and the latest,* Medicine and Society in France
> *(1980). The series is edited by Robert Forster and Orest
> Ranum. The historian Jean-Pierre Goubert is a member of the*
> Annales *group.*

Until very recently the history of medicine was, in France, the "private
domain" of physicians, just as the history of the Church has traditionally been the preserve of bishops and theologians. This tradition, which is still
powerful today, produces specialized and learned studies, for the most part
devoted to the history of medical science, epidemics, and "great physicians."
Its most serious shortcoming is self-absorption, at times even complacency.
A second, and also typically French orientation is related to the monopoly
claimed by the philosophers who are the only people qualified, or so they
say, to treat the history of ideas or of the sciences. Historians only broke into
this field—first by way of the related area of demography, then indirectly
through their work in anthropological and social history—in the wake of the
present critical attitude toward medicine, physicians, and "medical power."
The calls for a slowdown and, yes, the attacks launched by healthcare econ-
omists and certain sociologists given to tautological thinking and vague stir-
rings of the soul, have nonetheless brought the historian out of the ivory
tower, where scholars are often most comfortable.[1] As a result, we are wit-
nessing a revolution. Neither the weight of the institutional and sociological
status quo, nor the traditional—one might actually say ritual—resistance
present in any profession was able to prevent its burgeoning. Now that this
trend has become irreversible, it is clear that the role played by the group
that has become known as the "Annales School" has been considerable.[2] Yet
it must be acknowledged that the original impulse came from elsewhere;
namely, essentially from Michel Foucault and his *Birth of the Clinic* (1963).
However, under Fernand Braudel's stewardship, the biological aspects of the

157

human adventure were given a more prominent place than ever before.[3] In 1966 and 1967, thanks to the discovery—or rediscovery—of the archives of the Société Royale de Médecine, Jean Meyer, Emmanuel Le Roy Ladurie, and Jean-Pierre Peter brought back to life, each in his own style, a two-hundred-year-old survey concerning climatic conditions and epidemics. In 1969 the *Annales, E.S.C.* published a special issue entitled *Biologie et Société*.[4] Since then, the emphasis has shifted from historical demography, epidemiology,[5] and even climatology[6] toward the sociology of the medical profession,[7] historical epistemology,[8] the analysis of the medical "discours,"[9] and the history of anthropology,[10] historical ethnology,[11] and psychoanalysis.[12]

I myself became involved in the history of medicine in 1963 when I was a student. This amounts to saying that this paper is in the mainstream and pursues the objectives of the movement I have just described. Moreover, this paper makes use of findings elaborated by a collective study conducted for the most part under the direction of members of the former "sixième section." However, it results from my personal interpretation, for which I assume full responsibility. It is conceived, essentially, as an attempt at synthesis, even if it is an essay constructed on the basis of a small number of studies that have not, so far, been integrated. Its method consists of lining up and assessing the ingredients that have gone into the medicalization of French society in four areas: (1) the images of the medical discourse; (2) the legal principles involved; (3) the socioeconomic realities; and (4) the sociocultural effects.[13]

THE IMAGES OF THE PHYSICIAN AND OF MEDICINE

What was the collective image of the physician and of medicine current within the medical profession at the end of the Ancien Régime? Let us listen to testimony from three witnesses. Here, first and foremost among them is Vicq d'Azyr, secretary and spokesman of the Société Royale de Médecine who, between 1776 and 1789, delivered some fifty funeral orations.[14] In doing so, Vicq d'Azyr drew "the outline of a collective profile of the French medical elite that had reached the top of the profession."[15] At the same time, he also presented to the correspondents of the young society, more than 60 percent of whose members were provincials, a normative model of the "enlightened" physician.[16] This model, moreover, had a militant quality, in the sense that in these funeral orations Vicq d'Azyr described the "instant history" of the thrust of the Enlightenment: in the sense also that, since the academy had to choose a replacement for the deceased, the account of his life became a *topos*. Militant as well was Vicq d'Azyr's conception of biography. In choosing to mention certain facts because they would not hurt the feelings of his provincial correspondents, Vicq d'Azyr developed a strategy for conveying the praise of the academy that reconciled the *mediocritas* of the obscure practitioner with the renown of the illustrious men of learning. This is why he stressed education, the indispensable study of the "basics," professional training, and the advancement of talent that—in some cases—ensued from a family tradition. In passing, Vicq d'Azyr singled out medicine as an art that allows its practitioners to search for the truth, in other words, to cultivate the creative doubt and to be a "philosopher." Finally, he outlined for his audience and for his readers the main features of a highly desirable reform of the medical curriculum based on three principles: to wit, the oneness of the "art of healing," the scientific revolution in medicine, and the joining together of theoretical learning and practical experience in the hospital. He pointed out that the enlightened physician, divided between his study, his office, and the social duties imposed by his vocation, owes it to himself to be a patriot and a citizen useful to society. This is why in this discourse the ideal death for a physician was that of the practitioner who died in the pursuit of his task, a victim of duty and a laicized hero of the sacred ministry of medicine.

The features of this portrait, then, express the aspirations and the demands of the "enlightened" physician who, as a man of learning and experience, was determined to wield power over the material as well as over the social world, and who intended to make his voice heard in the affairs of his country by virtue of his unquestioned learning and merit.

Now let us find out whether "la défense et [l']illustration" of the art of healing presented by Vicq d'Azyr corresponded to the collective self-image and the wishes expressed in the revolutionary *cahiers de doléances* by the physicians, surgeons, and apothecaries in eight provincial towns.[17] A quantitative reading of these documents yields a very clearcut finding: what these provincial representatives of medicine wanted was the end of the Ancien Régime, a bourgeois revolution that would make room for a constitutional monarchy. They severely criticized the slow working, the expense, and the social inequity of the existing legal system. With respect to every issue they expressed their vivid desire for the end of arbitrary government and the overthrow of privilege; but they also demanded various liberties. In this manner, the medical profession, despite certain nuances of difference between towns and various corporations, manifested its basic unity and its political consciousness. However, opinions were still divided as to the form these changes should take. Some, for example, felt that all functions should be open to all, free of charge, on the basis of merit alone, while others demanded the abolition of venal charges with compensation for the owners. And, to give another example, certain physicians were hostile to the idea of parity between medicine and surgery, which was vigorously advocated by the surgeons.

One can see, therefore, that the model presented by Vicq d'Azyr must have had a profound effect in the countryside. The virtues it extolled, the bright prospects it held out, the "useful" reforms it foreshadowed, all of this had become not only highly desirable but, in the eyes of most medical practitioners, quite within the realm of the possible, provided that the "good king" would act upon the grievances expressed by a group of subjects that offered to march in the forefront of a society of citizens. And yet, the things that were not said by these physicians are just as significant as those that were clearly stated. What about charlatans? Not a word! And what about fees? Not a word about that either! These two topics were not part of the official discourse, of the plea *pro domo*. And was it not true, after all, that in a society "policed" or governed by an "enlightened" elite, including physicians, money was not (!) an important sign of talent and merit, while any trace of charlatanry had—must have—disappeared?

So the physicians of that time had nothing to say about charlatans? Come now, they certainly did!...In the many proposals for reform they drafted at the end of the Ancien Régime, and in their responses to surveys about surgery, medicine, or obstetrics, they were always quick to dip their pen in poison: "scourge of humanity," "venomous horde," "sect of cannibals"—a veritable hail of epithets was unleashed.[18] The vocabulary used by the lieutenants of the king's first surgeon is remarkable for its narrowness and confusion. These men used the word "charlatan" to designate a number of recognizable types representing traditional medical practices and a store of popular knowledge about the body quite simply in order to rid themselves of genuine competition. In their desire to medicalize all biological aspects of human life and thereby to promote their art, the patented surgeons acknowledged the flourishing of charlatanry only to the extent that it threatened their own position. Yet they were unable to state the number of charlatans in their district; and even those surgeons who reported a small number of charlatans had a great deal to say about the evils of charlatanry. In fact, they usually proved incapable of describing it, even in its external aspects, partly because they did not want, and partly because they were unable to do so. Their fierce desire to crush charlatanry, and the charges they leveled against it suggest that they viewed it as the negative mirror-image of their own profession. The characteristics applied to the charlatans—barbarians, criminals, swindlers—were term for term the exact opposite of the virtues the surgeons claimed for themselves as learned and enlightened men, benefactors of humanity, men who earned the just rewards of their talents and their merits. For the most part, they resigned themselves to the influence of charlatanry, feeling that there was no possibility of reducing or suppressing it, although some did call for more stringent repressive measures. Locked into their learned culture and seated on the high horse of their certainties and their pretentions, these enlightened blind men were ready to go to war. United in a pioneering effort, they launched a new crusade, the crusade for medicalization.

It is clear, then, that the enlightened segment of the medical profession shared a certain number of desires, feelings, and attitudes that contributed to giving it a certain cultural unity. At the level of the medical discourse, the failure to include three interrelated issues is indicative of a deep professional unity. The fact that money and profit, charlatans and popular culture, and a social revolution are absent from this discourse symbolizes the emergence of a unified professional, political, and social consciousness. These, then, are three symptoms that foreshadow the process of medicalization that has come into its own in contemporary French society. Yet one wonders whether the fortuitous presence of the mirror-model designed by Vicq d'Azyr to foster the social and symbolic reproduction of the medical profession was sufficient to set in motion and to *root* within French society itself the process of medicalization that existed *in the realm of words*, even before the fall of the Ancien Régime. In order to answer this far-reaching question, we must go beyond the analysis of the medical discourse and the area of utopian thinking. If indeed there was such a process, let us attempt to locate the legal, economic, and social bases that permitted it to "take off."

LEGAL STATUS AND SOCIAL POSITION OF THE MEDICAL PROFESSION

The legal and regulatory texts that governed the status of the medical profession, and the study and the practice of medicine, surgery, and pharmacy in the kingdom, unanimously suscribed to three principles.[19] First and foremost, the field of health care and the supervision of all matters concerning the body were considered the exclusive monopoly of the medical profession. Secondly, the rules pertaining to the study and the practice of medicine were identical throughout the kingdom. Thirdly, the various branches of the profession were assigned specific places where they could practice: on the basis of the practitioner's course of study, the degree he had obtained, and his membership in a corporation or guild. These texts thus established a correlation between and an (alleged) hierarchy of talents. For this purpose, the country was divided essentially into three categories of places: (1) towns with faculties, *collèges*, and corporations; (2) towns without *collèges*, faculties, or corporations; and (3) market towns and rural areas.

These laws and regulations made for an urban aristocracy and a rural mass of ordinary foot soldiers. As people lived farther away from a town, they were less and less likely to come under medical supervision. It is important to recognize this fact, which was to make its influence felt for a long time to come. Moreover, the city was considered, following a longstanding tradition, to be the bastion and the lighthouse of society. The only "full-fledged" physician was one who lived in that archetype of society, the city. The others were but benighted semiphysicians in a benighted, disorganized, and poorly "policed" world; they were the negative mirror-image of the model of perfection. In this manner the internal division within the world of medicine (two types of physicians: *régents* and *forains*, members and non-members of corporations, two types of surgeons, *internes* and *externes*; but three types of licenses: for practicing in towns with corporations, in towns without corporations, and in rural areas) symbolized the trend toward generalization and uniformity that attempted to devise an orderly structure for the medical professions, a trend that can be perceived in other professions as well.

How did the actual realities of life, such as today's historian is able to reconstruct them, fit into this legal framework? Was there any margin of nonconformity, any room in the space between its interlocking wheels? As far as medical education is concerned, we have already seen that diversity and inequality were the rule throughout the kingdom.[20] As for the spatial distribution of physicians and surgeons, the outline of an answer is suggested by the systematic analysis of the administrative survey of 1786 in selected *généralités*.[21] Here is a first, and rather striking finding: No legal distinction between categories of physicians and surgeons was made in the questionnaires sent to the subdelegates who, for the most part, adhered to the form of the questionnaire. This means that administrative usage was not in keeping with the existing legal principles. A second finding, resulting from calculations of density, indicates that the spatial distribution of the medical profession was far from even. Certain areas in northern and eastern France were more "medicalized" than others, especially in western France. The third phenomenon to emerge is the fact that there were four to ten times fewer physicians than surgeons. The medical profession thus had the shape of a pyramid. Finally, a fourth conclusion can be drawn from this body of material: the level of medicalization in urban areas was three times as high as in rural areas.

It is clear, therefore, that the statistical picture and the spatial distribution of the medical profession reflect the spirit that informed the legal texts: 78 percent of the physicians lived in towns, 74 percent of the surgeons lived in rural areas. However, 61 percent of the medical profession in towns was made up of surgeons. This latter fact softens the cliché somewhat and provides an inkling of the important role played by the surgeons, both in towns and in the countryside. The survey of 1786 thus permits us to observe a double cleavage between town and country on the one hand and physicians and surgeons on the other. But one phenomenon already looms very large: the fact that, in normal times, 50 percent of the medical profession provided medical care for 15 percent of the population, namely, that of the towns, while the other half took care of the remaining 85 percent, that is, the rural population. The figures provided by statistics thus lend substance—albeit in a rudimentary manner—to the criticism voiced by the enlightened elite, which claimed that the countryside was totally deprived of medical care, a claim that turns out to be based on more than idealized Rousseauist views. Under these circumstances it is easy to understand the feeling, expressed in the medical discourse, that there was a void out there to be filled, a space waiting to be conquered and medicalized. The proponents of the utopia of a medicalized society reacted strongly to a situation they considered intolerable, both for the welfare of society and the welfare of medicine. What, then, were the social preconditions for this *conquista*, at least within the medical profession? Was there not a danger that the diversified, even compartmentalized structure of its legal status, in conjunction with its obvious preference for cities, would prevent it from carrying out this ambitious project? And how would it overcome the resistance of the patients, indeed the resistance within its own ranks? In other words, was the medical profession sufficiently in tune with society to carry out its ambitious project, or would it have to change its ways? In the cultural domain, this question must surely be answered in the negative, for the physician's rejection of a popular culture concerning the body was likely to place him in a position of conflict.

From the social and more exactly socioeconomic point of view, the study of the assessments for the *capitation* in eleven towns of Brittany, at Angers, Lyon, and Paris brings to light considerable differentials at the end of the Ancien Régime.[22] The surgeons were split into three very distinct social groups: a small number of them paid only a few livres; the majority paid between 5 and 20 livres; and a minority had to pay 30 to 60, even 80 and up to 100 livres. The surgeons thus formed a heterogeneous category, akin either to the *petit peuple*, or, most frequently to the *petite bourgeoisie*, and in some cases to the *moyenne bourgeoisie*. In the absence of a prosopographical study, it is impossible to assert that these three social groups corresponded to the three legal categories of surgeons. However, this seems to be the most likely hypothesis. By contrast, the world of surgeons was divided into only two social groups. At Nantes, Angers, Lyon, and in nine towns of Brittany no physician paid less than 10 livres *capitation* at the end of the century. This shows that the physicians' pyramid started at a higher level than that of the surgeons. Moreover, the majority of the physicians of Brittany had higher incomes than the surgeons: while 48 percent of the surgeons paid between 5 and 19 livres, 53 percent of the physicians paid between 10 and 29 livres in *capitation*. Finally, 11 percent of the surgeons paid over 50 livres, while 32 percent of the physicians were in that bracket. There were, however, some exceptions to this rule. At Angers, Brest, and Rennes a minority of the surgeons paid as much *capitation* as the physicians, sometimes more. Likewise, and also at Angers, the average assessments of physicians and surgeons were roughly equal, while at Rennes they were very dissimilar (32 and 67 livres respectively). Socially speaking, then, the separation between the two branches of the art of healing, already legally attenuated by the edict of Compiègne (1756), had become less marked by the end of the eighteenth century.[23]

Not much is known about the tax assessments for apothecaries from recent studies, but we do know about two cases, those of Angers and Paris. The difference between these two cities was considerable as far as the average assessment (17 and 60 livres, respectively) and the affluence of a majority of the apothecaries are concerned: 9 percent at Angers and 0 percent at Paris paid less than 6 livres. At first sight, the world of apothecaries seems to be divided into three groups at Angers and two groups at Paris. The most humble were not found in the capital at all. The reason may be that social aspirations were a typical aspect of life in Paris; but in the absence of other comparisons, it is too early to come to any conclusion on this point.

To my knowledge, no study of the fortunes of the members of the medical profession has been made recently, even though there is abundant archival material for the eighteenth century. There is more to such a study, of course, then the mere indication furnished by tax assessments. In the case of Lyon, a global study refines the three-tiered stratification of physicians, surgeons, and apothecaries by showing average fortunes of 17,000 livres for the apothecaries, 14,000 livres for the physicians, and 4,700 livres for the surgeons. The two groups constituted by the apothecaries and the physicians were characterized by a comfortable affluence, while the surgeons as a group were further divided into two subgroups, namely the 40 percent who had fortunes of less than 1,000 livres and the small group of 2.5 percent who had fortunes between 2,000 and 5,000 livres. In the case of Paris, a study based on a sampling of the inventories after death of physicians and surgeons clearly shows the greater affluence of the physicians, since 50 percent of them, as opposed to 22 percent of the surgeons, had fortunes of over 50,000 livres. Moreover, great fortunes (over 500,000 livres) were found only among the physicians; the wealthiest surgeons barely reached 200,000 livres. Thirdly, 10 percent of the surgeons left negative balances of between 500 and 50,000 livres, compared to the 7 percent of physicians who left debts ranging from 500 to 1,000 livres. It should nonetheless be noted that in Paris a fortune of 5,000 livres was the "watershed" that marked bourgeois status, and that this line was crossed not only by 85 percent of the physicians but by *75 percent* of the surgeons as well.[24] Finally, and this is quite remarkable, a comparison between the surgeons' inventories at the time of marriage and their inventories after death indicates that they became rich more rapidly.

To be sure, the case of Paris is exceptional. Such factors as inherited wealth and revenues drawn from court charges explain much of the opulence of the Parisian medical profession. Yet even in Paris there were, *at that time*, poor practitioners, especially among the surgeons.[25] The inventories after death are a particularly useful source because they enable the historian to reconstitute the material circumstances and the life style of the medical world. The poorest among these practitioners lived very modestly, in one or two rooms, without servants. The middling group, that is to say, the majority, lived a bourgeois life, employed at least one or two servants, rented a fairly spacious apartment, and had well-stocked wine-cellars, libraries, and wardrobes. Better yet, they had a coach, if not a carriage. As for the wealthiest, their style of life was downright luxurious, affording them several conveyances, several residences, jewelry, books, and clothes in profusion, sometimes a bathroom, a billiard room, or a natural history collection.

The case of Paris thus clearly shows the social diversity within a—supposedly—unified legal category; it also shows the social advances made by a segment of the surgeons. This by and large adequate—and often more than adequate—material situation must be attributed to the continuous advances made by a profession whose aspirations were far reaching indeed. Recall that the edict of Marly (1707) was promulgated to promote the teaching of medicine, and that the edict of Compiègne (1756) had raised surgery to the status of a liberal art. In addition, the quality of the teaching—at least in certain places and in certain institutions—was raised, not only in Paris outside the ancient faculty of medicine and at the new College of Pharmacy (founded in 1777), but in the provinces as well. At Rennes and Angers, for example, new courses and a new School of Surgery were created in 1738 and 1740, respectively, and both were attended by sure success.[26] On the level of daily life, another indication for the advance of the profession is furnished by the rise in tax assessments for the *capitation* at Nantes and Rennes, and even in Paris in the case of the pharmacists. Does it not appear, therefore, that the French medical profession, bolstered by a phase of rising economic prosperity, improved social status based on better education, and a *discours* that promoted the emergence of a political consciousness, had acquired the principal characteristics that would enable it to carry out the medicalization of society? Yes and no. The fact is that in attempting to reconstitute the social realities involved in the practice of medicine and surgery, both among patients and in the hospital setting, one uncovers, on the one hand, a situation located midway between tradition and modernization and, on the other, a large area that was just being opened to the exercise of medical supervision, namely the area of public health.

THE ROAD TO MEDICALIZATION

Two concrete examples—and too few of them have yet been brought to light by scholarship—will show that private practitioners conformed to one or the other of these models. These two examples are a rural[27] and an urban[28] surgeon. To begin with, they differed in their education. The former had passed the *légère expérience* [that is, demonstrated his proficiency in the basic surgical techniques] and was certified to practice in market towns and rural areas; the latter had passed the *grande expérience* [that is, demonstrated his proficiency in advanced surgical techniques] and having studied at the Hôtel-Dieu at Reims and then in Paris under Levret, was certified to practice in a town that had a corporation. As for their social origins, one was the son of a tenant farmer and stayed in his province, while the other was the son of a city-dweller (and a city-dweller himself), a former student in Paris, and a former military surgeon. One gave up surgery and took up stock-farming as soon as he had come into an inheritance, the other specialized, became an *accoucheur*, and taught obstetrics. While both practiced within a narrow radius, one gave advice and treatment to peasants, the other to townspeople, and, after 1786, to the well-to-do vintners of the outlying areas. The rural surgeon practiced "pro-pharmacy,"[29] prescribing herbal remedies, mostly the traditional evacuants of "humoral medicine," while the urban surgeon intervened in "unnatural" confinements, studied his successes and failures, and was able to reduce the mortality rate at birth by his use of the forceps. In short, the practices of these two men can be considered symbolic of two worlds: the wooded, traditionalist countryside of western France; and the more urbanized, more literate milieu of northeastern France, no doubt a more favorable terrain for the advance of medicalization.[30]

Concerning the activities of the medical profession in the hospital setting, we also have two—and no more—concrete examples to show a widening gap and an increasing divergence between two kinds of medical practice.[31] These examples are the Hôtel-Dieu of Provins[32] and the hospice of the College of Surgery in Paris (founded in 1774).[33] Aside from its exceptional wealth, the Hôtel-Dieu of Provins was a traditional institution. Under secular management, it was administered by the town's "better people." Treatment was prescribed by the medical profession, and services were performed by religious personnel. A traditional haven for the needy, and a place of refuge, it played a crucial role in the periods of crisis that caused profound disruptions in the provincial society of the Paris Basin at the end of the century. Well-run, well-kept, and able to provide an abundant and varied diet for its inmates, it was a remarkably effective force for social stability, located as it was along the path of migration toward the capital in a grain-producing area where food shortages and epidemics were compounded by pervasive poverty. In such a situation, the role played by the medical profession was bound to be secondary. Rather poorly paid for their services, medical practitioners had no hand in the administration and the day-to-day management of the institution; they only looked in from time to time, but then their presence made no difference to the life of the hospital and its patients anyway. In periods of crisis the ineffectiveness of their art turned this Hôtel-Dieu into a veritable "dying place" for the forsaken, the lonely, the poor: in short, for those who were cast aside by society. Epidemics brought in from the outside swept through this closed environment with explosive force. Rather late in the century, that is, on the eve of the Revolution, the medical profession finally did make its influence felt by devising sanitary measures to deal with overcrowding, the faulty exposure of the rooms, and the pervasive humidity. Accordingly, floors were leveled, walls were patched up, and running water was installed. In the absence of any possibility to control disease itself, the hospital was ruled by hygienic considerations, to be more precise, by a set of sanitary rules.

The hospice of the College of Surgery in Paris was virtually at the antipodes from the Hôtel-Dieu of Provins. Planned and founded by a segment of the medical profession, it amounted to a seizure of power on the part of the profession, even if it was exceedingly small (22 beds in 1786) by Parisian standards. In comparison with the traditional hospital, it was profoundly original in three respects. First of all, it was specialized, that is, it admitted only certain kinds of *conditions* and hence, patients. Secondly, the medical profession was involved in its management. Lastly, it constituted a scientific and teaching environment, where clinical research and teaching were conducted "at the patient's bedside." It was thus one of the "curing machines" (*machines à guérir*) evoked by Jacques Tenon. And indeed, its strictly medical function had replaced the traditional hospital's functions in the area of welfare and social regulation. As a social institution and as a place devoted to the advancement of knowledge, this hospice gave expression to a revolution in the priorities of medicine when it brought medical science into the hospital setting, with all the consequences that were bound to ensue from this step. It foreshadowed the hospital as we know it today. Nonetheless, at the end of the Ancien Régime the traditional hospital was still predominant, at least as far as the number of medical beds is concerned.[34] In any event, the prevailing image was still—and would be for a long time to come—that of the dreaded hospital created for the dregs of society, a place that one left feet first.

Thus we see that, as far as their impact on society is concerned, neither the private practitioners of medicine nor the hospital were in the forefront of a medicalization to which they subscribed, even though a few advanced sectors had emerged into view. At the same time, however, ample opportunity to deploy the technical proficiency, the scientific zeal, and the ambition of the medical profession was opened up by the development of the public health sector.[35] Three examples will suffice to depict the advances made by the utopia of a medicalized society: "epidemic diseases," inoculation, and the use of mineral waters.

The "epidemic physician" was not, of course, an innovation of the eighteenth century. What was new was the creation of an institutional framework for his activity.[36] Henceforth, the medical profession no longer waited to see how a particular situation would develop before it decided to combat an epidemic; the medical structure was in place before the epidemic struck. At this juncture, the monopolies of the physician and the surgeon were officially recognized by the powers that be. Hence, a whole medical bureaucracy, working in close cooperation with that of the intendant and his subdelegates, as well as with the network of parish priests, who were considered to be in charge of the *biological*, and not only the spiritual, life of their flocks. The parish priest drew up the list of "needy patients," the physician diagnosed the illness and prescribed the treatment; the surgeon provided the actual treatment; and the State paid for the distribution of food and medical attention. Unlike the private practice of medicine, the public medicine that now came into being was primarily interested in the well-being of society and in the impact of disease on the human body itself. This orientation

greatly contributed to shaking up the rigid tenets of a theoretical body of
learning; it stimulated the physician to search for more widely effective
therapeutic measures in order to fulfill the expectations of the public authorities. Epidemics, the object of a major survey conducted by the Société
Royale de Médecine, propelled the physician into the public arena, instilled
him with epistemological zeal, and strengthened his ambition to be "useful
to society." In a certain sense the epidemic physician in the twilight years of
the Ancien Régime foreshadows nothing so much as the gropings, the successes, and the eventual triumph of the hygienic movement of the nineteenth century.

Another concern of public health, inoculation against smallpox, represents the first instance, and the first victory, of the physician's direct fight
against disease and death.[37] Yet this preventive weapon had a double edge.
Empirically arrived at, contrary to the medicine based on evacuants, and involving risks to the patient, it was at the time vigorously "debated" among
theologians and scholars. The medical profession was deeply divided and the
Société Royale de Médecine reticent on this issue. However, the manner in
which the inoculators conceived of their task clearly shows their desire to further the advance of medicalization. Their generalized use of a single technique, the arguments they advanced, the massive scale of their objectives,
their stated expectation that the procedure would prove immediately and
visibly effective, all this testifies to their intent. But the hostility of the parish
priests, in Brittany for example, the resistance of a population that preferred
to call on its own knowledge of the body, as well as the reluctance of patients
to forestall an uncertain and far-away danger by means of an immediate risk,
prevented the victory of a campaign that would have legitimized the desires
and the ambitions of the "enlightened" members of the medical profession
who were sympathetic to inoculation.

One last example, concerning the use of mineral waters, does testify to an
undeniable success of the movement toward medicalization at the end of the
eighteenth century.[38] To recapitulate: one of the tasks entrusted to the Société Royale de Médecine in 1768 was the gathering of information about
and the supervision of the kingdom's mineral waters. As far as the scientific
aspect of this twofold task is concerned, the Société's efforts clearly ended in
failure. The small number and the poor quality of the analyses made demonstrate that hydrology was still in its infancy, as yet unable to rise to a scientific level. As an immediate result of this situation, physicians remained in
the dark as to the reasons for the observable effectiveness of certain waters in
certain conditions. Mineral waters remained what they had always been,
namely, a last resort or even a "universal remedy" as we can see from the
crossing of hydromineral data with the prescriptions of the time. As in the
case of epidemics, the state of the art was patently inadequate. But as in the
case of inoculation, the strategy adopted and the arguments advanced permit us to discern the extraordinarily modern overtones that betray the trend

toward medicalization. First of all, and as one would expect, this trend is perceptible in the strict regulations that gave a complete monopoly to the physicians, the intendants, and the distributors of mineral waters: a monopoly, to be sure, that was soon broken by the pervasive laxity of the time. The trend toward medicalization is also evident in the practice of marketing mineral waters under a medical "label" designed to sell to a frequently well-to-do clientele a certain form of leisure-time activity, and even tourism; indeed to sell hope for recovery, often the last, by stressing the beneficial effects of a "natural remedy" that was being restored to a place of honor by the neo-Hippocratic movement. Finally, the medical profession's deep involvement in this area is shown by the dues paid to the Société Royale de Médecine, which showed little interest in the complaints, the abuses, and the profits made in this trade, but was always anxious to collect its money as soon as it was due.

Thus, we have seen how the utopia of a medicalized society found a first expression in the medical *discours* during the last years of the Ancien Régime. Thanks to the improved social position of the medical profession, thanks to the urban network it deployed, and because of an alliance concluded between the medical profession and the public authorities—much rather than by virtue of any particular breakthrough in medical knowledge—this utopia had spawned a certain number of accomplishments. Unequal in scope to be sure, but always tangible, these accomplishments often assumed the form of public institutions, especially in the field of public health. In short, the economic, social, and ideological foundations of the "medical imperialism" of the nineteenth and twentieth centuries were laid some time before the Revolution, at least in certain sectors, in certain regions, and in a large segment of the medical profession. The direction was charted, agreed upon, and marked. The physician's perception of the world underwent a gradual change; his horizon narrowed, his ambition expanded. The physician was to do his part in breaking both the Ancien Régime and the Revolution. In this manner, he prepared the way for the crowning of the new élites, whose reign had to be established before the physician, a new Caesar, could crown himself.

Translated by Elborg Forster

NOTES

[1] I am thinking here of certain aspects devoted to the past in the work of Ivan Illich and his successors.

[2] In presenting this communication for the fiftieth anniversary of the Institute of the History of Medicine of The Johns Hopkins University and of the *Annales, E.S.C.*, my purpose has been to present before an international audience the work accom-

plished by the *Annales* group. That said, there should be no question of neglecting or ignoring the essential work of pioneers in the field of medical history.

[3]See F. Braudel, *Civilisation matérielle et capitalisme* (Paris: A. Colin, 1967), and idem, *Civilisation matérielle, économie et capitalisme, XVᵉ–XVIIIᵉ siècles*, vol. 1, *Les structures du Quotidien* (Paris: A. Colin, 1979). Cf. J.-P. Aron, *Essai sur la sensibilité alimentaire à Paris au XIXᵉ siècle* (Paris: A. Colin, 1967); J. J. Hémardinquer, ed., *Pour une histoire de l'alimentation* (Paris: A. Colin, 1970). See also the numerous articles on the history of alimentation that appeared in the *Annales, E.S.C.*

[4]A number of the articles in this issue are available in English translation in R. Forster and O. Ranum, eds., *Biology of Man in History: Selections from the Annales, E.S.C.* (Baltimore: The Johns Hopkins University Press, 1975). Another *Annales* issue entitled *Les Médecins et la médecine en France aux XVIIIᵉ et XIXᵉ siècles* appeared in 1977.

[5]See F. Lebrun, "Les hommes et la mort en Anjou aux XVIIᵉ et XVIIIᵉ siècles..." (Paris-La Haye: Mouton, 1971); J. Meyer, "Une enquête de l'Académie de Médecine sur les épidémies: 1774–1794," *Annales, E.S.C.* 21 (1966): 729–49; J.-P. Peter, "Une Enquête de la Société Royale de Médecine (1774–1794); Malades et maladies à la fin du XVIIIᵉ siècle," *Annales, E.S.C.* 22 (1967): 711–51; M. D. Grmek, "Préliminaires d'une étude historique des maladies," *Annales, E.S.C.* 24 (1969): 1473–83; and J.-P. Peter, "Les Mots et les objets de la maladie," *Revue Historique* 245 (1971): 13–38.

[6]See E. Le Roy Ladurie, *Histoire du climat depuis l'an mil* (Paris: Flammarion, 1967); idem, ed., *Médecine, climat et épidémies à la fin du XVIIIᵉ siècle* (Paris: Mouton, 1972).

[7]See J. Leonard, *Les Médecins de l'Ouest au XIXᵉ siècle*, 3 vols. (Paris: H. Champion, 1978).

[8]See J.-P. Aron, *Essais d'epistémologie biologique* (Paris: Christian Bourgeois, 1969).

[9]Here the word *discours* is understood in the structuralist meaning; for this remark, see M. Foucault, *L'ordre du discours* (Paris: Gallimard, 1971).

[10]See E. Le Roy Ladurie, ed., *Anthropologie du conscrit français...: 1819–1926* (Paris: Mouton, 1972); cf. idem and A. Zysberg, "Anthropologie des conscrits français (1868–1887)." *Ethnologie français* 9 (1979):47–67.

[11]See F. Loux, *Le Jeune Enfant et son corps dans la médecine traditionnelle* (Paris: Flammarion, 1978), and idem, *Le Corps dans la société traditionnelle* (Paris: Berger-Levrault, 1979).

[12]See J.-P. Peter, "Le Corps du délit," *Nouvelle revue de psychanalyse* 3 (1971): 71–108, idem and J. Revel, "Le Corps: L'Homme malade et son histoire," *Faire de l'Histoire* 3 (1974).

[13]By medicalization I understand a process of long duration that took root during the second half of the eighteenth century (in the case of France) and is even yet continuing to this day. This process subsumes the changes of orders: scientific, technological, and sociocultural. It expresses access to scholarly medicine, whether or not it is "scientific," to a cross section of the population for everything that has to do with health; accordingly it often encounters resistance when all or part of this population clings to a specific knowledge about the body, whether this knowledge is "popular" or not. In the second half of the French eighteenth century, this process took hold following an alliance between the public authority and the medical elite: An alliance that strengthened the professionalization of health even before a "revolution" in the regulation of medicine was produced.

[14]Daniel Roche, "Talents, raison et sacrifice: L'Image des Lumières d'après les Eloges de la Société Royale de Médecine (1776–1789)," *Annales, E.S.C.* 37 (1977): 866–68. (English translation in Robert Forster and Orest Ranum, eds., *Medicine and*

Society in Eighteenth-Century France: Selections from Annales, E.S.C. [Baltimore: The Johns Hopkins University Press, 1980].)

[15]Ibid., p. 867.

[16]Daniel Roche, *Le Siècle des Lumières en province. . .* (Paris: Mouton, 1978), 1:316.

[17]According to Dominique Lorillot, "Les Cahiers de doléances des médecins, des chirurgiens et des apothicaires en 1789" (master's thesis, University of Paris I, 1975).

[18]Jean-Pierre Goubert, "L'art de guérir: Médecine savante et médecine populaire dans la France de 1790," *Annales, E.S.C.* 37 (1977): 908–26. (English translation in Forster and Ranum eds., *Medicine and Society.*) See also Toby Gelfand, "Medical Professionals and Charlatans: The *Comité de Salubrité Enquête* of 1790–91," *Histoire Sociale/Social History* 11 (1978): 62–97.

[19]Some of these texts have been published by Isambert in his *Recueil général des anciennes lois françaises* (Paris, 1822–28). The edict of Marly, for example, is found in vol. 20, pp. 508–17. Other texts can be found in the National Archives (Paris), for example under the call number AD XI, 21.

[20]P. Huard, "L'Enseignement médico-chirurgical," in *Enseignement et diffusion des sciences en France au XVIIIᵉ siècle*, ed. R. Taton (Paris: Hermann, 1964), pp. 508–17. See also J.-P. Goubert and François Lebrun, "Médecins et chirurgiens dans la société française du XVIIIᵉ siècle," *Annales cisalpines d'histoire sociale* 4 (1973): 119–36.

[21]J.-P. Goubert, "The Extent of Medical Practice in France around 1780," *J. Soc. Hist.* 10 (1977): 410–27.

[22]"Capitation": royal tax of incomes.

[23]The data for this development are taken from the following studies: Jean Meyer, "L'Enquête de l'Académie de Médecine sur les épidémies: 1774–1794," *Etudes rurales* 34 (1969): 7–69; François Lebrun, *Les Hommes et la mort en Anjou aux XVIIᵉ et XVIIIᵉ siècles* (Paris: Mouton, 1971), esp. pp. 199–235; Benedicte Dehillerin, *Les Maîtres-apothicaires de Paris au XVIIIᵉ siècle* (master's thesis, University of Paris I, 1976); Catherine Virole, *Les Médecins et les chirurgiens à Paris dans la seconde moitié du XVIIIᵉ siècle* (master's thesis, University of Paris I, 1976); also Nicole Barré, *Introduction à l'étude des médecins et chirurgiens bordelais du XVIIIᵉ siècle* (master's thesis, University of Bordeaux, 1969); Denyse Muller, *Les Médecins et les chirurgiens de Toulouse de 1740 à 1830* (thesis for the D.E.S., University of Toulouse, 1961); Maurice Garden, *Lyon et les lyonnais au XVIIIᵉ siècle* (Paris: Les Belles Lettres, 1970), esp. pp. 190 and 738–39.

[24]Five thousand livres according to A. Daumard and F. Furet, *Structures et relations sociales à Paris au milieu du XVIIIᵉ siècle* (Paris: A. Colin, 1961); 7,000 livres according to Steve Kaplan for the end of the eighteenth century.

[25]On this point, see Guy Chaussinand-Nogaret, "Nobles médecins et médecins de cour au XVIIIᵉ siècle," *Annales, E.S.C.* 37 (1977): 851–57.

[26]On the professionalization achieved in the eighteenth century see Toby Gelfand, "From Guild to Profession: The Surgeons of France in the Eighteenth Century," *Tex. Rep. Biol. Med.* 32 (1974): 121–34.

[27]See Edna Hindie Lemay, "Thomas Hérier—A Country Surgeon Outside Angoulême at the End of the Eighteenth Century: A Contribution to Social History," *J. Soc. Hist.* 10 (1977): 524–37.

[28]See Jacques Gélis, "La Pratique Obstétricale dans la France moderne: Les carnets du chirurgien-accoucheur Pierre Robin (1770–1797)," *Annales de Bretagne et des Pays de L'Ouest* 86 (1979): 191–210.

[29]For a physician or surgeon to practice "pro-pharmacie" meant to furnish medicaments to patients in the absence of an apothecary in the neighborhood.

[30]On the regional level, a significant correlation can be established between high

literacy rates and medicalization. See, in this connection, François Furet and Jacques Ozouf, *Lire et écrire* (Paris: Editions de Minuit, 1977).

[31]For the hospital in France at the end of the Ancien Régime, see Michel Foucault, ed., *Les Machines à guérir* (Paris: Institut de l'Environnement, 1976).

[32]See Françoise Lelu, *La Population des "pauvres malades" de l'Hôtel-Dieu de Provins de 1762 à 1791* (master's thesis, University of Paris I, 1975).

[33]See Toby Gelfand, "Les Caractères originaux d'un hospice parisien à la fin de l'Ancien Régime," in *Mensch und Gesundheit in der Geschichte*, ed. Arthur E. Imhof (Husum: Matthiesen Verlag, 1980), pp. 339–55.

[34]On this point, see Muriel Joerger, "La Structure hospitalière de la France sous l'Ancien Régime," *Annales, E.S.C.* 37 (1977): 1025–51, especially p. 1034 (English translation in R. Forster and O. Ranum, eds., *Medicine and Society*.)

[35]In this connection, see Michel Foucault, "La Politique de la santé au XVIIIe siècle," in *Les Machines à guérir*, pp. 11–21.

[36]See Michel Foucault, *Naissance de la clinique* (Paris: Presses Universitaires de France, 1963), p. 24. In Poitou this institutional framework was established in 1784, in Brittany in 1787.

[37]For inoculation, see Jean-Claude Perrot, *Genèse d'une ville moderne. Caen au XVIIIe siècle* (Paris: Mouton, 1975), vol. 2, pp. 1048–49; also Robert Favre, "Les Mémoires de Trévoux dans le débat sur l'inoculation de la petite vérole (1715–1762)," *Etudes sur la presse au XVIIIe siècle* 1 (1973): 39–57; Jean-Pierre Peter, "Les Médecins français face au problème de l'inoculation variolique et de sa diffusion (1750–1790)," *Annales de Bretagne et des Pays de l'Ouest* 86 (1979): 251–64.

[38]See Pascale Muller, *Les Eaux minérales en France à la fin du XVIIIe siècle* (master's thesis, University of Paris I, 1975).

Commentary

Caroline Hannaway

Dr. Goubert has given us a suggestive and informative paper which synthe-
sizes the results of work carried out by a number of French scholars but
which offers his own distinctive interpretation of the meaning of that work.
While the facts he reports are now fairly well known, the themes he develops
offer considerable scope for comment.

I wish to begin my discussion by first considering the introductory section of the paper which offers an overview of the current focus of interest in
the history of medicine in France. Dr. Goubert characterizes his study of
"The Medicalization of French Society at the End of the Ancien Régime" as a
contribution to the mainstream of French medical history. Younger French
historians, and also some of their American and British counterparts, have
recently focused their attention upon topics such as the sociology of the
medical profession, the analysis of medical language, and the history of attitudes towards the body, often under the influence of anthropology, historical ethnology, and psychoanalysis.[1] While none of this may seem new to a
number of medical historians in this audience, some of whom began the exploration of these approaches up to thirty or forty years ago,[2] in France, according to Goubert, this was not the case. Prior to the 1960s, he believes,
the history of medicine languished in the hands of physicians and philosophers, two groups that have had a circumscribed outlook on the subject. Like
all generalizations, this statement overlooks the efforts of certain individuals. Such hardworking scholars as Paul Delaunay, on whose wide-ranging
publications all who investigate this area still depend, and who was both
physician and historian, seem to me obvious counterexamples to this claim.[3]
Be that as it may, according to Dr. Goubert it was only with the advent of
the new demographic, anthropological, and social perspective of the sixties
that the history of medicine in France received a new Enlightenment and es-
caped from being a parochial and complacent area of scholarship. Now while
there are obviously elements of truth in this description, and interesting and
influential new studies are certainly being produced, a survey of current
work in the history of medicine in France does not lead one to be quite as
sanguine as Dr. Goubert that the limited and parochial outlook of the past
has been entirely overcome.[4] One continuing weakness of medical history by
French scholars is the relative lack of comparative reference to medical events
beyond the bounds of France which might enable historians to see develop-

ments within the country in a broader context. Another difficulty is the little recognition given to the substantive and ever-growing body of work on the medical history of France being produced by other European and American scholars.[5] Satisfaction on having managed to move from Paris to the provinces, from bourgeois perceptions of control to the peasant mentality of suffering, and the dread tyranny of official medicine to the sympathetic and helpful attitudes of the folk healer, should not obscure this lack of dialogue. Let us hope that a symposium such as this will help to promote a new awareness for all concerned.

In the main body of his paper, Dr. Goubert offers a contribution to the fashionable debate on the process of what has been termed the "medicalization" of society. In his discussion, Dr. Goubert seems to subscribe to the meaning of the term given wide currency by Ivan Illich in his book *Medical Nemesis*.[6] Society, in this view, has become increasingly dependent on medicine and the medical profession in organizing everyday life. In fact, the medical profession has perpetrated a fraud on society by persuading it that it cannot make decisions about matters of health, hygiene, and life and death without reference to medical expertise. Dr. Goubert accepts the validity of this thesis and his task, given that this process has occurred, is to determine when it started. He argues that this "medical imperialism," another catch phrase of the nineteenth and twentieth centuries, had its origins in a late-eighteenth-century vision of medicine. Professional gains, both social and economic, the urban concentration of personnel, and an alliance between the medical profession and the public authorities laid the groundwork for the power developed by the bourgeois physician in the nineteenth century. This line of argument is of course related to the general historical thesis of the rise of the bourgeoisie to social dominance at this time with the associated gains made by all the professions.[7] In a more secular society, medicine becomes the new priesthood. In this regard, Dr. Goubert's initial comparison of medical history to ecclesiastical history is surely no accident.

As outlined by Dr. Goubert, the eighteenth-century vision of medicine which set the stage for nineteenth-century developments is that ascribed to the Société Royale de Médecine. Far from presenting a radical outlook, Dr. Goubert's argument fits into the conventional historiographical view that this medical society anticipated in many respects the development of nineteenth-century French medicine. Already the Society has been characterized by other historians both as the advance guard of the new scientific medicine as manifested in the early-nineteenth-century Paris hospital and as the forerunner of the professional institutions that developed in the post-Revolutionary period.[8] In Dr. Goubert's account we are now invited to see it as providing the storm troops of the new medical profession who were going to invade all corners of the French countryside, wrest control of all health and medical matters from local providers of care and advice, and fill the void where no such sources existed.

All of these ways of using the Société Royale de Médecine in historical discussion have certain problems, and to understand why this is the case we need to consider a little more closely several aspects of eighteenth-century French medicine. In my commentary I propose to focus on three: the nature of this medical society; the question of professional autonomy, and the significance of rural medicine.

The Société Royale de Médecine was in conception, organization, and activity an institution of the Ancien Régime. It came into being as an agency of the State with a twofold charge: firstly, to collect and systematize all the available data on epidemics; and secondly, on the basis of the information thus collected, to render advice and assistance to the royal administration on the management of epidemics, both human and animal. Although the basis of its interests broadened over the years, this concern with epidemic disease remained central to its activities and its continuing advisory role to the French government.[9] It was for carrying out this function that the Society wished to bring its concerns to the attention of the provincial intendants and to integrate its program with the administrative network of the state in the provinces. In this role as an agency of the government, it is not accurate to portray the Society's activities as a self-expression of bourgeois professionalism or as an autonomous expression of medical dominance. It was the servant of an absolutist state.

The Société Royale de Médecine also sought to be accepted and to gain public recognition as an Academy of Medicine. This other major aspect of its activity was also very much linked to an eighteenth-century outlook. By the time the Society was instituted in 1776, many young physicians felt that they were losing status in the medical world in a way that contrasted sharply with the social and professional gains achieved by some surgeons. As far back as 1731, the surgeons had developed their own learned society, the Académie Royale de Chirurgie. They had freed themselves to a large extent from the teaching and supervision of the medical faculties and colleges and upgraded their own educational requirements. Finally their independence and prosperity had received public recognition with the building, at government expense, of the splendid new Schools of Surgery in Paris, which were opened in 1772.[10] In emulation of the surgeons, the physicians of the Society sought to forge an alliance with the government to obtain support and funding, with some loss of the corporate autonomy enjoyed by the medical faculties and colleges.

There was more to this, however, than a question of royal patronage in exchange for usefulness for the royal administration. The vehicle or institution by which they sought to elevate the standing of medicine was a characteristic eighteenth-century one; namely, through a learned Academy. The public symbol of the Society was a body of learned physicians devoted to the advance of medical science through observation and experiment. It is a mistake to underestimate the value that the early members attached to the scientific function of the Society and make this subservient to purely professional goals. The image of the eighteenth-century Parisian savant is a more dominant image than that of the proto-nineteenth-century physician in the provinces.

Unless this eighteenth-century context is kept in mind, it is all too easy to characterize the Société Royale de Médecine's plans as forerunners of broader nineteenth-century professional development. Dr. Goubert seems to see a transformation of one into the other but anyone who really wants to make this argument has to explain exactly how the Society's approach was transformed into the new bourgeois professionalism. It is not sufficient to say that a program existed and therefore it was an augur of things to come. The historical reality, that the Société Royale de Médecine was perceived by contemporaries as one of the elitist and royalist institutions of the Ancien Régime and was therefore abolished like them in 1793, cannot be wished away. Traditional or old-fashioned history of medicine has often been decried for its anticipatory vision: its penchant for seeing too readily in earlier medical developments the portent of things to come. Those who advocate the sociological approach should also tread warily to avoid falling into the same traps.

Let us now look a little more closely at this whole question of professional autonomy. To what degree do late eighteenth-century views represent a new professional outlook? The medical profession of the eighteenth century in France was scarcely a united front. The divisions between physicians, surgeons, and apothecaries or pharmacists were very real. The rise of the surgeons, as I have already indicated, was a source of concern to many physicians and a number of different strategies were developed to counter this threat. Moreover, the physicians themselves were deeply divided on the best means to advance medicine and further the interests of the profession. Far from contributing to the autonomy of the medical profession, in the eyes of many physicians the Société Royale de Médecine and its proposals represented a distinct threat. For the development of an alliance with the royal government by some physicians was a challenge to the corporative control exerted by the medical faculties and colleges and to their position as medical authorities and founts of medical wisdom. Many physicians were far more concerned about preserving their independence from outside interference in professional activities than with provision of medical care to all the French population regardless of whether it was wanted or needed.[11]

To describe the Société Royale de Médecine as a purveyor of a normative vision that set the scene for nineteenth-century developments seems overstated. It did serve to ally some physicians with the new scientific medicine but by no means all of them.

Again if we wish to demonstrate how the bourgeois physician developed a position of authority and power, we really need far more discussion of developments in the early nineteenth century. What was the structure and the status of the new groups and professional institutions after the Revolution? Still not nearly enough is known about this period and the tendency to write medical history as if the Revolution makes no difference to outlook or professional aspirations and ambitions is becoming perhaps too common and is obscuring a number of real historical developments.

Another claim made by Dr. Goubert is that, in the utopia of a medicalized society dispensed by the Société Royale de Médecine, the countryside of France was seen as an area devoid of medical care wide open for invasion by an aggressive medical profession. I too have argued elsewhere that through the Society physicians sought to gain some influence in rural medicine, but I feel Dr. Goubert's portrayal simplifies the position too much.[12] In the first place, the Society's concern with medical care in the countryside was part of an agronomic vision of medicine and society that constituted an integral part of its outlook. Too little attention has been paid to the fact that animal epidemics were one of the key reasons that this Society was founded and a concern with animal and crop diseases constituted an essential part of its continuing program of research. In addition to Vicq d'Azyr, Turgot was instrumental in the establishment of this medical society. Himself not a physician but a minister of state, he articulated the physiocratic philosophy that the land and its products were the primary source of wealth for a state, thereby influencing the entire Society program. The unification of medicine that was of primary concern to Vicq d'Azyr was the unification of human and animal medicine. He exhorted physicians to become concerned with the latter not primarily to further "medicalization," but rather to foster a scientific vision and research program rooted in a comparative anatomy and pathology. In short, what Dr. Goubert sees as a monolithic professional imperialism is composed in my view of a number of complex strands: administrative response to social and economic crisis; professional insecurity; and a well-articulated scientific program.

The physicians of the Society did not in fact seek to go out in the countryside themselves to extend their professional sphere. Rather they tried to become involved in the training of veterinarians and establish the latter as a rural medical corps for more systematic care of diseased animals. As a study of this process has shown, many veterinarians, instead of encountering a void, found it difficult to make a living at all in rural areas: encountering great local resistance to innovation in healers and also resentment from already established guilds of farriers.[13]

The overwhelming reason, however, for the interest by Society physicians in the Veterinary School at Alfort was to gain research facilities for their scientific program. Research ideals were more at stake than medical dominance.[14] The programmatic statements governing Society activities as well as the eulogies of Vicq d'Azyr need to be considered for any rounded account of a normative vision.

At the beginning of his paper, Dr. Goubert cited two main sources as the inspiration for the new French medical history. On the one hand is the highly theoretical, one must say philosophically inspired, writing of Michel Foucault: on the other, the very different aim of tracing the material conditions of existence represented by the Annales School. The major problem confronting the use of these traditions in medical historiography is bringing the insights of these two very different approaches together. Dr. Goubert's paper today represents a significant attempt to achieve just such a synthesis. While I have been critical of some aspects of his interpretation, there can be no doubt that the problem he has confronted and the issues he has raised will remain important in the history of medicine for some time to come.

NOTES

[1]The work of Michel Foucault has greatly influenced these younger French scholars. See *Madness and Civilization: A History of Insanity in the Age of Reason*, trans. Richard Howard (New York: Pantheon Books, 1965); idem, *The Order of Things: An Archaeology of the Human Sciences* (New York: Pantheon Books, 1970); idem, *The Birth of the Clinic: An Archaeology of Medical Perception*, trans. A. M. Sheridan Smith (New York: Pantheon Books, 1973); idem, *Les Machines à guérir* (Paris: Institut de l'Environnement, 1976). The other influence is the work of the *Annales* school. See the many articles on medical topics in recent years in the journal *Annales: Economies, Sociétés, Civilisations*. English translations of a selection of these have been made available in Robert Forster and Orest Ranum, eds., *Biology of Man in History* (Baltimore: The Johns Hopkins University Press, 1975) and idem, *Medicine and Society in France* (Baltimore: The Johns Hopkins University Press, 1980). For examples of the work of some American and British scholars see Patricia Branca, ed., *The Medicine Show: Patients, Physicians, and the Perplexities of the Health Revolution in Modern Society* (New York: Science History Publications, 1977).

[2]See, for example, the work of Erwin H. Ackerknecht in the *Bulletin of the History of Medicine* in the 1940s and also his *Medicine and Ethnology: Selected Essays*, ed. H. H. Walser and H. M. Koelbing (Bern: H. Huber, 1971). See also Ackerknecht, "A Plea for a 'Behaviorist' Approach in Writing the History of Medicine," *J. Hist. Med.* 22 (1967): 211–14.

[3]Paul Delaunay, *Le Monde médicale parisien au dix-huitième siècle* (Paris: J. Rousset, 1905); idem, *La Vie médicale aux XVIe, XVIIe et XVIIIe siècles* (Paris: Editions Hippocrate, 1935); idem, *Etudes sur l'hygiène, l'assistance et les secours publics dans le Maine sous l'ancien régime* (Le Mans: Imprimerie Monnoyer, 1922–23); idem, *La Maternité de Paris* (Paris: J. Rousset, 1909).

[4]See, for example, J.-P. Goubert, *Malades et médecins en Bretagne: 1770–1790* (Paris: Librairie Klincksieck, 1974); François Lebrun, *Les Hommes et la mort en Anjou aux 17e et 18e siècles* (Paris: La Haye, 1971); François Loux, *Le Jeune Enfant et son corps dans la médecine traditionelle* (Paris: Flammarion, 1978).

[5]For example, Toby Gelfand, *Professionalizing Modern Medicine: Paris Surgeons and Medical Science and Institutions in the Eighteenth Century* (Westport, Connecticut: Greenwood Press, 1980); idem, "Medical Professionals and Charlatans: The *Comité de Salubrité enquête* of 1790–91," *Histoire Sociale/Social History* 11 (1978): 62–95; William Coleman, "Health and Hygiene in the *Encyclopédie*: A Medical Doctrine for the Bourgeoisie," *J. Hist. Med.* 29 (1974): 399–421; Dora Weiner, "Le Droit

de l'homme à la santé: Une belle idée devant l'Assemblée Constituante, 1790–1791," *Clio Med.* 5 (1970): 209–23; idem, "The French Revolution, Napoleon, and the Nursing Profession," *Bull. Hist. Med.* 46 (1972): 274–305; Caroline Hannaway, "The Société Royale de Médecine and Epidemics in the Ancien Régime," *Bull. Hist. Med.* 46 (1972): 257–73; idem, "Veterinary Medicine and Rural Health Care in Pre-Revolutionary France," *Bull. Hist. Med.* 51 (1977): 431–47; Louis Greenbaum, "Jean-Sylvain Bailly, the Baron de Breteuil and the Four New Hospitals of Paris," *Clio Med.* 8 (1973): 261–84; Matthew Ramsey, "Medical Power and Popular Medicine: Illegal Healers in Nineteenth-Century France," *J. Soc. Hist.* 10 (1977): 560–87; Harvey Mitchell, "Rationality and Control in Eighteenth-Century Medical Views of the Peasantry," *Comp. Stud. in Soc. and Hist.* 21 (1979): 82–112.

[6]Ivan Illich, *Medical Nemesis: The Expropriation of Health* (New York: Bantam, 1977).

[7]W. J. Reader, *Professional Men* (London: Weidenfeld and Nicolson, 1966); M. Larson, *The Rise of Professionalism* (Berkeley: University of California Press, 1977).

[8]Erwin H. Ackerknecht, *Medicine at the Paris Hospital: 1794–1848* (Baltimore: Johns Hopkins University Press, 1967), p. 27; Paul Ganière, *L'Académie de Médecine: Ses origines et son histoire* (Paris: Librairie Maloine, 1964), pp. 15–30.

[9]Hannaway, "Société Royale de Médecine and Epidemics," pp. 257–73.

[10]See Gelfand, *Professionalizing Modern Medicine*, chaps. 4, 5, and 6.

[11]Caroline Hannaway, "Medicine, Public Welfare and the State in Eighteenth-Century France: The Société Royale de Médecine of Paris, 1776–1793," (Ph.D. diss., The Johns Hopkins University, 1974), chap. 7 "Corporate versus Academic Medicine."

[12]Hannaway, "Veterinary Medicine," pp. 431–47.

[13]Ibid., pp. 442–43.

[14]Ibid., pp. 439–40.

THE INFLUENCE OF THE NINETEENTH-CENTURY VIENNA SCHOOL ON ITALIAN MEDICINE: THE ROLES OF PADUA AND TRIESTE

Loris Premuda

In this essay I shall try to condense the results of my previous studies, offering a general picture of the influence of the nineteenth-century Vienna School of Medicine on Italian medicine and detailing the twofold function—assimilation and cultural mediation—that characterized the medical life of Padua and Trieste during this period.

Padua is a very old center, a place where the roads of Veneto and Trentino-Alto Adige and those of northeast Italy and Emilia meet. It is an important rural, trade, and industrial center.

Trieste, whose origins are old too, emerged as an important port and commercial center during the early decades of the eighteenth century, when the Habsburg Empire began a period of great reforms. Padua had been the seat of a university since 1222, Trieste only for some decades. The former prospered under the Venetian Republic from 1405 to 1797; its control was then contested by Austria and France until 1813, and it remained thereafter under the Austrian Empire until 1866. Trieste remained almost uninterruptedly under the protection of Austria—from 1399 until the end of World War I. For more than five centuries, most of its population has been bilingual—both Italian and German being spoken—whereas in Padua there were greater difficulties with German. Only a small part of the population, in fact, was able to speak it properly in the last century.

Between the fourteenth and fifteenth centuries, it was Vienna that absorbed the first elements of a modern medical science from Padua; in 1404, Paduan Galeazzo da Santa Sofia (1368–1427), professor of medicine in Vienna between 1398 and 1406, performed the first formal post-mortem examination before the public.[1] The nineteenth century, however, saw Italy become the recipient. Italian medicine drew upon the experience and thought of the teachers of "*Alma Mater Rudolphina,*" and was influenced—though to a lesser extent—by the period of "*Wiener Medizin der Stifft-Zeit*" (1803–1836) and that of the "*zweite medizinische* Schule" and of the "*neuer Spezialismus.*"[2] At the beginning of that century, Italy had just weathered the Napoleonic storm and was heading towards its national identity; its commitments, therefore, essentially followed political and military objec-

180

tives. Italy, which had in the previous centuries been magistra of arts and sciences, saw itself forced to lag behind, to become a tributary of other countries. Given the times, for Padua and Trieste, as well as for Pavia, the political circumstance of living under the hegemony of the Habsburg Empire represented a fortunate opportunity from the point of view of medicine. The relationship with the Medical School of Vienna, just at the apogee of its greatness, developed that much more directly, swiftly, and easily.

The roles of Padua and Pavia in receiving and transmitting the Vienna medical philosophy have usually been neglected by critics, and that of Trieste often simply ignored. Political elements of nationalistic nature clearly prevailed over historical objectivity, and, for one reason or another, they arrested the work of many valuable scholars. Arturo Castiglioni (1874–1953), a native of Trieste, was an Italian irredentist with liberal-nationalistic ideals whose work dealt briefly with some aspects of the nineteenth-century medicine of Trieste. Characteristically, it did not go as far as a direct analysis of the rich relationship between Trieste and the Medical School of Vienna.[3] In his short monograph on Padua, he confined himself to a treatment of Bassini (1844–1924), renowned surgeon and hero of the Risorgimento, and De Giovanni (1838–1916), while ignoring other personalities who were somehow linked to the Vienna school.[4] Massalongo (1857–1920), Tanfani (1882–1953), F. Pellegrini (1883–1960), and the keen and versatile Davide Giordano (1864–1954): all were occasionally interested in the history of Paduan medicine, but never dwelt upon the Padua-Vienna aspect *ex professo*. In Austria, at the other end, even the famous Neuburger acted similarly. Recently, Lesky pointed out the value of any study aimed at better defining the influence of the Vienna Medical School of the nineteenth century on international medicine. She also very kindly referred to the work we conducted precisely in this sector.[5]

As early as the first decades of the century in question, an interesting cultural exchange took place, involving the migration of Paduan physicians to Vienna and vice versa. Winners of scholarships from Padua were sent to Vienna for a two-year period in order to attend there the K. K. Operateurinstitut, which according to Lesky's judgment was "the springboard for future Austrian surgeons," in the framework of "Stifft's surgical reform program."[6] They operated first under the direction of von Kern (1760–1829) and later von Wattmann (1789–1866), with the objective of obtaining the qualification of *Magister der Chirurgie und Geburtshilfe*, the latter designation referring to their having attended lessons in obstetrics as well. Young and worthy collaborators belonging to the modern Viennese clinics moved to Padua and held different, newly instituted chairs in that university. At the same time, in Trieste—whose links with Vienna and the monarchy dated back considerably—there were several physicians who had the qualification of *Magister der Chirurgie und Geburtshilfe* stemming from the "Alma Mater Rudolphina": many were indigenous practitioners, while others came from Austria, Hungary, Bohemia, or Poland.[7] Among their number it suffices to cite Teofilo Koepel (or Koepl) (ca. 1795–1862), whom Corradi remembered as a pioneer among Italian surgeons as regards the ligature of the carotid.[8]

Let us go back to those Paduan physicians who had moved to Vienna in order to specialize. Many of them were to hold chairs at Padua: Francesco Cortese (1802–1883), Vincenzo Fabeni (1799–1861), Giacomandrea Giacomini (1797–1849), Bartolomeo Signoroni (1796–1844), Luigi Gianelli (1789–1872), Tito Vanzetti (1808–1888), and Lodovico Brunetti (1813–1899). Officially, specialization courses were centered on surgery or, as in the instance of Brunetti, extended to obstetrics at most. In practice, however, students in the great European center of studies moved from institute to institute and hence attended different subjects and listened to the lessons of some of the most noted scholars of that time. Cortese, for example, a qualified military surgeon, had the opportunity of attending anatomy courses in Vienna under the guidance of Joseph Berres (1796–1844), teacher of the renowned Joseph Hyrtl (1811–1894), and firm supporter of the didactic importance of an anatomy museum.[9] Cortese, who in 1838 was called to the chair of human anatomy, improved on this idea and conceived of an anthropological museum. Simultaneously, the experience at the Vienna school stimulated his interest in morphological research on blood vessels by means of intracapillary injections.[10] During his residency in Vienna, Vincenzo Fabeni had, besides the tenets of specialist surgery, acquired an excellent training in biology. In 1836 he was called to succeed Gallini (1756–1836), a forerunner of the scientific concept of "tissue" (1792),[11] and in Padua he imported the latest acquisitions in the fields of histology, physics, and organic chemistry that were of great interest for the progress of physiology.[12] The teaching and the research of Giacomini and Gianelli show the fermenting presence of new ideas transmitted from Viennese circles.[13] The former advocated a renewal of experimental pharmacology while the latter preached a more up-to-date statistical and comparative approach to medical and hygienic issues in collaboration with the other European countries.[14]

Clear evidence of the deep doctrinal and methodological connections of Signoroni with the school of von Kern is found in the specific action of the Viennese teacher in supporting Signoroni's appointment as regular professor of the surgical clinic at the University of Pavia, a post that Signoroni held until 1830 when he transferred to Padua.[15] As regards Vanzetti, the pupil of Signoroni in Padua and of von Wattmann in Vienna, it is well to remember that already in 1837 he was called to direct the surgical and ophthalmological clinic at the University of Karchoff, and that in 1852 he had come back to Padua to take over his teacher's chair, thereby acting as mediator of the new ideas he had acquired during his stay in Vienna and in his European travels, both on the level of clinical organization and of surgical techniques.[16] In reference to Brunetti, it should be pointed out that, after having completed his specialization in Vienna, he had the fortunate opportunity to explore the field of pathological anatomy under the expert direction of Rokitansky, for whom he acted as temporary assistant. Subsequently, in 1855, he returned to the university of his origin and held there the first chair of pathological anatomy.[17]

The academic year 1818–19 marked the arrival at the Paduan *Studium* of several professors of the Vienna school. First among them was Anton Rosas (1791–1855), disciple of Georg Joseph Beer (1763–1821), head professor of the ophthalmology clinic in Vienna. Rosas introduced a new approach in the evaluation of eye affections in Padua on the basis of careful and precise objective examinations.[18] In illustrating the eye affections to his pupils, Rosas, among other things, made use of valuable wax models that were prepared by J. H. Hofmayr, a sculptor as well as a renowned surgeon who was active in Vienna; these have recently been described by the present writer.[19] In 1819, after almost a four years' stay in Trieste, where at the Spedale Civico he had held lessons of *ars obstetricia* to midwives, Rodolfo Lamprecht (1781–1860), former pupil of Johann Lucas Boër (1752–1835) at the Vienna University, was appointed professor of theoretical and practical obstetrics at the Paduan *Studium*.[20] He introduced the *ars obstetricia per expectationem* he had derived from his teacher first in Trieste and then in Padua. He was a firm and fervent advocate of this notion and was soon able to report on the effective results achieved in childbirth assistance.[21] Lamprecht's teaching was one of the most successful channels for the transmission of Boër's approach in Italy. Martin Steer (ca. 1800–1850), a Hungarian physician, also stemmed from the Vienna school. In Padua he was responsible for the chair of general pathology and pharmacology in 1827, a post he held until 1842.[22] Wilhelm Lippich (1799–1845), disciple of von Raimann (1780–1847), assumed in 1834 the direction of the medical clinic and brought a fresh impetus of objectivity in the medical circles of Padua (even if only within certain limits, since the excesses of Brownianism were still to be felt). After an independent experience as codirector at the Ljubljana Hospital, he was able to stir up the interest of his colleagues in Padua. Furthermore, it was under his guidance that Vincenzo Pinali (1802–1875), his assistant, began the seminars of physical semeiology in the academic year 1835–36.[23]

At this point an entire new chapter is open to our consideration: that concerning the problem of the reintroduction of Morgagni's anatomical-clinical method in Padua, after its analytical and perfective filtration by the Paris school. What are the channels of this operation? As early as in 1974, we were able to draw the clear conclusion that, as regards cultural information, Brera (1772–1840), medical clinic director, had written of *"percussione toracica ed auscultazione"* (thoracic percussion and auscultation) in 1823, that is, four years after the publication of the treatise of Laennec; and that in

1825, Amadeo de Moulon (1796–1879) had published, during his final year, a work of mere compilation on the lines of Laennec himself "on the way of using Laennec's stethoscope in order to state the affections of the lungs and heart by means of mediate auscultation."[24] As has already been said, Pinali, Lippich's disciple, was the pioneer in the organization of seminars for the students where he employed the auscultatory method: he reported the fact, yet without giving it much publicity. Indeed, rather marginally and unpretentiously he wrote: "At the end of this introduction I discharge my debt of gratitude toward D. Vincenzo Pinali, the expert assistant in my course for both this and the previous year, because in the examination of the patients he always performed his duties most excellently, above all with the stethoscope, as well as all the other means at his disposal."[25] However important the successful approach of Pinali to physical semeiology might be, obviously it was not tantamount to a complete adoption of the anatomical-clinical method. Pinali's contribution, rather, was a necessary stage in the edification of anatomical clinicians. The breaking off with the links of romantic-vitalistic ideals is epitomized by the call of Francesco Saverio Verson (1805–1849) to the chair of medical clinic for surgeons "by appointment of H.I.R. Majesty, dated July the 23rd, 1842, from Vienna."[26]

But let us first see who this Verson was: a figure almost ignored, even forgotten, by histories of medicine.[27] Verson received his education in Vienna where he graduated in July 1830, "Excellent First in all Subjects." In 1834 he became medical chief physician at the Trieste hospital where he was able to examine a considerable number of patients. We can call upon the words of Carlo Bonafini, I. R. assistant at the clinic directed by Verson in Padua. In a detailed evaluation of the lesions induced by fever in the cardiovascular system, Bonafini reports his teacher's ideas. "In the numerous postmortem examinations he performed...in the great hospital of Trieste... [Verson] stated that he had sometimes found traces of inflammation on the internal surfaces of the vena cava and in the principal arterial tracts; sometimes he could not find the least indication either of existing or of previous inflammation."[28] This brief reference and the very words of Verson in 1844 about a necroscopic experience on the basis of more than one thousand autopsies of cases that had been thoroughly followed on the clinical level,[29] present us with a systematic use of post-mortem examinations carried out both on hospital cases, in Trieste, and in cases from the clinic in Padua. Bonafini, in his detailed report on the cases examined in the clinic in the school year 1842–43,[30] reminds us of the customary utilization of "*soccorsi diagnostico-acustici*," in other words, the systematic resort to percussion and auscultation. Yet, beside the precise evidence of the disciple, the entire treatise by Verson makes clear reference to a more modern physical semeiology and to the stethoscope as early as 1838. In *Der Arzt am Krankenbette der Kinder und an der Wiege der Säuglinge*, dedicated to Raimann and published in Vienna in that year, a systematic reference occurs to a thorough clinical examination supported by anatomo-pathological reports, providing clear evidence of the mature conviction and the confidence that Verson placed in the methods of the *anatomische Klinik* in the 1830s, and, what is more significant, even before the appearance of *Abhandlung über Perkussion und Auskultation* by Skoda (1805–1881). The direct sources of Verson's knowledge were those of Vienna. The fact that his teacher at the medical clinic, Raimann, would advise "percussione ad modum Auenbruggeri, sthetoscopo (sic!) Laennecii probe examinare" is well known.[31] As regards anatomical-pathological education we know that the years of Verson's residency in Vienna marked his activity as *Prosektur* under the direction of Lorenz Biermayer (1780–1830?), assisted by Johann Wagner (1800–1833) and Karl Rokitansky (1804–1878), who was then *Praktikant*. To judge from the picture emerging from these data of the *anatomische Klinik*, it does not appear to have been very prosperous in Vienna either, since the approach to the method was rather hesitant, which corroborates our straightforward positive judgment on the efficacy and accuracy of Verson's achievements. In fact he had been able to develop and improve upon the initial trend of the Viennese school by means of sound and solid arguments, and to transmit it to the southern areas of *Mitteleuropa*.

These premises enable us to highlight certain aspects and moments of a phase of great importance in the diffusion of Viennese medical thought: we can observe, within the framework of the revival in Trieste, Padua, and Italy in general, Morgagni's anatomical-clinical method, being extended and perfected. Firstly, we may say that the first direct, if timid, moves towards Laennec's doctrine by Breda and de Moulon in Padua had remained "dead letter." A bolder incentive proved more successful. The early work carried out by Pinali in his seminars in physical semeiology, combined with the riper achievements of Verson, were able to break the ties with vitalistic romanticism in medicine, thereby establishing positive and solid bases for future scientific work. Furthermore, it should be made clear that Verson's presence, first in Trieste and then in Padua, enabled the medical circles of Trieste, which was not yet a university seat, to assimilate the anatomico-clinical approach before Padua. A further matter of interest is the fact that the Paris school had comparatively little influence in the eastern area of northern Italy, which, on the contrary, was prevalently influenced by the activity of the Vienna school. That all clinical innovations and improvements then elaborated in Padua were swiftly channeled and spread out into the rest of Italy is easily understandable, bearing in mind that the Paduan surgical *Studium* numbered roughly 500 students around 1830 and continued to enjoy a considerable renown.[32]

It appears to be a general admission that the 1840s and 1850s were marked by the fundamental activity of the team of Skoda and Rokitansky and represented the apogee of the Vienna Medical School. Its didactic, methodological, and operative accomplishments had obtained a new impetus by the appointment of Johann von Oppolzer (1808–1871) to the direction of the Second Medical Clinic in 1849. Sigerist acutely pointed out: "Thus in the middle decades of the nineteenth century there was a widespread feeling that no European doctor's education was complete unless he had spent a considerable period of study in Vienna."[33] As a matter of fact, Paduan physicians did attend Skoda's clinic and Pinali is very likely to have been one of his disciples in the 1840s. Vittore Dal Canton, clinical assistant in Padua, was certainly present as temporary assistant of von Oppolzer at the beginning of the 1850s. We may recall his translation of *Lehrbuch der Krankheiten des Herzens*, which was authored by his teacher.[34] It is certainly to be stressed that the 1850s and the 1860s recorded the peak of the activity of the team of Pinali and Brunetti in Padua, clinician and anatomical pathologist respectively. On a smaller scale, the two were the reflected image of the Vienna-based team of Skoda and Rokitansky. Pinali's anatomical-clinical conception fully emerges from the minute of his appointment at the medical clinic. It is important to notice the acceptance of the new clinical approach, semeiological method, on the one hand, and the unquestioned confidence in the value of anatomical-pathological report as "surer guide and direction" in the medical profession on the other.[35] Brunetti's approach is unquestionable. It goes hand in hand with Rokitansky's, whose assistant Brunetti had been.

Trieste, before Padua, recorded Verson's presence in its medical circles. We are led to think that Skoda's doctrine and methodology were certainly conveyed by him to the Adriatic town. The best known among Skoda's disciples in Trieste was, however, Alessandro Manussi de Ochabitza (1836–1914). First- and second-class aide at the Allgemeines Krankenhaus of Vienna from June 1858 to May 1862,[36] then chief physician at the Spedale Civico of Trieste, he seized the opportunity of his position to mold several generations of physicians on the basis of anatomical-clinical method.[37] At this point a correction should be made in Plitek's statement crediting Giacomo Benporat (1836–1898), a pupil of Pinali in Padua, with having carried the method of physical diagnosis to Trieste during the 1860s.[38] As has already been said, the indisputable contribution of Verson as early as in the 1830s and the further-reaching and more authoritative accomplishments of Manussi have, in fact, been exhaustively demonstrated. Having come so far, it should be pointed out that the second half of the century witnessed an even more accentuated influence from Italian exponents of the Viennese school in all sectors of the public and cultural life of Trieste; nor were physicians wanting. Trieste, in fact, was the only important Italian town that had direct contacts with the culture of *Mitteleuropa*, and of Vienna in particular.

Theodor Billroth (1829–1894) is certainly the most conspicuous personality among the nineteenth-century surgeons. He was responsible for a significant turning point and a fresh impetus in the evolution of surgery. At the end of his life he wrote: "What has given me joy in a diversified life has been the foundation of a school which is continuing the trend of my activities alike in scientific and in humanitarian directions, so that it seems destined to have a fair measure of durability."[39] This school developed and spread out to all Europe, becoming a significant reality in nineteenth-century medical life. The contribution of Billroth's Trieste disciples in the diffusion of his scientific doctrine and of his surgical techniques in Italy was essential to this process. It occurred through two generations of surgeons, shaping Billroth's direct disciples and the pupils of those disciples. Among the disciples of the first generation who most distinguished themselves, we can cite: Arturo Menzel (1844–1878), who had been Billroth's favorite assistant in the first years of Viennese teaching and then became chief surgeon in Trieste in 1872; and Gustavo Usiglio (1855–1933), who for more than five years attended the clinic of Billroth and the school of Leopold von Dittel (1815–1898) alternately.

Arturo Menzel was at first *operateur* and then clinical assistant of Billroth until August 1872, when he was called to the direction of the IV Surgical Department of the Spedale Civico of Trieste. Pagel writes that he was "a daring, enterprising, deliberate, assured and elegant operator."[40] In a letter to Brettauer, president of the Spedale of Trieste, Menzel's teacher wrote that Menzel was "not only one of my most esteemed students, but also one of my most faithful friends."[41] He published forty-five works. One of these which deserves special attention is the research work, "On the Resorption of Food-Stuffs from the Subcutaneous Cellular Tissue," completed in 1869 in collaboration with H. Perco, aide at the Allgemeines Krankenhaus.[42] This study prepared the foundations for the investigation of parenteral nutrition and was therefore a clear prelude to the forthcoming requirements of patients undergoing stomach or intestine operations. The scientific production of Menzel is marked by a great variety of interests—ranging from studies of necrosis of bone in different parts of the skeleton, of ovariectomy and osteopathology to studies of esophagostomy, neoplasias, and the surgical therapies in different affections. All these scientific works appeared partly in *Wiener medizinische Wochenschrift* and in *Archiv für klinische Chirurgie*, and partly in *Gazzetta Medica Italiana Lombardia*. In the *Centralblatt für Chirurgie*, Menzel summarized Italian studies in surgery. All this "made him the interpreter in the exchange of ideas between two cultures, the architect of an international mission to which he was particularly suited, being a master of the two languages."[43] Gustavo Usiglio was, in turn, the Italian translator of the fundamental monograph by Wölfler (1850–1917), "Ueber die von Herrn Professor Billroth ausgeführten Resektionen des carcinomatösen Pylorus."[44] Thus, only a short time after the significant surgical accomplishment, he brought the news of the resection performed for the first time in the history of surgery by the Viennese teacher to the Italian public. Usiglio, besides, had great scientific talent but, for many reasons, he did not enjoy the recognition he deserved. He was author of several scientific notes. To one of these special consideration should be given: a monograph on thyroid tumors, which, in 1895, shortly after its first edition, was published for a second time, structured on the guidelines of the celebrated school of surgery from which Usiglio stemmed. Among Billroth's disciples who enjoyed renown in Trieste and in Italian cultural circles, we may also cite Theodor Escher (1847–1923), the master's pupil in Vienna and the clinical assistant of Rose (1836–1917) in Zürich. He succeeded Menzel in Trieste and was the initiator of abdominal surgery on a large scale: operations such as gastroentero-anastomosis in ulcers with pyloric stenosis, removal of large segments of intestine in the case of tumors, and, in 1900, a circular resection of the esophagus with immediate and permanent suture of the stumps to avoid stenosis.[45] The X Surgical Department—of recent creation—recorded the activity of another among Billroth's disciples: Vittorio Massopust (1857–1944), a gifted *operateur*.

Among the disciples of the second generation, Billroth's "grandchildren," our consideration should be directed to an entire squad of valuable surgeons, all of whom shared a deep and meticulous knowledge of human anatomy, in line with the principles of the Vienna school of surgery. They were pupils of von Eiselberg (1860–1939) like Almerigo d'Este (1880–1959), successor of Escher; Renato Gandusio (1887–1930), whom the teacher held in high esteem and affectionately recalled in his *Lebensweg eines Chirurgen*;[46] and Ettore Nordio (1889–1977), director of a surgical nursing-home. As a disciple and assistant of Karl Gussenbauer (1842–1903), successor to Billroth's chair, we recall Emilio Comisso (1875–1954), who was first surgical assistant of Escher in Trieste and, in 1909, founder, and for thirty years director, of the Ospizio Marino di Valdoltra, an important health resort near Trieste that was well known for the treatment of osteoarticular affections. Between 1910 and 1940 the center became the meeting point of many Italian surgeons who went there to learn from Comisso. He had been a disciple of the famous Lorenz (1854–1946) in Vienna and was operating along the lines of the fundamental principles preached by Billroth. Thus he was able to teach all those refined techniques of osteoarticular surgery which were then radiated to the universities and the hospitals of the rest of Italy.

Ettore Oliani (1878–1956), a friend of Sauerbruch (1875–1951) and chief surgeon in Trieste, was the one who in 1929 was able to make reference to an extremely wide range of cases—almost 782—of surgery on gastroduodenal ulcers. This was the richest experience from a statistical point of view in Italy at that time,[47] obviously conducted along the lines of the specific interests of the Vienna School. It must be said, in fact, that Oliani had been the disciple, in Graz, of Viktor Hacker (1852–1933) who directed the surgical clinic and was one of the last eminent disciples of Billroth. Still further, always referring to the excellent results achieved in Trieste by the descendants of the famous Billroth school of surgery, let us focus on the two instances of heart sutures effected by Adolfo de Dolcetti (1866–1928), disciple of

Wölfler,[48] and by Adolfo de Grisogono (1874–1945), disciple of Gussenbauer.[49] These were two accomplishments which have been practically ignored in the history of cardiac surgery, but which, on the contrary, deserve great consideration.

It should be made clear that the Paduan school of surgery remained almost untouched by the influence of Billroth's achievements, although to trace the causes of this phenomenon would take us too far off the track. Suffice it to say that it was Trieste that proved the essential link in the promulgation of the philosophy of Billroth's school in Italy, through the work of a number of highly qualified representatives.

It has already been pointed out that, around the mid century, both in Padua and in Trieste, the *anatomische Klinik*—that is, the combination of clinical observation and autopsy, two pillars of hospital medicine—had achieved the maximum benefit possible from the association of the two methods at that time. This occurred through the work of the Skodian, Manussi, in Trieste. Further progress was to depend on the more or less swift assimilation of the remarkable progress achieved in the field of basic sciences by the various medical branches. Once more Padua and Trieste extended the foundations of further progress derived from Viennese scientific knowledge. Disciples of Hyrtl (1810–1894) and Brücke (1819–1892) brought to their places of origin the principles of the new histology and microscopic anatomy, the use of vital dyes, the principles of the organization of a laboratory for biological research, and the pedagogy that focused exclusively on observation and experiment. Thus were they instrumental in radiating Viennese scientific thought to the rest of Italy.

The chair of human anatomy once held by Vesalius and by Morgagni passed to a twenty-seven-year-old Dalmatian, Giampaolo Vlacovich (1825–1899), a graduate from Vienna who had come from three years of experience at the Institutes of Anatomy and Physiology, first as Hyrtl's, then as Brücke's assistant. Vlacovich held that post for over forty-seven years; he did not, however, produce great things on the scientific level but, notwithstanding, he proved an eminent and capable teacher who introduced the thousands of pupils flocking to the celebrated University of the "Veneto" to dissection techniques and to the new and delicate skills of microscopic preparations. Biographers[50] agree in attributing the lack of fertility in the scientific field to a certain degree of hesitation accompanied by profound moral rectitude and by the scruple of publishing data which might not have undergone a thorough critical scrutiny. His teacher's great talent, in our view, may have played a role in arousing doubts in the pupil and may have kept him back from writing. Thus Vlacovich did not accomplish great discoveries and yet, as a convinced Darwinist, he left us writings of myological interest concerning, for example, the sterno-cleido-mastoid, and an anomalous muscle situated in the perineal area, and other structures. These findings were published in the *Atti* of the Istituto di Scienze, Littere e Arti between 1860 and 1875[51] along with two works carried out in collaboration with the pathologist Vintschgau on the measurement of heartbeat in the framework of physiological research on the vagus nerve and the sympathetic nerve, and other works on comparative anatomy, history of anatomy, anthropology, and even silkworm breeding.[52]

The ambitious and animated antivitalistic program of the "Berliner Avantgardisten" for a "mechanische Analyse der Natur" (Virchow) was echoed even in Padua. It arrived there through the work and the word of two of Brücke's assistants: Raffaele Molin (1825–1887) and Maximilian Vintschgau (1832–1902). The former occupied the chair of natural history at Padua, the latter that of physiology. Incidentally, it must be said that both Vlacovich and Molin are numbered also by Lesky among non-Austrian assistants of the eminent physiologist,[53] together with Vintschgau who, a native of Innsbruck, was one of the main Austrian assistants.[54] Molin brought a breath of fresh life in that he introduced a new approach to naturalistic problems, having proved himself an excellent biologist and a systematic expert in the field of zoology.[55] Vintschgau brought a limpid scientific-experimental vision to his teaching and his research. When he was called to Padua, in 1857, he founded there the Istituto Fisiologico, which was made up of a "chemical-physiological laboratory," a "physiological laboratory" and a "lesson room." In applying for some equipment, he asked at least for a "little stove" for a "heater" and a "cupboard for the equipment and the anatomo-microscopic preparates and physiological preparates," and for tables and chairs.[56] Apparently, he intended to create an institute in Padua similar to the recent one of Brücke in Vienna. He imprinted his teaching with a strict experimentalism and denied any kind of speculation. In his Paduan institute, Vintschgau had the opportunity of completing experimental research work on the action of saliva on blood, frog eggs, and the like.[57]

Alexander Lustig (1857–1937), also a disciple of Brücke and later of Recklinghausen (1833–1910) and Hueppe (1852–1938), carried out a research work on "timed observations on the perception of the self-developing positive image of an electrical signal" (1884) in collaboration with Vintschgau. Together with Vincenzo de Giaxa (1848–1928), who came also from the Vienna School, Lustig was to introduce the newly revised criteria for the functioning of a laboratory covering the fields of biology, pathology, and hygiene in Trieste between the 1870s and 1890s: this, in the light of his interest in the struggle against infectious diseases. Lustig, later a professor of general pathology at Florence, became the leader of Italian pathology.

The first hesitant steps on Paduan ground of the flowering laboratory medicine, so closely intertwined with the achievements of the basic sciences, took place in the Medical Clinic of the already mentioned Pinali, whose relationship with the Viennese medical world had been rich and fruitful. A biographer of Pinali wrote in 1875: "When he took on the direction of the clinic its conditions were extremely poor; it lacked almost everything. A stethoscope was almost the sole instrument in the equipment for organo-pathological investigations. Whoever visits the clinic at present will find it thoroughly outfitted, so as to be able to compete with any of the principal and best-equipped clinics of Europe."[58] Clearly, apart from the mere aspect of the equipment, a complete operation in the wake of the physiopathological principles was in progress. The real leap forward in the field of laboratory medicine, however, was to be accomplished later by Luigi Lacatello (1863–1926), who was scientifically related to the German schools.[59]

The early approaches of Trieste to laboratory medicine have already been recorded. The structuring of real laboratory medicine developed with the summons of Adriano Sturli (1873–1964) to the direction of the II Medical Department at the Ospedale Civile of Trieste, which was considered second only to Vienna's medical facilities as regards its scientific value and its numerical capacity. Sturli had been a collaborator of Landsteiner (1868–1943) and a clinical assistant of von Neusser (1852–1912) at the II Medical Clinic in Vienna. Sturli, who, among other things, discovered the blood group IV in collaboration with Decastello (1872–1960), introduced modern hematology in Trieste, along with a perfect organization of the laboratory that was connected to the medical department; he subsequently introduced electrocardiography. On the whole, he preached a completely new conception for Trieste and, in a more limited sense, for Italian medical circles in general; he envisaged a systematic resort to functional and laboratory tests within the clinical activity—a doctrine he had learned during his short stay at Vienna.[60] At the end of the 1940s, the influence of Vienna and the air of the Allgemeines Krankenhaus still emanated from his department when the present author had the good fortune to work as Sturli's aide: the last of the line, in a sense.

It is a common observation that Vienna and Paris, and later Berlin, all played a key role in the history of medical and surgical specializations. Padua and Trieste were in the position of being influenced by the celebrated schools at their very early stages. Some disciplines—obstetrics and pediatrics for example—were already being taught separately in Padua before the nineteenth century; the remainder were instituted either in the nineteenth or in the twentieth centuries.

It has already been pointed out how Lamprecht, in Padua, happened to be the faithful interpreter of the *ars obstetricia per expectationem* of J. L. Boër.[61] After the death of Lamprecht, the relationship of Padua with Vienna in this sector stagnated. Viennese obstetrics and gynecology were guarded by a number of noted physicians from Trieste and transmitted to the Italian scientific world through their work. The major Viennese personalities spanning the two centuries in this field were Carl Braun (1822–1891) and Friedrich Schauta (1849–1919), directors of the I Clinic, and Rudolf Chrobak (1843–1910) and Ernst Wertheim (1864–1920), directors of the II Clinic. Trieste could boast one of the most devoted and qualified pupils of all these eminent teachers: Egidio Welponer (1848–1933), Braun's assistant, mentioned by Lesky,[62] who at the end of the 1870s was author of a significant contribution with his "Contribuzione alla statistica dell'ovaroisterectomia cesarea-metodo Porro."[63] In this field he was to become a major Italian representative. Roberto Cristofoletti (1874–1940), also particularly well prepared, had been clinical assistant of Schauta and had come to Trieste in 1921 in order to direct a gynecology department at a nursing-home. He was a skilled performer of Schauta's vaginal hysterectomy in cases of cervical cancer (1908). Between 1903 and 1955 he published a number of monographs on cystic congenital lymphangioma, on the pathogenesis of osteomalacia, with a rich illustration of laboratory data, on the pathogenesis and therapy of malign chorionepithelioma and on other interesting aspects of gynecology. He carried out independent teaching activities at Rome University. Among the multitude of Chrobak's disciples there was Sebastiano de Gattorno (1864–1945), an excellent surgeon who introduced Wertheim's panhysterectomy (1897) in Trieste (probably in Italy too) as early as in 1900. In 1903, he reported on twenty-six cases treated successfully.[64] Adolfo de Grisogono (1874–1945), head gynecologist at the Ospedale Civico, known all over Italy for his operative skills, was invited to draw up the fundamental monograph on vaginal operations for the *Trattato di Ginecologia* edited by Clivio (1868–1945).[65] Romolo Liebmann (1874–1931), disciple and assistant of Wertheim, was a convincing advocate of the radical operation named after his teacher, offering to his Italian and Trieste colleagues a detailed exposition[66] of the various operative phases of a surgical maneuver that was conceived and executed by the Viennese after various unsuccessful attempts by American, French, Belgian, and German surgeons. It can be maintained that the principles preached by Viennese teachers of obstetrics and gynecology reached Italian ground via the bridge provided by Trieste and through the active and direct participation of worthy and well-trained specialists.

Let us now turn to ophthalmology. Padua drew on the Viennese tradition, specifically on the teaching of Rosas and Arlt (1812–1887) through the contributions of Giuseppe Torresini (1790–1848) and Giovanni Gioppi (1818–1872). Torresini had been an assistant of Rosas in Padua for one year and succeeded him in 1821; Gioppi, in turn, had taken postgraduate training at the surgical school of Franz Schuh (1804–1865), Billroth's predecessor, and attended at the same time the clinic of Rosas. There is also a great likelihood he attended Arlt's school in Prague. It was Gioppi who, having obtained the chair in 1852, was responsible for significant progress in the techniques of operating for cataract and dacriocystitis. He also introduced a precise classification of the various symptoms on an anatomical basis and equipped his institution with modern devices such as the ophthalmoscope. Lesky mentions his name as a valid collaborator of Schuh; Sudhoff considers him a capable ophthalmologist.[67] Trieste was the scientific heir both of Arlt and, to a greater extent, of Fuchs (1851–1930). Joseph Brettauer (1835–1905), Arlt's assistant, a skillful histologist also renowned for his medal collection, imported the major accomplishments of the Viennese school as regards operative techniques and scientific doctrines.[68] He was also an excellent ophthalmoscopist; in Trieste he founded a good school of ophthalmology that was attended by pupils coming from all Italian regions. There were at least five of Fuchs's direct disciples operating in Trieste, circulating the wide range of theoretical principles, critical clinical observations, and operative techniques for the different structures of the eye they had learned at the famous Jaegers Klinik. Let us mention a few names: Giuseppe Manzutto (1869–1947), chief oculist at the Ospedale Civico and successor to Brettauer; Carlo Heinzel (1868–1903), Edoardo Horniker (1870–1943); Emilio Oblath (1877–1941) and Alberto Botteri (1879–1955). Horniker provided a valuable description of the symptomatology he called "retinite capillarospastica," which is today better known as central serous corioretinopathy.[69] The relationship of the teacher with his pupils was very close; Fuchs was the preferred consultant in difficult cases. He was honored on several public occasions. The ophthalmology department of Manzutto was intermittently attended by Italian oculists who wished to perfect their skills in the clinical examination of the eye and in other specialized fields.

Guthrie wrote: "Every otologist owes an immense debt of gratitude to Adam Politzer (1835–1920)."[70] Paduan otorhynolaryngology did not avail itself of this noted creator of the First Viennese Clinic. Trieste, in contrast, had among its specialists several of Politzer's pupils and assistants, those whom the teacher himself remembered in his classic *Geschichte der Ohrenheilkunde*.[71] Among them we find Eugenio Morpurgo (1839–1916), close friend of his teacher, who had the merit of disclosing the work of Politzer among Italian physicians through publications, reviews, and conferences.[72] Another, Edmondo Rimini (1867–1948), founded a specialist department in Trieste where several Italian physicians met in order to learn the operative techniques and the refined details of a true specialist examination. He was also the author of many distinguished works on pathology of the ear and related clinical techniques. An excellent review of cases of laryngectomy was that of Guglielmo Danelon (1877–1938), a disciple of Victor Urbantschitsch (1847–1921) and director of the Politzer Klinik between 1907 and 1918. As with other pupils of the Vienna school, once having come back to his birthplace he was not especially compelled to publish memoirs or divulge the results of his work. This phenomenon might have some psychoanalytical explanation, but it can also easily be understood in terms of the often close teacher-pupil relationship. The disciples were frankly dazzled by the work of their teachers; when they departed the courage to draw publicly upon the results of that special experience could well have failed them.

The dermatological doctrine of Fedinand von Hebra (1816–1880) had a progeny both in Trieste and in Padua. The Paduan dermatological clinic was

founded by Achille Breda (1850–1934), collaborator and disciple of the celebrated teacher and of his assistant, Heinrich Auspitz (1835–1886). Breda,
with only a few other Italian colleagues, imported the best fruits of a modern
dermatology that had developed on a morphological basis.[73] His and his
pupils' works are illustrated by pictures, some in color, and by fine micro-
photographs. The accomplishment of Breda, whose devotion to the Vienna
school remained unchanged during his almost fifty years of teaching, was of
major importance to the progress of studies on cutaneous pathology, and on
venereal diseases and their treatment. As early as 1872, Antonio Suttina
(1834–1886), from Zara, a disciple of von Hebra later to be active in Trieste,
circulated his teacher's treatise in Italian medical circles and served as editor
of its Italian translation.[74] It can be maintained that northeast Italy bene-
fitted from the spiritual legacy of von Hebra.

Italian urology, of which the founder may well be Giorgio Nicolich, Sr.
(1852–1925), from Trieste, is related to the Paris urological school of Guyon
(1831–1920) and Albarran (1860–1912). Among its initiators, however,
there is Gustavo Usiglio, whom we have already mentioned as assistant to
Leopold von Dittel, the father of Viennese urology. Usiglio was the author
of worthy monographs dating back to the 1870s and the 1880s during his
specialist activity.[75]

Trieste represented the driving force of radiology in Italy. The starting
point is once again Vienna. Immediately after the announcement of Roentgen
(1845–1923) in Würzburg, two willing physicians, Ventura Romanin (1844–
1942), former assistant of Dumreicher (1815–1880), and Edoardo Menz
(1862–1908), began experimenting with a small Ruhmkorff device connected
to a small tube and with other rudimentary equipment. But on 14 November 1904, Massimiliano Gortan (1873–1938), who had been the first assistant of Guido Holzknecht (1872–1931), founder of Viennese radiology, at
the Neusser Clinic in Vienna, opened the first Istituto Radiologico Italiano,
the first independent radiological institute whose director enjoyed equal status
with other hospital directors. Gortan was an earnest, generous, and modest
teacher. Among the many people who learned the foundations of radiology
from him was Antonio Busi (1874–1939), leader of Italian radiologists during the 1930s.[76] It is almost rhetorical to mention that Italian radiology was
born with Gortan, who had been trained in Vienna and other German centers. He investigated every aspect of radiological diagnosis and radiotherapy.
His name was authoritatively present in his branch of medicine during his
entire professional life. Paduan radiology, although Vienna inspired, developed independently and outside the Vienna school.[77]

The first Paduan psychiatrist, the noted professor Ernesto Belmondo
(1863–1931), was trained in Italy and in Berlin. Trieste, once more, deserves
a different consideration. The town can boast an old and valid tradition as
regards mental hospitals, which naturally took inspiration from the Viennese medical experience. Several figures deserve praise in this specialty. Here

we should mention Constantin von Economo (1876–1931), who received his premedical education in Trieste,[78] a city to which he remained affectionately bound. Giovanni Sai (1880–1947), disciple of Krafft-Ebing (1840–1901) in Vienna, and of Ziehen (1862–1950) in Berlin, was a lifelong advocate of the Austro-German methodology and directed the Ospedale Psichiatrico Provinciale of Trieste for more than twenty years. He also founded the highly-respected neurological department there. His scientific work is remarkable both from the neurological and psychiatric points of view. He enjoyed international recognition, and the recollection of his accomplishments is still vivid in Trieste and elsewhere.

We must not ignore the congress of the Società Italiana di Neuropsichiatria, which took place in Trieste in 1925. On that occasion, Eduardo Weiss (1889–1970), a native of Trieste and also a disciple of Freud (1856–1939), and Paul Federn (1871–1950), officially introduced psychoanalysis on the Italian scientific scene with a detailed exposition of more than forty pages.[79] A new era was inaugurated in Italy. Weiss, who spent the second part of his life in the United States, had been familiar with the Viennese Freudian circles; he was active in Trieste from 1919 to 1929 as the director of the Ospedale Psichiatrico.

In ending this exposition, we should summarize a few essential points:

1. Important and onerous political and military commitments hindered a swift and regular development of medical disciplines in Italy in the nineteenth century.
2. The direct exchanges of the universities of Padua and of Trieste with the renowned school of Vienna contributed to a lively and fruitful evolution, Vienna being was one of the great European centers where modern medicine was being "produced."
3. The role of Padua and Trieste in the promulgation of Viennese medicine has been of major importance.
4. The purpose of this exposition was to give official credit to historical facts which, for various reasons, have hitherto received little or no consideration.

NOTES

[1] L. Premuda and G. Ongaro, "I primordi della dissezione anatomica in Padova [critical review]," *Acta Med. Hist. Patavina* 12 (1965–66): 117–42, 132.

[2] We were glad to follow the order proposed by E. Lesky in *The Vienna Medical School of the Nineteenth Century* (Baltimore: The Johns Hopkins University Press, 1976).

[3] Here we refer to the following writings of A. Castiglioni: "Precursori ed

iniziatori della vaccinazione a Trieste," *Rivista Sanitaria* 14 (1921): 5, 7; and idem, "Medici e Medicine a Trieste al principio dell' Ottocento (Trieste, 1922). No mention is made in these of the Trieste-Vienna link (not even marginal), nor in "The Medical School of Vienna," *Ciba Symposia* 9, nos. 3–4 (1947), either.

[4]A. Castiglioni, "La Scuola Medica Padovana attraverso i secoli," *Annali Merck* 1 (1930).

[5]E. Lesky and H. Wyklicky, "1900–1930: Eine Epoche österreichischer Medizin," in *Oesterreichische Aerzte Zeitung: Sammlung der Titelblätter des Jahres 1975* (Vienna: Sonderdruck des Verlags der Oesterreichischen Aerztekammer, Institut für Geschichte der Medizin der Universität Wien, 1975).

[6]Lesky, *The Vienna Medical School*, pp. 43–44.

[7]*Elenco dei Signori Medici e Chirurghi che esercitano la libera practica nella città di Trieste: Pubblicato dal Gremic Farmaceutico nel 1844* (Trieste, 1844).

[8]A Corradi, *Della chirurgia in Italia dagli ultimi anni del fino al presente commentario* (Bologna, 1871), p. 131.

[9]L. Schönbauer, *Das medizinische Wien: Geschichte — Werden — Würdingung*, 2d ed. (Vienna: Urban & Schwarzenberg, 1947), pp. 201–2.

[10]G. Vlacovich, *Commemorazione del Prof. Francesco Cortese letta il 7 dicembre 1884 nell' Aula Magna della R. Università di Padova* (Padua, 1887).

[11]L. Premuda, *Storia della Fisiologie* (Udine: Del Blanco Editore, 1966), pp. 217–32.

[12]F. Argenti, *Il Prof. Vincenzo Fabeni* (Padua, 1862).

[13]G. Giacomini, *Trattato filosofico-sperimentale dei soccofsi terapeutica*, 5 vols. (Padua, 1833–39).

[14]B. Panizza, *Sul merito di Giuseppe Gianelli rispetto alla medicina civile* (Padua, 1874).

[15]V. Bianchetti, *Elogio del fu Bartolomeo Signoroni...scritto per l'I.R. Accademia medico-chirurgica* (Brescia, 1845); *Elogio funebre del Prof. Bartolomeo Signoroni recitato nella Chiesa degli Ognissanti in Padova il 30.11.1844* (Venice, 1845).

[16]E. Bassini, *Commemorazione del Prof. Tito Vansetti letta nel giorno 8 dicembre 1888 nell'Aula Magna della R. Università di Padova* (Padua, 1889).

[17]P. Maffeis, *L'attività didattica e scientifica di Ludovico Brunetti (1813–1899), anatomo-patologo a Padova* (Padua: Thesis on Medicine and Surgery, University of Padua, 1973–74).

[18]Lesky, *The Vienna Medical School*, pp. 60–62; G. Ovio, *Storia dell' oculistica* (Cuneo: Ghibaudo, 1950, I:610.

[19]L. Premuda, "The Waxwork in Medicine," *Image* 48 (1972): 17–24.

[20]G. de Laurentiis and L. Premuda, "Rodolfo Lamprecht (1781–1860): Professore di Ostetricia Teorica e Practica all'Università di Padova — Nota biografica," *Acta Med. Hist. Patavina* 22 (1976–77): 23–24.

[21]Idem, "L' 'ars obstetricia per expectationem' di J. L. Boër (1751–1835) tra Vienna e Padova," *La Riforma Medica* 94 (1979): 185–89.

[22]J. Pagel, "Steer Martin," in *Biographisches Lexikon hervorragender Aerzte aller Zeiten und Völker*, ed. A. Hirsch, E. Gurlt, and A. Wernich, 2d ed. (Berlin: Urban & Schwarzenberg, 1929–35), 5:401.

[23]L. Premuda, "Die Einführung der Perkussion und der Auskultation in das 'Studio medico' von Padua," in *Circa Tiliam* (Leiden: Brill, 1974), pp. 230–55; also see pp. 243–49.

[24]Ibid., pp. 235–39.

[25]*Annales scholae Medico-Clinicae Patavinae edidit Fr. Guil. Lippich, M.D. Praxeos Med. Prof. P. O. — Annus 1834–35* (Padua, 1837), p. 19.

[26]L. Premuda, "The Revival of the Anatomical-Clinical Method in Padua: The Fundamental Contribution of F. S. Verson (1805–1849) from Trieste, a Disciple of the Vienna School of Medicine," *Janus* 67 (1980) 31–39.

[27]We feel that we were among the first, or actually the first, to mention Verson's name in a communication to the 20th International Congress for the History of Medicine in Berlin, 22–27 August 1966. L. Premuda, "Einflüsse der Wiener Medizinischen Schule auf die Medizinschule von Padua im 19. Jahrhundert," *Verhandl. der XX. Intern. Kongr. f. Gesch. d. Med.* (Berlin, 22–27 August 1966, Hildesheim, 1968), pp. 750–57, see p. 752.

[28]C. Bonafini, *La Clinica Medica pei chirurghi nella I. R. Università di Padova durante l'anno scolastico MDCCCXLII-XLIII* (Padua, 1844), p. 18.

[29]F. S. Verson, *Trattato di Medicina Pratica* (Venice, 1844), 1:xi.

[30]Verson, *La Clinica Medica pei chirurghi nella I. R. Università di Padova*.

[31]Ibid., p. 74.

[32]M. Saibante, C. Vivarini, G. Voghero, "Gli studenti della Università di Padova dalla fine del '500 ai nostri giorni (Studio statistico)," *Netron* 4 (1924–25): 163–223; see also pp. 211–12).

[33]H. Sigerist, *The Great Doctors: A Biographical History of Medicine*, trans. Eden and Cedar Paul (New York: W. W. Norton, 1933), p. 302.

[34]*Manuale delle malatie (!) del cuore e delle arterie del dottore Enrico Bamberger, tradotto dal Dott. Vittore Dal Canton*, Gia assistente alla Clinica Medica dell' I. R. Università di Padova, ora Assistente straordinario alla Clinica Medica del Prof. Oppolzer in Vienna (Padua, 1859).

[35]Archivio Antico of the Paduan University. Facoltà Medico-Chirurgico-Farmaceutica, Concorsi, Busta 9, Fasc. 48 (Session of 11 August 1856).

[36]V. Plitek, *L'Associazione Medica Triestina in cinquant'anni di vita* (1875–1926) (Trieste, 1926), p. 92.

[37]V. Cominotti, "Allesandro de Manussi 1862–1919: Nel cinquantesimo anno della sua operosità professionale," *Rivista Sanitaria* 6 (1919): 121–22.

[38]Plitek, *L'Associazione Medica Triestina*, p. 87.

[39]Quoted from Sigerist, *The Great Doctors*, p. 383.

[40]J. Pagel, "Menzel Arthur," in *Biographisches Lexikon hervorragenden Aerzte*, Bd. 4, p. 168.

[41]T. Billroth, *Briefe* (Hannover: Hahnsche Buchhandlung, 1922), p. 182.

[42]A. Menzel and E. Perco, "Ueber die Resorption von Hahrungsmitteln vom Unterhautzellgewebe aus," *Wien. Med. Wochenschr.* 19 (1869): 517–18.

[43]G. Brettauer and Arturo Menzel, *Resoconto Sanitario dell'Ospitale Civico di Trieste per l'anno 1877* (Trieste, 1879), 5:v–xii; see also p. vii.

[44]Billroth, *Resezione del piloro per carcinoma esposta del Dott. Antonio Wölfler, medico assistente nella Clinica Chirurgica del Prof. Billroth e docente di Chirurgia nell'Università di Vienna*. Traduzione con aggiunte autorizzate dal Dott. G. Usiglio, operatore nella Clinica stessa (Bologna, 1881).

[45]L. Premuda, *Cento anni di chirurgia a Trieste (1840–1940)*. (Trieste: Grafad, 1975), pp. 9–11.

[46]A. von Eiselberg, *Lebensweg eines Chirurgen*, 2d ed. (Innsbruck-Vienna: Tirolia-Verlag, 1949), p. 392.

[47]E. Oliani, *L'ulcera gastrica e duodenale nella chirurgia moderna* (Bologna: Cappelli, 1929).

[48]A. de Dolcetti, "Sutura del cuore," *Boll. Assoc. Med. Triestina*, 9 (1905–1906): 113–16.

[49]A. de Grisogono, "Ferita da punta ledente il cuore," *Resoconti Sanitari degli Ospedali Civici di Trieste: 1909–1910* (Trieste, 1914), pp. 148–52.

[50]D. Bertelli, *Commemorazione del Prof. G. P. Vlacovich, letta il giorno 14 gennaio 1900, nel'Aula Magna della Regia Università di Padova* (Padua, 1900); G. Solitro, *Maestri e Scolari dell'Università di Padova nell'ultima dominazione austriaca* (Venice, 1922).

[51]G. Vlacovich, *Atti delle Reale Istituto Veneto di Sci., Litt. ed Arti*, 3rd Series, T. X. Dispensa X (Venice, 1864–65), pp. 1294–1323.

[52]This work dates back to 1871 and was published in *Atti delle Reale Istituto Veneto di Sci., Litt. ed Arti*, together with others between the 1860s and 1880s.

[53]Lesky, *The Vienna Medical School*, p. 231.

[54]Ibid., p. 259.

[55]The title of the major work in this regard is *Elementi di storia naturale per uso dei Ginnasi e delle Scuole Tecniche Superiori delle Provincie Austro-Italiche* (Vienna, 1852).

[56]R. Molin, *Caratteristica del Regno Animale* (Padua, 1858); idem, *Prodromus Faunae Helminthologicae Venetae* (Vienna, 1861).

[57]As regards Vintschgau, besides Lesky, *The Vienna Medical School*, and K. E. Rothschuh, *Geschichte der Physiologie* (Berlin, Göttingen, and Heidelberg: Springer Verlag, 1953), pp. 123, 141, 143; see L. Bizzotto and G. Rialdi, "L'attività didattica e scientifica del fisiologo Maximilian Vintschgau (1832–1902) all'Università di Padova," *Acta Med. Hist. Patavina* 22 (1975–76): 9–20.

[58]A. Luzzatto, "Vincenzo Pinali," *L'Isonzo*, 15 December 1875.

[59]L. Premuda, *Luigi Lucatello a cinquant'anni dalla morte* (Padua: La Garangola, 1976).

[60]For greater detail about Sturli see L. Premuda, "Adriano Sturli (1873–1964) als Forscher und Arzt," *Medizinische Diagnostik in Geschichte und Gegenwart: Festschrift für Heinz Goerke zum sechzigsten Geburtstag*, ed. C. Habrich et al. (Munich: W. Fritsch, 1978), 327–39.

[61]De Laurentiis and Premuda, "Rodolfo Lamprecht (1781–1860)."

[62]Lesky, *The Vienna Medical School*, p. 426.

[63]In *Lo Sperimentale* 43 (1879): 607–27.

[64]A contribution discussed during a report by R. Liebmann, *Boll. Assoc. Med. Triestina* 6 (1902–1903): 257–68.

[65]A. de Grisogono, "La tecnica operativa negli interventi sull'utero ed annessi per via vaginale," *Trattato di Ginecologia*, ed. I. Clivio; 3d ed. (Milan: Vallardi, 1944), ch. 6 (in this edition the monograph is published with the name of Massazza as well, who was not mentioned in the previous two editions).

[66]R. Liebmann, "L'operazione radicale di Wertheim nel trattamento chirurgico del cancro dell'utero," *Boll. Assoc. Med. Triestina* 6 (1902–1903): 257–68.

[67]Lesky, *The Vienna Medical School*, p. 171 (mention is made of Giannantonio, but is it the same person?); K. Sudhoff, *Kurzes Handbuch für Geschichte der Medizin* (Berlin: 1922) p. 442; cf. F. Marzolo, *In morte del Prof. Giovanni Gioppi* (Padua, 1872).

[68]Lesky, *The Vienna Medical School*, p. 198, n. 30; E. Holzmair, *Katalog der Sammlung Dr. Josef Brettauer "Medicina in nummis"* (Vienna: Selbstverlag, 1937).

[69]E. Horniker, "Su una forma di retinite centrale vaso-neurotica (Retinite capillarospastica)," *Annali di Oftalmologia e Clinica Oculistica* 55 (1927): 578–600, 689–88, 830–40, 865–83.

[70]R. S. Stevenson and D. Guthrie, *History of Otolaryngology* (Edinburgh: E. & S. Livingstone, 1949), p. 113.

[71]A. Pollitzer, *Geschichte der Ohrenheilkunde*, intro. by E. Rothschuh (Stuttgart, 1913; reprint ed. Hildescheim: G. Olms, 1967), pp. 302–3.

[72]Politzer's treatise was reviewed in *Bollettino delle malattie dell'orecchio della gola e del naso* 11 (1893): 140–45.

[73]Among the other Italian colleagues: Casimiro Manassei (1824–1893) and Giuseppe Profeta (1860–1910). — A. Bellini, "Storia della dermatologia e venereosifilolgia in Italia," *Giorn. Ital. di Dermatologia Sifilogia* 13 (1934): 1091–1205; see also pp. 1132 and 1188. On Breda, see L. Premuda, "Un secolo di ricerche padovane sulla sifilide," *Acta Med. Hist. Patavina* 11 (1964–65): 145–75; see also pp. 146–62.

[74]F. von Hebra, *Trattato delle malattie della pelle*. Italian translation by Antonio Suttina (Milan, 1872).

[75]Usiglio's urological interests went from kidney surgery to lithotripsy, from cystotomy to urethrotomy. The monograph *Litotrissia e litolapassia con tre or otto atti operativi e tre tavole litografate*, 3d ed. (Trieste, 1882), is dedicated to Billroth.

[76]L. Premuda, "Die vermittelnde Funktion von Triest für die Verbreitung des medizinischen Denkens der Wiener Schule in Italien," *Wien und die Weltmedizin*, ed. Erna Lesky (Vienna, Cologne, and Graz: Verlag Hermann Böhlaus, 1974), pp. 99–115; see esp. pp. 105–6.

[77]S. Sirica, *La scoperta Roentgen (dicembre 1895) e i primordi della Radiologia nel Veneto (1896–1916)*, Thesis, University of Padua, 1956.

[78]L. Premuda, "La formazione intellettuale e scientifica di Constantin von Economo," *Rassegna di Studi Psichiatrici* 66 (1977): 1326–36.

[79]E. Weiss, "Psichiatria e psicoanalisi (II Relazione)," Arch. Ital. per le malattie nervose e mentali LI, *Riv. Sperim. di Freniatria* 50 (1927): 442–83.

Commentary

Jerome J. Bylebyl

In his paper, Dr. Premuda has documented very thoroughly the extensive ties that linked nineteenth-century Italian medicine to the second Viennese school, with the aim of demonstrating that, at a time when Vienna was the actual political capital of large areas of Italy, Italian medicine became largely a provincial offshoot of that school. It is thus a most unchauvinistic piece of historical research.

More than 10,000 Americans also went to study in the Viennese clinics during their heyday, and American medical historians are quite accustomed to singing the praises of these and other young doctors who went abroad in quest of better training than they could obtain at home.[1] It may therefore come as something of a surprise to learn that their Italian counterparts have been, according to Premuda, reluctant to acknowledge such indebtedness. However, the difference becomes more understandable when we consider how this phase of study abroad fitted into the national and medical history of the two countries. For Italy, the dependence upon a foreign school followed a long period in which she herself had been the place to which so many medical students from other countries, including Austria, had turned. Moreover, this reversal of roles was linked with the national humiliation of political disunity and domination by foreign powers. By contrast, international relations were of little or no importance in determining the need of American medical students to go abroad, or in influencing their choice of where to go. Furthermore, Americans can examine their own phase of medical dependence content in the knowledge that greater things were yet to come here at home.

In the remarks that follow, I have chosen to focus on the earlier period when Italy was an importer of medical students and an exporter of medical ideas. I hope that this will add an element of perspective to the developments that Dr. Premuda has discussed, as well as make it clear that the Italy into which the Viennese influence diffused was not exactly a medical vacuum, but had her own rich heritage of clinical teaching and investigation.

Let me begin by noting that broad cultural and social factors had much to do with the earlier attractiveness of Italy as a place for foreigners to study medicine. Italy was well prepared for the training of physicians largely because the university-educated physician had been thoroughly assimilated into Italian culture and society at an earlier time than in other parts of Europe. Thus, as Carlo Cipolla has shown, in 1630 the grand duchy of

Tuscany, with a population of about 770,000, supported a total of more than 100 physicians.[2] And Cipolla points to further qualitative evidence which suggests that a relatively high physician/population ratio had existed in this and other parts of Italy since the late Middle Ages. By contrast, by as late as 1780 there were still only about 500 graduate physicians in all of Great Britain, whose population was then about 7 million.[3]

To educate this large number of physicians the Italians had numerous medical universities, and, more important, the individual medical faculties in Italy were much larger than those in northern Europe. The largest of the Italian medical universities was at Bologna, where by the sixteenth century as many as fifty physicians would lecture on one or another of the major medical subjects every year, while at Padua the number of medical professors was usually about twenty-five.[4] By contrast, the entire teaching faculty of contemporary northern European medical schools might consist of only two physicians, and generally did not exceed six or eight.[5] Moreover, not only was Italy better prepared to educate physicians through theoretical lectures, but the Italian medical profession was also strongly oriented toward providing practical training through bedside precepting.[6] Indeed, for the leading physicians of the large cities, whether or not they also lectured on medicine, it appears that no sharp distinction was made between practice and teaching. Thus when patients, even well-to-do ones, engaged the services of a prominent physician, they were apparently quite content for him to arrive with a group of students in tow, with whom he would actively interact during the course of his examination and treatment.

It seems to have been this ready availability of practical precepting that was the major factor in drawing so many foreign medical students to Italy during the Renaissance.[7] Many of these students would acquire the theoretical part of their training at the smaller universities in their native lands, then round this off with two or three years in Italy, where they could concentrate on following the great physicians in their practice. A clear indication of these priorities is provided by an incident that occurred at Padua in 1597.[8] The moderators of the university, apparently concerned that the students were neglecting their attendance at the formal public lectures, proposed severe restrictions on all outside activities, including the visiting of the sick. The foreign students saw this as being especially inimical to their interests, for, as the annalist of the German students put it, "how few among us are there who, putting aside all the rest, have not come to this famous university for the sake of practical training alone? But how can we gain knowledge and experience of [medical practice] without constant inspection of the sick, and careful observation of the daily changes of diseases and their symptoms." The student representatives went to the syndic of the university and put it to him bluntly: "Few or none of us have come here only for the sake of lectures, and all of us have come to learn practice. We do not lack for lecturers in our own country, and we also have books at home which we can just as well read there as here. It is the study of practice that has led us to cross so many mountains, and at such great expense." The student annalist also noted that the move had provoked unusual unanimity among the foreign students, who continued their attendance on practice in defiance of the ruling. Eventually a compromise was worked out whereby those who had in fact completed their philosophy and medical theory could pursue their practical training as before.

As part of this broader practical orientation, Italian physicians were, by the latter part of the sixteenth century, already quite accustomed to using hospitals as places of medical teaching and research, both clinical and anatomical. This included not only having the students visit hospitals together with their teachers, both to see patients and to witness dissections, but in some cases young doctors would go through a period as an assistant hospital physician before entering into private practice. For example, at Florence in 1560 a recent medical graduate applied for a license to practice but was told by the examining physicians that he "must practice for another six months in the Hospital of Santa Maria Nuova and during this period he is not allowed to treat patients outside the Hospital unless in the company of another physician."[9] There is evidence of similar stints of hospital work by young doctors at Bologna and Padua around the same time,[10] though it is not clear to me how common it was to actually require a period of active hospital service as a condition for licensing.

Undoubtedly the greatest product of this native Italian clinical tradition was G. B. Morgagni's *On the Seats and Causes of Diseases*, which appeared in 1761 but was based on research by Morgagni and his teachers stretching back into the seventeenth century. And in an interesting passage in *De sedibus*, Morgagni himself traced this hospital tradition back even further:

> [When I reflect on] how much greater an opportunity hospitals offer for the observation of rare diseases, but especially of the more common ones, the more regret I feel for the ancient physicians, who necessarily lacked this [opportunity], because hospitals were first established only shortly before the time of Justinian.... And if from the time of their institution it had been permitted to use hospitals to study diseases, both in living patients and through the post mortem, one can imagine how much progress medicine would have made over the following ten centuries by considering how much it has accomplished since around the beginning of the sixteenth century when these two modes of investigation began to be permitted.[11]

Thus Morgagni had a clear conception of hospital research as a distinct and important historical phenomenon, but he regarded it as an invention of the sixteenth century rather than of the eighteenth.

Three years after the appearance of *De sedibus*, the hospital at Padua where Morgagni carried out so much of his teaching and research took on a new measure of importance in relation to the university. For in 1764, the Venetian Senate approved the establishment of a new chair of clinical medicine to be conducted in the hospital.[12] The first incumbent of this chair was

Giovanni dalla Bona, and the terms of the appointment gave him an un-
usually generous salary, because "his position requires the complete sacrifice
of his own person, because of the attention, diligence, and seriousness of his
obligation, so that he cannot expect from his profession that private income
which accrues to other physicians."[13]

In his inaugural lecture for this chair delivered in 1765, dalla Bona outlined the program that he proposed to follow.[14] Every morning he would
visit ten or twelve of the patients in the hospital, "accompanied by all the
youths who wish to come and who have some reason for being there." For
each patient he would deliver a "continuous oration" in which he would
declare what things are not according to nature and prescribe which remedies are to be used. More specifically, he would discuss what is the genus of
the disease, what hope of recovery there is, which of the evident (external)
causes gave rise to the disease, what is its proximate (internal) cause, how all
the phenomena of the disease arise from this cause, what changes for the
better are required, and how these might be brought about by therapeutic
means.

In his fuller explanation of his approach, dalla Bona particularly emphasized semeiology in the Hippocratic mode, as well as the determination of
the external causes of disease according to the doctrine of the non-naturals.[15]
On the other hand he would eschew the vain search for the hidden causes of
disease, and wherever possible he would pursue the proximate internal
causes through the only reliable means, namely the autopsy.[16] Here he made
it abundantly clear that he would be following in the footsteps of his senior
colleague, Morgagni, whose book on the seats and causes of disease had been
published just a few years before. Dalla Bona confessed to some trepidation
at having to confront his own diagnoses with the results of autopsy—his
powers of judgment and prediction would be put to the test every time—
and he fully expected that some mistakes would be made. However, his ability to rely on Morgagni's work now gave him much greater confidence in the
possibility of making accurate judgments in this regard, and he even hoped
that he might be able to add something new to the subject. Indeed, he suggested that the practice of conducting autopsies might prove to be the most
useful aspect of this new clinical chair the moderators of the university had
established.

Earlier in his lecture dalla Bona made equally flattering reference to Morgagni's continuing role as professor of normal anatomy and physiology at the
University of Padua.[17] He regretted that Morgagni was unable to attend the
lecture in person, but he congratulated both himself and the students that
they had all had the great man as their teacher, and expressed the hope that
he would continue among them for a long time to come. He also expressed
confidence that the students had been thoroughly grounded in the human
body in a state of health, and were thus well prepared to go on to the phenomena of disease.

However, while dalla Bona freely took on the mantle of Morgagni's prestige and authority, he did not mention the probable model for the establishment of a major chair devoted exclusively to clinical medicine. For it was just
ten years previously, in 1754, that Maria Theresa and van Swieten had
founded the teaching clinic at Vienna that was conducted by Anton de Haen
on a full-time basis.[18] Indeed, in his inaugural lecture de Haen had declared
to his students, "I give myself up to you, and all my being will be devoted
and sacrificed to you."[19] Thus in establishing their own clinical chair on a
similar basis the Venetian authorities were probably just following the prece-
dent set at Vienna, and other major Italian medical schools soon did the
same.

Nevertheless, it is scarcely surprising that the students and colleagues of
Morgagni should wish to emphasize their own independent heritage of hospital teaching and research. In fact, it was a group of Italian clinicians of the
late eighteenth and early nineteenth centuries who were responsible for
bringing to light a much earlier phase in the development of bedside teaching in the hospitals. The common view during the eighteenth century was
that such formal clinical teaching had first been instituted at Leiden during
the seventeenth century, with Franciscus Sylvius the leading candidate for
the prize of invention. This was the view taken by Simon-André Tissot, the
Frenchman who had briefly held the chair of clinical medicine at Pavia from
1781 to 1783, and who discussed the origin of clinical teaching in his essay
on the improvement of medical studies, published in 1785.[20] However,
Tissot also mentioned the possibility that formal clinical teaching had occurred at Padua even earlier than that at Leiden, but discounted it.[21] Nevertheless, this very rumor was soon confirmed by Andrea Comparetti, another
student of Morgagni's and the second incumbent of the chair of clinical
medicine at Padua. In 1793 Comparetti published an essay on the latter
chair in which he pointed out that in 1578 the Venetian Senate had indeed
formally authorized two Paduan professors to conduct bedside lectures in
the Hospital of St. Francis.[22] Moreover, in 1809 the clinician Giovanni Rasori
of Pavia and Milan was able to take the story back even further on the basis
of evidence that G. B. da Monte, the most celebrated medical teacher of the
mid sixteenth century, had lectured at the bedside in the Paduan hospital as
early as 1543.[23]

The evidence on which Rasori and others drew is quite remarkable in
itself. It consists primarily of a fairly large group of transcripts of da Monte's
bedside discourses, which were taken down by students who attended
them.[24] These transcripts were published during the sixteenth century
together with da Monte's formal written consilia. A fair number of these discourses are explicitly identified as having taken place in the Hospital of St.
Francis, and in one of the latter we are also told that "this was our 17th visit
to the hospital...in the year 1543."[25] Moreover, some of the transcripts
record the progress of the same patient visited on successive days.

In one of the latter, da Monte gave an interesting indication of the special role of the hospital in introducing students to the world of medicine. The case was a continued fever, and on the first two visits da Monte reviewed the manifest signs and symptoms in some detail, both to identify the underlying humoral cause of the disease and to predict its future course.[26] He was therefore quite anxious to examine the excreta to see if his deductions would be confirmed, but on the third day he returned to find that contrary to his orders they had been discarded. The transcript reports his opening remarks as follows:

> In the hospital, two things can be seen and practiced: First, diseases and symptoms, but there is also a second kind of practice which is very useful, and habituates us to being tolerant. Because nothing is done here as we order, and that is true not only here, but you will also find it everywhere else, that neither is the patient obedient, nor do those who attend him do what they ought. Last night the patient had eight spontaneous bowel movements, but we cannot judge what was the offending material, or whether it was concocted, that is, whether the movement indicated a crisis, because we have not seen the excreta.[27]

Thus all the evidence would seem to support the conclusion of the early-nineteenth-century Italian clinicians, that a true clinical school did indeed exist at Padua in the middle of the sixteenth century.

But did da Monte really inaugurate the first such clinical school, as his latter-day advocates further maintained? In other words, can we safely conclude that the earliest clinical lectures of which we have a record were necessarily the first to have been given? Here I am afraid that in their zeal to find a distinct inventor of the clinic, the clinician-scholars fell all too easily into such fallacious reasoning, and ignored some evidence which might have pointed them in different directions. Most notably, in one of the transcripts da Monte related that in his own student days he had himself attended such discourses by the great physicians of the time, although he had found the experience to be quite unsatisfactory:

> For first they would declare the [internal] temperament of the patient, before they had even pointed out the manifest signs, and so were trying to demonstrate the known through the unknown, which is a preposterous order. And when they had considered the temperament, they would go on to name the disease. And after that they would list the symptoms of that disease as they are described by Avicenna, whether or not they were actually present in the patient. And sometimes they would declare twenty signs, but when I approached the patient I could scarcely find two of them.[28]

Of course, da Monte does not indicate whether these discussions took place specifically within a hospital, but this scarcely weakens the point that his own discourses represented an effort to do properly that which had long been done, but in his view had been done improperly. He particularly emphasized that the very first thing to be done was to "make a catalogue" or to "construct a simple history" of just those things that can be directly perceived.[29]

Shall we then award to da Monte's teachers the prize for having invented the clinical lecture? Hardly so, for what they were doing had been part of routine medical practice for centuries, namely the formal bedside consultation, in which each of several physicians took his turn at offering a formal analysis of the case before them.[30] Prospective physicians had to master this particular skill along with the others that made up the practice of medicine, so that it was quite natural for students to attend such consultations, and so in turn for the consultations to become displays of learning directed as much to the students as to the other physicians. In fact, many of da Monte's own discourses were carried out in such a context, as is clear from the transcripts themselves, as well as from the remarks of Hieronymus Donzellini, an early editor of da Monte's consilia. According to Donzellini,

> In holding [such consultations da Monte] showed so much mental acumen, clarity, prudence, doctrine, erudition, and wisdom, that wherever he went numerous students followed him, so that not a single word would escape from his mouth which they did not religiously collect. I remember that some of [his former students] at Venice told me that in such medical consultations he was so dominant and triumphant that all who heard him were left in a stupor out of admiration.[31]

Donzellini emphasized that the publication of these transcripts would be particularly important for showing the rest of the world how medicine is commonly taught and practiced at Venice and Padua.

However, Donzellini also made a clear distinction between this kind of transcript that shows da Monte in consultation with other physicians, and those in which da Monte alone lectured on cases in the hospital. According to Donzellini, da Monte's intention in the latter was "to provide something that was prescribed by Galen as highly necessary, namely that the universal precepts which he had clearly explained from the lecture should be applied to particular instances, and it was for this reason that [da Monte] exercised his students [at the bedside]."[32] But while the distinction between the bedside consultation and the solo bedside lecture is not a trivial one, in da Monte's own mind there continued to be an organic relationship between the two, for one of the primary aims of the solo lecture was precisely to teach the students how to conduct a proper bedside consultation. This is made clear in the opening words of one of the hospital lectures:

> Let us approach this patient, and let us regard him as if he were a nobleman, since he differs in no respect from the latter except by fortune. What should be done? Consultations are gatherings of upright men for the sake of understanding and curing diseases, and for considering the prognostic signs of the outcome of the disease. They do not take place for the sake of boasting and ostentation. Those who only want to show off are imposters and deceivers, and nothing will succeed for them. But whatever is done without guile will lead to success. . . . Therefore in every disease you ought to converse with learned men, or with yourself, so that having understood the nature [of the patient] or the disease,

you will find the cure. And you should try to express your true opinion. And if to this, someone is able to add beauty and eloquence of speech, he will not do wrong.[33]

Thus in an age when the routine practice of medicine depended heavily upon verbal skills, no clear distinction could be made between the internal process of reasoning from manifest symptoms to diagnostic, prognostic, and therapeutic conclusions, and the external process of consultation in which the observations and deductions were set forth in a formal speech. The didactic bedside lecture, in turn, was a kind of practice consultation carried out on a charity patient, and was intended to teach the students both how to reason correctly in relation to an individual patient and, at the same time, how to formally verbalize the reasoning in the event of consultation.

And so if da Monte really did invent the hospital lecture, he did so in a context in which the formal analysis of individual cases had long been a routine part of medical teaching and practice. However, let me reiterate that while the transcripts of da Monte's discourses do provide superb insights into what he himself actually did in the way of bedside teaching, they do not serve as a very reliable index as to what others before him may or may not have done.

Our next glimpse of the hospital lecture at Padua is provided by the Venetian Senate decree of 1578, referred to above. Its terms were as follows: "Two of the professors of the practice [of medicine] will visit the hospital at established times, there to hold forth about the diseases presented by the occasion, for the utility of the students."[34] The initiative in securing this decree was taken by the German students, which again underscores the particular concern of the foreign students to maximize their opportunities for practical training during their limited time in Italy. The legislation may have been intended to revive a form of teaching that had lapsed since the time of da Monte; but it may also have been aimed simply at regulating an ongoing practice, since it coincided closely with a bitter dispute as to whether physicians other than the two attending physicians of the hospital had the right to teach there.[35] From the annals of the German students we learn that the hospital demonstrations were carried out on a daily basis, immediately following the morning lectures on the practice of medicine.[36] From the same source we also learn of efforts to link the presentation of live patients with the autopsy of those who died, but this practice was discontinued (probably only temporarily) because of the protests of the other patients.[37]

For many years after 1578 these daily hospital rounds seem to have persisted as a major feature of the medical teaching at Padua, and one which continued to be particularly attractive to the foreign students who lacked such opportunities in their native lands. For example, a German student at Padua reported in 1624:

I did not miss the occasion of going around mid-day to the Hospital of St. Francis, when Sr. Aldrighetti visited the sick, of which there were many there. In every room there was an attendant, an assistant at the hospital, who led Sr. Aldrighetti from bed to bed. Aldrighetti himself then discussed the patient and informed the students of the cause and circumstances of the disease. He then ordered the necessary medicine which the hospital assistant then had made in the hospital pharmacy.[38]

Aldrighetti was the senior attending physician at the hospital,[39] and it is possible that the assistants in question were the kinds of young medical graduates referred to above.

As is well known, it was at Leiden in the seventeenth century that the first important clinical school was established outside of Italy. A proposal to inaugurate formal hospital teaching at Leiden had been made as early as 1591 by two medical graduates of Padua, but it was not until 1636 that approval was given to a similar plan submitted by Otto van Heurne, the son of one of the earlier proponents.[40] Among other points, van Heurne argued that the provision of such instruction would eliminate the need for medical students to go abroad for their practical training, so it seems reasonably clear that he based his clinic on a foreign model, most probably that of Padua.

However, if the Leiden clinic was indeed an imitation of the Paduan model, it was in several respects a rather poor imitation.[41] For one thing, the hospital teaching in Italy was just part of a much broader spectrum of practical training that was available from the large university faculties and associated colleges of physicians. By contrast, the faculty at Leiden was very small, and apparently the clinic was intended to carry the main burden of practical training. It was conducted not by the attending staff of the hospital, but by a member of the medical faculty who would visit the hospital on Wednesday and Saturday afternoons, rather than on a daily basis. And eventually the clinical teaching was confined to two wards of six beds each, which were provided with galleries to accommodate the large number of students.

Nevertheless, the very poverty of the opportunities for practical training at Leiden seems to have made the clinic stand out there as something much more distinct and important than it had been in its original Italian context. Thus it happened that as Leiden emerged as the most important European medical school, under the leadership of Boerhaave, the clinic seemed to become a uniquely Dutch institution; and it was the Leiden model that was to be copied in so many other cities of Europe.[42]

The most famous offspring of the Leiden clinic was, of course, the one established at Vienna in 1754 as part of the general medical reform instituted by van Swieten. However, as Erna Lesky has shown, even before van Swieten's arrival from Leiden in 1745 there had been repeated efforts to institute hospital teaching at the Austrian capital.[43] Indeed, as early as 1554 two students of da Monte had attempted to use the civic hospital as a place for training students, but without lasting success. Furthermore, as Lesky has again pointed out, when van Swieten first arrived in Vienna the kind of clinic he had in mind was the rather modest sort that he had experienced under Boerhaave.[44] Only subsequently did this evolve into the more ambitious conception that was put into effect in 1754, with de Haen devoting all of his efforts to the teaching clinic. It was at this point that the clinic clearly became something more substantial than the practical precepting that had long been readily available in the Italian schools, and, as we have seen, Padua was quick to follow the new model in 1764. And I might add that at this time the Venetian Republic was still an autonomous country, so that the new Paduan clinic was not something that was simply imposed upon a possibly unwilling subject.

In 1797 the armies of Napoleon brought an end to Venetian independence, and after a period of time under Austrian rule, the Veneto joined the rest of Italy as part of the Napoleonic empire in 1805. This brought the university of Padua under the national plan for all the Italian universities which the French had imposed in 1803. In the area of medicine this had the effect of reforming all the medical faculties along the lines of the new French Schools of Health.[45] In particular the clinic was now divided into two distinct phases, with the students spending one year in the clinic as auditors, followed by a second year as practitioners.

With the defeat of Napoleon northern Italy returned to the polyglot Austro-Hungarian empire, where it remained for two generations. This coincided with the period when the Vienna medical school emerged as a major influence even outside the empire, and so it is not surprising that other schools within the empire, including those in Italy, should be especially affected by it. Now it was not just a matter of importing a Viennese teaching method, as happened at Padua in 1764, but of the Italian schools being staffed by individuals who were trained at Vienna, including a few who were not Italians, but ethnic Germans. Dr. Premuda has documented this Viennese influence in such detail as to place it beyond dispute, and one hopes that in his future work Dr. Premuda will address the further question of how the imported tradition may have interacted with the native one. It might be, of course, that Italian academic medicine was so weakened by the political turmoil of the late eighteenth and early nineteenth centuries that it was simply swept aside by the Viennese trends, which were so powerful for both medical and political reasons. Or it might be that these trends were somehow modified for the better or for the worse in their new environment, as when the Paduan clinic was transferred to Leiden, or when the Leiden clinic was imported to Vienna.

NOTES

[1]Thomas Neville Bonner, *American Doctors and German Universities: 1870–1914* (Lincoln: University of Nebraska Press, 1963), p. 69.

[2]Carlo M. Cipolla, *Public Health and the Medical Profession in the Renaissance* (New York: Cambridge University Press, 1976), pp. 79–93.

[3]A.H.T. Robb-Smith, "Medical Education at Oxford and Cambridge Prior to 1850," in *The Evolution of Medical Education in Britain*, ed., F.N.L. Poynter (London: Pitman Medical Press, 1966), pp. 50–51.

[4]J. J. Bylebyl, "The School of Padua: Humanistic Medicine in the Sixteenth Century," in *Health, Medicine and Mortality in the Sixteenth Century*, ed. C. Webster, (New York: Cambridge University Press, 1979), p. 337.

[5]T. Puschmann, *A History of Medical Education* (New York: Hafner, 1966), pp. 235, 314–18.

[6]Bylebyl, "The School of Padua," pp. 339, 346–51.

[7]Ibid., pp. 351–52.

[8]Ibid.

[9]Cipolla, *Public Health and the Medical Profession*, p. 4.

[10]M. T. Gnudi and J. P. Webster, *The Life and Times of Gaspare Tagliacozzi, Surgeon of Bologna* (New York: H. Reichner, 1950), p. 37; A. Favaro, ed., *Atti della Nazione Germanica artista nello studio di Padova*, 2 vols. (Venice, 1911–12), 2:111.

[11]Morgagni, *De sedibus et causis morborum per anatomen indagatis*, 2 vols. (Venice, 1761), 2:255.

[12]G. Cervetto, *Di Giambatista da Monte e della medicina italiana nel secolo XVI* (Verona, 1839), pp. 169–70.

[13]Ibid., pp. 119–20, n. 54.

[14]dalla Bona, *Observationes medicae…praemissa oratione prima in Gymnasio habita* (Padua, 1766), pp. iii–iv.

[15]Ibid., pp. viii–x.

[16]Ibid., pp. x–xiv.

[17]Ibid., pp. vi–vii.

[18]Erna Lesky, "The Development of Bedside Teaching at the Vienna Medical School from Scholastic Times to Special Clinics," in *The History of Medical Education*, ed. C. D. O'Malley (Berkeley: University of California Press, 1970), pp. 222–24.

[19]Ibid., p. 224.

[20]Tissot, *Essai sur les Moyens de perfectionner les études de médecine* (Lausanne, 1789), pp. 102–3.

[21]Ibid., p. 102.

[22]Comparetti, *Saggio della scuola clinica nello spedale di Padova* (Padua, 1793), pp. 6–7.

[23]Rasori, *Opere complete* (Florence, 1837), pp. 293–96. A much fuller account of da Monte and his hospital teaching was published in 1839 by the clinician Cervetto in his *Di Giambatista da Monte*, cited above.

[24]Bylebyl, "The School of Padua," pp. 346–49.

[25]da Monte, *Explicatio eorum, quae pertinent, tum ad qualitates simplicium medicamentorum, tum ad eorundem compositione* (Paris, 1554), p. 238 r.

[26]da Monte, *Consultationum medicarum opus absolutissimum* (Basel, 1565), cols. 900–907.

[27]Ibid., col. 905.

[28]Ibid., col. 939.

[29]Ibid.

[30]D. W. Amundsen, "History of Medical Ethics: Ancient Greece and Rome," in *Encyclopedia of Bioethics*, 4 vols. (New York: Free Press, 1978), 3:935.

[31]da Monte, *Consilia medica omnia* (Nuremberg, 1559), editor's preface, p. ix.

[32]Ibid.

[33]da Monte, *Consultationum* (1565), col. 938.

[34]J. Facciolati, *Fasti Gymnasii Patavini*, 3 parts in 1 (Padua, 1757), p. 215. See also Favaro, *Atti della Nazione Germanica*, 1:138–39: J. P. Tomasini, *Gymnasium Pata-*

vinum (Udine, 1654), pp. 420–21; L. Münster, "Die Anfange eines klinischen Unterrichts an der Universität Padua im 16. Jahrhundert," *Med. Monatsschr.* 23 (1969): 172.

[35]Favaro, *Atti della Nazione Germanica*, 1:138–39.

[36]Ibid., p. 138.

[37]Ibid., pp. 143–44.

[38]G. Fichtner, "Padova e Tübingen: la formazione medica nei secoli XVI e XVII," *Acta Medicae Historiae Patavina*, 19 (1972–73): 54, citing Walter G. Brieger and John W. S. Johnson, eds., *Otto Sperlings Studienjahre* (Copenhagen, 1920), p. 57.

[39]A. Antonelli, *Cenni storici sull 'origine e sulle vicende dello Spedale Civile di Padova* (Padua, 1885), pp. 157–58.

[40]G. A. Lindeboom, "Medical Education in the Netherlands: 1575–1750," in O'Malley, *History of Medical Education*, pp. 204–5.

[41]Ibid., pp. 205–6.

[42]Ibid., pp. 207–12.

[43]Lesky, "The Development of Bedside Teaching," pp. 220–22.

[44]Ibid., pp. 222–24.

[45]L. Belloni, "Italian Medical Education after 1600," in O'Malley, *History of Medical Education*, pp. 111–12.

Robert S. Morison

> *"The difficult art of giving," to use John D. Rockefeller's phrase, is an art with which Dr. Robert S. Morison became thoroughly familiar in the service of the Rockefeller Foundation. The phrase was adopted in 1967 by Dr. Wilder Penfield for his biography of Alan Gregg.[1]*

I have not been in the difficult art of giving for fifteen years or so, but my memory is that it is indeed difficult. As a matter of fact, my career has been divided into about ten years at Harvard as a research worker, twenty years in the difficult art of giving, ten years in the difficult art of administering the division of Biological Sciences at Cornell, and ten years as a free-lance writer and teacher at M.I.T. Contrary to what you might suppose, I have to confess that the twenty years spent in the difficult art of giving turned out to be the least satisfactory ones in my life. It really is not easy, and it is not as much fun as you might think. Perhaps it is partly because you have to rely on so many other people for the success of what you are trying to do. Fortunately in the particular case we are celebrating (with which I had almost nothing to do) the difficult art of giving turned out to be a success, even though at the time, as I will try to show, nobody in the foundation really knew what they were doing when they made the grant, beginning with Abe Flexner and Richard Pearce and continuing with Alan Gregg and others.

When Professor Stevenson called to ask me to review the early history of the Institute of the History of Medicine, he hinted rather strongly that all I would have to do would be to summarize the material in the Rockefeller Archives. Knowing something of the meticulous record keeping of the Rockefeller Boards, I accepted the invitation without further reflection and waited until summer to consult the archives.

If you have never been to the Rockefeller Archives at Pocantico Hills, I recommend that you get yourself a project that would require that you do so. They are kept in a house that the second wife of Mr. John Rockefeller, Jr., built for herself. Her very good taste is evident in the pleasant surroundings. Now some very nice archives have been added, with some very nice people to help you with them. As a result one may spend a good week there looking into the background of the Rockefeller Boards. Somewhat to my surprise, however, the files in relation to the founding of this institute are curiously incomplete. For example, nowhere is there a formal memo by a member of the staff of either the Rockefeller Foundation or the General Education Board setting forth the reasons for believing that the history of medicine should be supported on such a substantial scale. That surprised me, because, at the time that I worked in this particular vineyard (from 1944 to 1964), whenever we launched a new program of any kind we developed memoranda saying exactly why we did so. I can remember for example an absolutely brilliant memorandum by Warren Weaver saying why the foundation should support an Institute of Agriculture in the Philippines to work on the breeding and cultivation of rice. This, of course, led directly to the International Rice Institute, which in turn started the "Green Revolution." I could not find anything similar in the archives about the history of medicine. Indeed the subject first appears in 1923 simply as part of a package request for major support for a medical library. In addition to space for what was then called a department, the very tentative budget included mention of, but no definite funds for a professorship of the history of medicine. Revised requests submitted in 1925 were, however, a little bit more definite on this point.

At the same time, another line of thought was represented more richly in the file. This concerned the future of Popsy Welch who was to become seventy-five in April of 1925 and who quite properly felt that it was time to turn over his administrative duties as dean of the School of Public Health to Professor Howell. Howell had done an excellent job as associate dean and in Popsy's view deserved the opportunity for a freer hand. The university trustees were loath to accept his retirement, but understood his feelings about the deanship. The solution appeared to lie in the establishment of a chair in the history of medicine that Welch might ornament, at least for a few initial years. The idea seems to have occurred more or less simultaneously to the officers of the General Education Board, especially to Abe Flexner, who felt personally indebted to Welch for a number of reasons, and to various members of the Hopkins community, notably Professor McCollum. There is, in fact, a very touching letter from Professor McCollum, who had succeeded Welch as professor of pathology some years earlier.

It is impossible to tell from the written record how the motivations were divided between the desire to provide an appropriate position for the revered Welch and a more general interest in forwarding teaching and research in the history of medicine. It is even more difficult, without further research or somewhat gratuitous prying (the two are often confused), to discover what was said by whom, and to whom, about the timing and magnitude of future support for a separate enterprise in the history of medicine.

Perhaps the best place to leave this technically intriguing point is where Robert Lambert put it in his diary note of a conversation with Dean Lewis Weed in June 1930. By then, the grant had been made and Lew Weed had come up to express his appreciation in a formal way. We were very much more formal in those days. Thus Weed felt it necessary to take a four-hour trip on the B&O, cross the Hudson on the ferry, and so to the Rockefeller Foundation to say how happy Hopkins was that the board had made the grant, even though he felt compelled to confess that he himself had not been particularly enthusiastic about such a large proposal. Lambert closes his note with a characteristically cryptic, and at the same time revealing, parenthesis. "There are confidential exchanges on certain features of the negotiation with the G.E.B. (General Education Board), which Weed and R.A.L. agree in regretting."

In spite of some more or less explicit disclaimers elsewhere in the files, it seems likely that in the more personal, expansive days of the middle 1920s, suggestions had been made and perhaps overinterpreted about the possible size of support for the history of medicine. In this connection it may be appropriate to note that the negotiations covered a five-year period marked by the retirement of Abraham Flexner from the General Education Board, and the taking over of its medical responsibilities by the recently reorganized Rockefeller Foundation. As everyone knows, the Flexner era was primarily one of institution building, and it was carried on with a personal assurance and dash worthy of an Elizabethan explorer. By 1929 it had become obvious to others that the middle years of the twentieth century called for a different strategy. For one thing, the resources of the private foundations were no longer such a predominant slice of the total educational budget of the country. For another, some symptoms of resentment could be discerned from those who did not like having university policy dictated by outsiders, however rich, wise, or dogmatic they might be. Incidentally that is a part of the difficult art of giving that we did not mention earlier: how far can you go in asking people to do something they don't really want to do. Abe sometimes went pretty far.

For whatever reasons, the Rockefeller Foundation program in medical education became at this time much more focused on particular projects. In a very few years, the emphasis shifted from endowing institutions "forever" to helping particular parts of institutions to get started. The hope was that permanent support would be found elsewhere, and I am sure that almost all of you here are aware of some of the less happy results of that change in policy. As St. Paul said of the Athenians, foundation officers are always in search of "some new thing." As a result universities are left trying to find permanent financing after the "new thing" is no longer new.

It was doubtless the need to review the expansive notions of the early twenties in the light of the sobering guidelines of the depression years that gives the Rockefeller Foundation file in the history of medicine what, one hopes, is a quite unusual, bureaucratic flavor. Reading between the lines on the basis of later experience in the same office, one cannot help feeling that the principal motivation of the officers in considering the 1930 grant was the wish to find the least expensive, but still decent, way of meeting the obligations expressed or implied by their predecessors.

But we are getting ahead of the actual course of events. Way back in the fall of 1925, the Trustees of the General Education Board considered a proposal for a medical library including a department of the history of medicine. Welch had by then definitely decided to leave the deanship and was therefore at liberty to take a new job. On the other hand, the board felt that more needed to be done to refine and perhaps reduce the library request per se. The proposal was therefore separated into two parts. Two hundred thousand dollars was immediately appropriated for a professorship of the history of medicine, while the library proposal was left to be further incubated.

Welch entered into the duties of the chair in November of 1926, and immediately set about removing any ambiguity about how the position was to be regarded. Far from accepting Abraham Flexner's undoubtedly exaggerated suggestion that he "should spend your loafing years lolling about in the Chair of the History of Medicine," Welch immediately assumed an activist role. On the other hand, he had no illusions about becoming a professional historian. In fact, his delay in accepting the post was in part due to his fear that "for me to take such a Chair at my age would merely emphasize the spirit of dilettantism, in which the subject is regarded and pursued generally in this country." I must say that I admired his insight and self-awareness when I came across that passage. On the other hand, he knew, perhaps better than many historians, what a knowledge of history might mean to the future of medicine. Above all, he had every reason to be confident of his entrepreneurial powers. Thus, he finally accepted the post for what would obviously be only a few initial years, in order, as he said "to get the ball rolling."

In pursuit of this objective he left in May 1927 for Europe and did not return until November 1928. His first stop was in Leipzig, where, as I'm sure you all know, Karl Sudoff had founded what Welch described as "the only well developed Institute of the History of Medicine." He had recently turned it over to Henry Sigerist, and its obvious success convinced Welch that nothing less than a full-fledged institute would do for Hopkins. He held to this view in spite of clearly expressed doubts by many of the Hopkins faculty, administration, and somewhat surprisingly, even by Abe Flexner, all of whom explicitly preferred the less pretentious "department." The latter preference is not explained, at least in the files that I saw, but I could guess that there was some worry on the part of people who had studied in Europe that the term *institute* might encourage the head to act like a German *Geheimrat*. But Welch insisted, and it was indeed called an institute as it is today, although I do not think that it has exactly the kind of status that some university institutes have in Europe. Nevertheless, it is interesting that there was that much controversy about the term and it is interesting that Welch won.

Much of the year abroad was spent in meeting other historians and in buying books for a historical library. He returned full of enthusiasm for his enlarged concept of what the Institute should do. As set forth in the Flexners' biography, Welch was not an antiquarian, nor was he primarily interested in the development of the history of medicine for itself or as a branch of the history of science. All this is quite clear in the file. Although scarcely a materialist-determinist, he is what today would be called an externalist (if Professor Webster will allow me to use that term) in his approach to the history of science. He was thus much interested in how the development of medicine related to simultaneous events in the culture as a whole. As a further consequence, in putting together his library, he felt that "there is scarcely any subject which for the study of the History of Medicine does not present significance." The books he chose reflect this catholic approach.

As hinted above, there is nothing in the written record that shows that the officers of the General Education Board or the Rockefeller Foundation fully shared or even understood this expanded vision when they finally made the grant of a capital sum of $250,000 plus $12,500 a year for five years, to get the program started. On the contrary, the staff memorandum of the discussion on which the final grant was based is concerned largely with such procedural matters as the following; and the comments are almost all negative in tone:

1. In the four years since the establishment of the chair, nothing has been done by Johns Hopkins, up to six months before, to stimulate either undergraduate or graduate interest in the History of Medicine.
2. Although the budget of the medical school has increased over a million dollars in the past five years not one dollar of undesignated funds has been allocated to the History of Medicine. (It would be interesting to know how many undesignated dollars are allocated today.)
3. The future leadership of the Institute is very uncertain.
4. The Institute idea has grown considerably since it was originally put forward.

All these misgivings are understandable enough to professional foundation officers, as they were to me. They also justify the cautious approach to financing that was ultimately adopted. But they also show that the foundation was far from recognizing that a knowledge of history might be just as important to future physicians as a knowledge of biochemistry. It is also obvious that the administration of Johns Hopkins was equally unconvinced. It was, in fact, many years before the university made more than token contributions to the Institute.

So that is the end of that story as I read it in the files. It is interesting to me in part because it shows how people who make decisions do not always see what the results are going to be, and may indeed be influenced by quite extraneous reasons. Nobody can read this file without feeling that the primary considerations were personal and historical rather than an unequivocal vision of the place of the history of medicine in the future development of the profession.

As far as the foundation was concerned, the appointment of Henry Sigerist in 1932 marked the beginning of a new era. Everyone was impressed, and not only with his almost immediate success in attracting students. In any case, Alan Gregg, who became director for medical education about the time the original grant was made, was himself deeply interested in the broader social and historical relationships of medicine, with which Sigerist was so fully engaged. Support for the Institute thus continued through the Sigerist regime and well into that of his successor, when more permanent arrangements could be made. But this is another story, which many of you know better than I.

Since history, as Professor Temkin has recently reminded us in his magnificent book, is like Janus, two-faced, perhaps I may be allowed to close with some personal reflections. From looking back at the past I will turn, Janus-like, to the future. Although I was a member of Dr. Gregg's staff during the postwar period, I had nothing to do with the Hopkins grant until the period after Sigerist's departure. Indeed, I fear that during most of my life, my relation to the history of medicine in general has been that of an onlooker, if not, indeed, of a Philistine. My reactions are clearly those of a nonexpert, but may be worth recording simply for that reason. In a way they may serve to answer the question: Why should the history of medicine be of interest to people not interested in it as such? The answer is related, of course, to an argument that has gone on for a long time within your profession. But recent events have, for me at least, given the history of medicine and its social relevance a new note of urgency.

In the first place, it is now obvious to everyone that medicine is "doing better and feeling worse," as elaborated in the Daedelus issue put together by the late John Knowles. It is doing better in the narrow sense of understanding, diagnosing, and to a certain extent, treating disease. But people in general are feeling worse, in a number of complex ways that we cannot examine in detail here. Many of them clearly have to do, however, with the economic and social context in which medicine is practiced. As I look back upon the last half century and ask myself what the foundations did—or might have done—in the difficult art of giving, to anticipate our current troubles, I find that their record is somewhat, though not very much, better than that of organized medicine, or of most medical schools. Thus, the Commonwealth Fund had a very early program in rural hospitals and the regionalization of medical care. Others, including the Rockefeller Foundation, supported early experiments in group practice and, of course, innumerable *studies* beginning in 1929 with the famous Committee on the Cost of Medical Care, chaired by Ray Lyman Wilbur. If I have regrets, and I have many, about my career as a Foundation Officer the biggest probably concerns the number of studies that we supported and nobody read. In retrospect, many of the experiments and most of the reports were too episodic and ad hoc. What was clearly lacking was any kind of solid intellectual base, any continuing philosophy of medical care, any coherent rationale for the equitable distribution of care in a society such as ours.

It therefore gives me a certain ironic pleasure to note that during the early period, the most significant, perhaps the only, center for such studies was right here at Hopkins under the inspired Henry Sigerist. The ironic part, of course, is that Johns Hopkins had long been a citadel of scientific medicine, a little self-consciously proud, perhaps, of its purity and lack of a relationship to the everyday needs of society. Indeed, I have been told that there were some members of the faculty who were less pleased at the presence of Henry Sigerist than I seem to be today.

Most of all perhaps, one finishes this appraisal of the place of the Institute with a heightened appreciation for the vision of Popsy Welch. As a Harvard man I must confess that I was never quite sure about the sainthood of Popsy Welch. In fact, there were times that I laughed at a story about the three most overrated things in the world, one of which was The Johns Hopkins Medical School. And also, when I read the biography of Popsy Welch, as a Harvard man again, I was turned off by the advice that he gave to a lady, who wrote asking where her son should best enroll in college. He wrote back, "If he's the kind of boy who has a chance of making Skull and Bones, then he should go to Yale. If he is not that kind of boy it doesn't make much difference where he goes." This, if I may say so, rather turned me off, but after I read the record we have just reviewed I must confess I ended with a gool deal of admiration for the man.

Certainly there is no need to review the evidence that Welch is one of the two or three most important founders of modern scientific medicine, at least in the United States. More interesting is the fact that just as his planting was reaching its first flowering in the 1920s, we find him warning of the dangers of the narrowly scientific training given to contemporary medical students. He viewed his proposed institute as a counterbalance to this limited view of medical responsibility. The proposal to the General Education Board, which he must have supervised if not actually written, reads as if it had been prepared in the 1960s, when other medical educators finally awoke to the constricting effects of the so-called Flexnerian Revolution.

How refreshing and, indeed, how humbling it is to go back and see that one of the leading revolutionaries of the early Scientific Revolution saw the dangers of a purely technological reign of terror and began to erect defensive structures. Nevertheless, and in spite of the clear vision of one of our forefathers, neither the history of medicine, nor any other humanistic discipline, has yet provided the medical establishment with the basic philosophy, the sophisticated self-image, and the historical perspective that it now obviously needs. Let me give a couple of examples of what I mean, very briefly, very sketchily, drawn from my recent experience as a superannuated administrator trying to understand what he was trying to do during his active life.

First and foremost, it turns out that we know surprisingly little about the relationship between medical care and health. There are at least two quite different reasons for being interested in this. The first is the growing interest in population dynamics. Demographers have displayed great ingenuity in reconstructing family structures, birth and death rates, in various periods. But there is still much argument about whether the extraordinary changes in the last two hundred years are due to changes in agriculture, in industry, in the technology of medical care, or to more subtle changes in life style. We heard something about this in the preceding essays, and the British epidemiologist, McKeown, has done a good deal to correct naive notions accepted by some historians that medicine and public health played a very important role in the growth of the European population during the eighteenth and nineteenth centuries.

A great deal more needs to be done before we understand the whole picture. Certainly changes in life style, especially in relation to public and personal hygiene, played a role. Today, as we grow more conscious of the importance of life style for the health of our own middle-aged population, it would be interesting to know how those earlier changes, which affected younger people, were brought about. How, for example, did the youth of the reckless regency turn, in a couple of decades, into the orderly, sober, more-or-less incorruptible, self-righteous, and often hypocritical dignitaries of the Victorian Age. More specifically, what role did John Wesley and his followers have in finally improving the health and decreasing the infant mortality rate of the English lower-middle class? It may seem puckish of me to pick John Wesley, but as far as I know, he was the first person to introduce into Christianity the idea that cleanliness is next to Godliness. He picked it up from some earlier Jewish scholar, and his followers started weekly meetings to change people's life style. In many ways, these were like the group therapy sessions now carried on by Alcoholics Anonymous. It would be interesting to go back and review that history in the light of what is known about the vital statistics of the period.

Secondly, and on a quite different level, I have found very little systematic thinking about the origins of the social obligation to provide health services for everyone. It has become fashionable in these days to regard health care as a right, like habeus corpus; but the idea does not stand close examination, as Charles Fried and others have recently shown. The revival of interest in distributive justice under the leadership of John Rawles has tempted some philosophers to bring medical care into this abstract framework; but the results so far, are unimpressive. In the Western world there seems no doubt that St. Paul's ideas about charity played an important idea in the establishment of institutions for the care of the unfortunate; and many modern high-technology hospitals still are somewhat incongruously named for Christian saints. Still other threads can be traced in the origins of the modern welfare state, both in its Brandenburgian, paternalistic form and in the more egalitarian mode followed by the utilitarians and evangelicals in laying its Victorian foundations.

There are numerous individual historians that know a great deal about various parts of this complicated picture. No one, so far as I know, has brought it all together in a way that puts our present predicament in true historical perspective, much less in a form that might have some hope of influencing policy. As the practical difficulties of devising a scheme that will be effective, equitable, and affordable become ever more obvious, the reexamination of the philosophic base for making every man the keeper of his brother's health seems less and less a luxury and more and more a necessity.

As a kind of footnote to this broader interest in medical care, I personally must confess to a possibly useless curiosity as to why we, as a people, place such a very high value on medical care per se. For some time now, people like Victor Fuchs have been telling us that the relationship between medical care and health is really not very close. There are even some voices, like that of Ivan Illich, that suggest the correlation is actually negative. I suspect, but cannot prove, that the historian who tells us how we came to put such a high value on health care will at the same time tell us something important, but perhaps not very pleasant, about the rest of our value system.

So, to recapitulate, although there may have been, and probably was, a general recognition among the officers of the two foundations that the growing emphasis on medicine's scientific base ought to be balanced by more attention to its social and historical contexts, the actual decision to make a grant to Johns Hopkins for this purpose was based on much more immediate and, to a certain extent, purely bureaucratic considerations. High on the list certainly was the general respect and affection for Popsy Welch, if not indeed, a sense of indebtedness to him for the constructive role he had played in the founding of the Rockefeller Boards and Institute. Second come rather more mixed feelings about Abe Flexner and the commitments he may have made in his enthusiasm for seeing to it that Welch would spend his declining years as gracefully as possible. Third was the entirely legitimate, if slightly irritated, feeling that if the project was as important as Johns Hopkins kept saying it was, then the university ought to be willing to put some of its other money into it.

In the event, both the foundation and the university probably achieved rather more than they had expected or planned, simply by following what was then a cardinal principle of action in the foundation. Choose the best man and help him to do his best. The Institute managed to bring to this country, in the person of Henry E. Sigerist, perhaps the one person who could effectively acquaint us with the changes taking place in Europe in regard to the distribution of medical care. That we have not yet been able to use this information to devise our own peculiarly American solution is no criticism of him. At least we are now a good deal more sophisticated than we would have been without him. Although I have perhaps unduly stressed his social interests, I do not have to remind this audience that he was a very great scholar in the traditional European sense, with his dawn-to-dusk industry and his frightening command of languages. As such, he established, with the tremendously important collaboration of Professor Temkin and others, what I would call medical history per se on a sound foundation here at Hopkins. Finally, he flashed a brilliant, sometimes rather blinding, light on what history and sociology might do for the future relations of medicine and sociology. Although I can no longer speak for the foundations, I feel that they should be grateful for the way things have turned out.

NOTE

[1]Wilder Penfield, *The Difficult Art of Giving: The Epic of Alan Gregg* (Boston and Toronto: Little, Brown and Company, 1967). Several pages (340–42) are devoted to Gregg's relationship with Henry E. Sigerist during, and also after, Sigerist's Johns Hopkins period. On p. 384 appears this biographical sketch of our speaker: "*Dr. Robert Morison* carried out significant work on the brain as a neurophysiologist at Harvard. He came to the Rockefeller Foundation in 1946 to be Gregg's assistant, was subsequently appointed Associate Director in the Division of Medical Sciences, and took charge of the work when Gregg retired. Morison later retired from the Foundation to return to his physiology as Director of Basic Biology, Cornell University, Ithaca, N.Y." This has been followed by his present work at M.I.T.

APPENDIX: DEGREES GRANTED UNDER THE AUSPICES OF THE INSTITUTE OF THE HISTORY OF MEDICINE

1939   Genevieve Miller, M.A.: "Albrecht von Haller's Controversy with Robert Whytt." Associate Professor Emeritus of the History of Science, Case Western Reserve University School of Medicine; Research Associate, The Johns Hopkins University Institute of the History of Medicine.

1947   Ilza Veith, Ph.D.: "Huang Ti Nei Ching Su Wen: The Yellow Emperor's Classic of Internal Medicine." Professor and Vice-Chairman Emeritus, Department of the History of Health Sciences and Professor Emeritus, Department of Psychiatry, University of California, San Francisco.

1949   Lloyd G. Stevenson, Ph.D.: "A History of Lead Poisoning." William H. Welch Professor and Director, The Johns Hopkins University Institute of the History of Medicine.

1951   William B. Walker, M.A.: "Dr. John Crawford of Baltimore (1746–1813)." Gstaad, Switzerland.

1964   Samuel Greenblatt, M.A.: "John Hughlings Jackson: The Development of his Main Ideas to 1864." Associate Professor of Neurological Surgery, Medical College of Ohio, Toledo.

1966   Robert P. Hudson, M.A.: "Patterns of Medical Education in Nineteenth Century America." Chairman, Department of the History and Philosophy of Medicine, Kansas University Medical Center, Kansas City.

1968   Gert H. Brieger, Ph.D.: "Stephen Smith, Surgeon and Reformer." Professor and Chairman, Department of the History of Health Sciences, University of California, San Francisco.

1969   Chester R. Burns, Ph.D.: "Medical Ethics in the United States Before the Civil War." James Wade Rockwell Professor of the History of Medicine and Professor, Department of Preventive Medicine and Community Health, University of Texas Medical Branch, Galveston.

1970   Dennis G. Carlson, M.A.: "African Fever and British Response; A Study of European Medicine, Technology, and Science in a Non-Western Environment, 1787–1864." Associate Professor, Department of International Health, The Johns Hopkins University School of Hygiene and Public Health.

1971   Kenneth M. Ludmerer, M.A.: "Genetics and American Society;
            An Historical Appraisal." Assistant Professor of Medicine,
            School of Medicine and Assistant Professor of History, Fac-
            ulty of Arts and Sciences, Washington University, St. Louis.

1973   Toby Gelfand, Ph.D.: "The Training of Surgeons in Eighteenth-
            Century Paris and Its Influence on Medical Education."
            Associate Professor, The Hannah Chair of the History of
            Medicine, Faculty of Health Sciences and Associate Profes-
            sor, Department of History, Faculty of Arts, University of
            Ottawa.

1974   Donald Peterson, Ph.D.: "Galen's 'Therapeutics to Glaucon'
            and Its Early Commentaries." Assistant Professor, Depart-
            ment of Pathology, Marshall University; Chief, Laboratory
            Service, Veterans Administration Medical Center, Beckley,
            West Virginia.

1974   Edward C. Atwater, M.A.: "Financial Subsidies for American
            Medical Education Before 1940." Associate Professor of
            Medicine and Associate Professor of the History of Medicine,
            University of Rochester School of Medicine and Dentistry.

1975   Donald G. Bates, Ph.D.: "Thomas Sydenham: The Development
            of his Thought, 1666–1676." Thomas F. Cotton Professor
            of the History of Medicine and Chairman, Department of
            Humanities and Social Studies, McGill University.

1976   Pauline M. H. Mazumdar, Ph.D.: "Karl Landsteiner and the
            Problem of Species, 1838–1968." Jason A. Hannah Profes-
            sor of the History of Medicine, University of Toronto.

1978   Douglas Price, M.A.: "The Phantom Limb Phenomenon: A
            Medical Historical and Comparative Folklore Study." Clin-
            ical Assistant Professor of Psychiatry, Georgetown Univer-
            sity School of Medicine and Staff Psychiatrist, Washington
            Veterans Administration Medical Center.

1978   W. Bruce Fye, M.A.: "Henry Pickering Bowditch; A Case Study
            of the Harvard Physiologist and his Impact on the Profes-
            sionalization of Physiology in America." Chairman of the
            Department of Cardiology and Director of the Cardiograph-
            ics Laboratory, Marshfield Clinic; Adjunct Assistant Professor
            of the History of Medicine and Clinical Assistant Professor
            of Medicine, University of Wisconsin, Madison.

1979   Robert J. Miciotto, Ph.D.: "Carl Rokitansky: Nineteenth Cen-
            tury Pathologist and Leader of the New Vienna School."
            Assistant Professor of the History of Medicine, Louisiana
            State University Medical Center, New Orleans.

1979   Edwin R. Wallace, IV, M.A.: "Freud and Anthropology: A His-
            tory and Reappraisal of *Totem and Taboo*." Assistant Pro-

fessor, Department of Psychiatry, Yale University School of Medicine.

Addendum: In 1974 The Johns Hopkins University awarded a Ph.D. in the History of Science to Caroline Hannaway for a dissertation entitled: "Medicine, Public Welfare, and the State in Eighteenth-Century France: the Société Royale de Médecine of Paris (1776–1793)." Assistant, The Johns Hopkins University Institute of the History of Medicine.

List of Contributors

ERWIN H. ACKERKNECHT, M.D.
Ottikerstrasse 42
CH 8006 Zurich, Switzerland

DONALD G. BATES, M.D.,
PH.D.
McGill University
Montreal, Quebec, Canada H3G
1Y6

WHITFIELD J. BELL, JR., PH.D.
American Philosophical Society
Philadelphia, Pennsylvania 19106

JEROME J. BYLEBYL, PH.D.
Institute of the History of
Medicine
The Johns Hopkins University
Baltimore, Maryland 21205

ROBERT G. FRANK, JR., PH.D.
UCLA Medical School
Los Angeles, California 90024

JEAN-PIERRE GOUBERT, DOCTEUR
ÈS LETTRES
Centre de Recherches Historiques
Ecole des Hautes Etudes en
Sciences Sociales
75270 Paris, Cedex 06, France

CAROLINE HANNAWAY, PH.D.
Institute of the History of
Medicine
The Johns Hopkins University
Baltimore, Maryland 21205

COL. ROBERT J. T. JOY, M.D.
Uniformed Services University of
the Health Sciences
Bethesda, Maryland 20014

JANET KOUDELKA, M.L.S.
Institute of the History of
Medicine
The Johns Hopkins University
Baltimore, Maryland 21205

NIKOLAUS MANI, M.D.
Medizinhistorisches Institut der
Universität Bonn
5300 Bonn 1, West Germany

GENEVIEVE MILLER, PH.D.
Institute of the History of
Medicine
The Johns Hopkins University
Baltimore, Maryland 21205

ROBERT S. MORISON, M.D.
P. O. Box 277
Peterborough, New Hampshire
03458

PETER H. NIEBYL, M.D., PH.D.
Institute of the History of
Medicine
The Johns Hopkins University
Baltimore, Maryland 21205

LORIS PREMUDA, M.D.
Istituto di Storia della Medicina
Università di Padova
35100 Padua, Italy

L. J. RATHER, M.D.
Stanford University School of
Medicine
Stanford, California 94305

FRANK B. ROGERS, M.D.
1135 Grape Street
Denver, Colorado 80220

CHARLES ROSENBERG, PH.D.
University of Pennsylvania
Philadelphia, Pennsylvania 19174

LLOYD G. STEVENSON, M.D.,
    PH.D.
Institute of the History of
    Medicine
The Johns Hopkins University
Baltimore, Maryland 21205

CHARLES WEBSTER, M.A., D.SC.
Wellcome Unit for the History of
    Medicine
University of Oxford
Oxford OX2 6PE, England